THE Men'sHealth® LONGEVITY PROGRAM

THE Men's Health® LONGEVITY PROGRAM

A 12-WEEK PLAN TO

- **Bolster Your Health**
- **Get Lean**
- **Boost Your Brainpower**
- **Power Up**
- **Feel Great Now and Later**
- **Keep the Sex Hot**

From the Editors of Men's Health Books
with Kenneth A. Goldberg, M.D.
Founder and Director of The Male Health Center

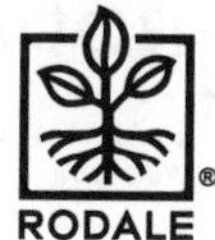

Notice

This book is intended as a reference volume only, not as a medical manual. The information given here is designed to help you make informed decisions about your health. It is not intended as a substitute for any treatment that may have been prescribed by your doctor. If you suspect that you have a medical problem, we urge you to seek competent medical help.

Printed in the United States of America
Rodale Inc. makes every effort to use acid-free ♾, recycled paper ♻

The questions in "How Are You Doing?" on page 165 are adapted from *Fighting for Your Marriage: Positive Steps for Preventing Divorce and Preserving a Lasting Love* by Howard Markman, Scott Stanley, and Susan L. Blumberg, quiz on pages 5–6. Copyright 1994 by Jossey-Bass, Inc. Reprinted by permission of John Wiley and Sons, Inc.

Library of Congress Cataloging-in-Publication Data

Goldberg, Ken (Kenneth A.)
The men's health longevity program : a 12-week plan to bolster your health, get lean, boost your brainpower, power up, feel great now and later, keep the sex hot / from the editors of Men's Health books ; with Kenneth A. Goldberg.
p. cm.
"Men's health books."
Includes index.
ISBN 1-57954-317-0 hardcover
ISBN 1-57954-366-9 paperback
1. Men—Health and hygiene. 2. Longevity. 3. Aging—Prevention. I. Title.
RA777.8 .G647 2001
613'.04234—dc21 00-010989

Distributed to the book trade by St. Martin's Press

2 4 6 8 10 9 7 5 3 1 hardcover
2 4 6 8 10 9 7 5 3 1 paperback

Visit us on the Web at www.menshealthbooks.com, or call us toll-free at (800) 848-4735.

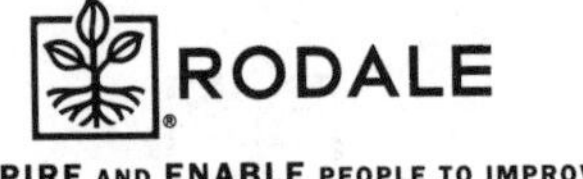

WE INSPIRE AND ENABLE PEOPLE TO IMPROVE THEIR LIVES AND THE WORLD AROUND THEM

The Men's Health *Longevity Program* Staff

Editor: Neil Wertheimer
Contributing Editors: Kenneth Winston Caine, Stephen C. George
Writers: Jennifer Bright, Kelly Garrett, Larry Keller, Eric Metcalf, Christian Millman
Associate Art Director: Richard Kershner
Interior Designer: Stephanie M. Tarone
Cover Designer: Charles Beasley
Photo Editor: James A. Gallucci
Interior Photographer: Mitch Mandel/Rodale Images, Svend Lindback, Beth Bischoff
Associate Research Manager: Anita C. Small
Lead Researcher: Molly Donaldson Brown
Editorial Researchers: Jennifer Bright, Rebecca L. Theodore
Permissions Coordinator: Lois Guarino Hazel
Senior Copy Editor: Kathryn C. LeSage
Editorial Production Manager: Marilyn Hauptly
Layout Designer: Bethany Bodder
Manufacturing Coordinators: Brenda Miller, Jodi Schaffer, Patrick T. Smith

Rodale Active Living Books

Vice President and Publisher: Neil Wertheimer
Executive Editor: Susan Clarey
Editorial Director: Michael Ward
Marketing Director: Janine Slaughter
Product Marketing Director: Kris Siessmayer
Book Manufacturing Director: Helen Clogston
Manufacturing Manager: Eileen Bauder
Research Director: Ann Gossy Yermish
Copy Manager: Lisa D. Andruscavage
Production Manager: Robert V. Anderson Jr.
Digital Processing Group Managers: Leslie M. Keefe, Thomas P. Aczel
Office Manager: Jacqueline Dornblaser
Office Staff: Susan B. Dorschutz, Julie Kehs Minnix, Tara Schrantz, Catherine E. Strouse

Contents

Week 3: The Save-Your-Body Supplement Plan

Week 4: Learn the Low-Stress Lifestyle

Week 5: Get Happy

Week 6: Activate Your Medical Support Team

Introduction

When your mother counseled you, "One day at a time, dear," it's unlikely that either of you ever expected anyone to take that phrase as seriously as have the editors of *Men's Health* Books. Laid out before you in the following pages is a comprehensive, scientifically proven calendar for self-improvement—one day at a time. In easily digestible steps, you'll fix your diet, develop an effective exercise program, learn what supplements you should be taking, reduce stress, cheer up, enlist health-care partners, shift your brain into high gear, look better, improve your outlook on life, plan to live longer, and much more.

More? More than living longer? Indeed. Erasing some of the 6-plus-year gap in life expectancy between men and women is a noble goal and the right thing to do. But I argue that it's even more important to pack as much value as possible into every year, regardless of how many you're dealt. And frankly, guys, that's what I like most about what you're holding in your hands. This book is a ticket to a life that's not only longer but also more fulfilling and fun.

Granted, there's not much happiness in life without good health. That's why diet, exercise, and disease prevention must form the foundation of a good life. And, true enough, there may not be much that's inherently fun about, say, broccoli. Still, when you understand what broccoli is for and why eating it works, it feeds your brain twice: once with the nutrition it packs and again with the knowledge that empowers your life. And empowerment is what you're really looking for.

In this age of information, the data that you need to take control of your health are all around you. But whose spiel should you believe? Frankly, there's some real junk being hawked out there, and with managed care taking over the health-care system, it's more important than ever that you look out for number one. With this program, the fellas at *Men's Health* Books make that easy for you, boiling down the information to its essence and translating it into a readable and guy-friendly form. Working with them has been a pleasure, and I wholeheartedly endorse this plan and its goals.

Those goals may be lofty, but they're not out of reach. True, historically, it hasn't been easy to be a man. We've been expected to fight and die, work and die, play and die. That was in the previous millennium, though, and I see every sign—this book being one of them—that manhood is finally being promoted to a full-time position. There has never been a better time to be a man and make the most of it.

In the more than 20 years that I've been practicing medicine, I've seen the changes—big ones. They're etched in my memory as the faces of men who've grown taller by embracing their health and their manhood. Jerry may be one of the best examples, though certainly not the only one. He was referred to me by his family practitioner after a suspicious prostate exam. He was concerned, and it turned out that he had some reason to be. Further tests confirmed prostate cancer, and I scheduled him for surgery. His fear turned to disbelief. You've heard the expression "Denial is not just a river in Egypt"?

Mostly through the graces of a supportive spouse, Jerry managed to survive until surgery and came through it just fine. Even by the end of the first post-op day, I could see the change. Jerry had learned that the fear was worse than the reality. Life gradually returned to normal, but Jerry didn't. Within weeks, he was on the phone asking if there were other men facing what he had faced. "I think I can make it easier for them," he said. "Ask them if they'd like someone to talk to." That was 10 years ago, and Jerry still visits men facing surgery and regularly addresses the local prostate cancer support group.

Men can talk and care, even to and for each other. When they do, they become much taller men in all eyes, including their own. A man who cares for others cares for himself. And when he cares for himself, he cares for his body too. More and more men are doing it, and I encourage you to tag along. Turn the page and take the first step. It's not difficult, and each step you take will move you closer to the best you can make of yourself and your life. Follow the plan 6 days a week (hey, everybody needs a day off) for 12 weeks, and I guarantee that you'll not only add years to your life but also have a great time doing it.

Finally, remember that the joy in our lives comes from those around us. Pass this book along to your partner, who can help you along, and to your sons. Spread health, and you cultivate joy. Enjoy!

Kenneth A. Goldberg, M.D.
Founder and Director
The Male Health Center
Dallas

WEEK ZERO

GETTING PREPARED

The Plan

What We're Trying to Accomplish

The Preparation

Appointments to Make, Money to Spend

The Mindset

How to Keep Yourself on the Program

What We're Trying to Accomplish

Our goal with this book is exquisitely simple. We want to add a decade, maybe two or three, to your life. We're not talking about old-guy, sitting-around years. We want those years to be marked by health, adventures, sex, good times, energy, and success.

Isn't that nice of us? But that's not all. We want you to have better health, adventures, sex, good times, energy, and success starting, say, this Monday. We bet that even your mother doesn't have such high hopes for you. But it is within your reach if you embrace the *Men's Health* Longevity Program.

Until recently, civilization defined health as the absence of illness. Now a new type of thinking has emerged. Health, under this new paradigm, isn't merely not being sick. Health is living well. It's having energy, feeling strong, being connected, coping well with stress. This is not the realm of doctors and pharmaceuticals, where issues of disease still reign, but the realm of daily living, with nary a doctor in sight. You control whether you have good health, not some guy or gal with a stethoscope.

Behind this thinking is an extraordinary body of research. Here are the topics of the new science of health and longevity.

Nutrition. You would think that food would be a simple subject for science to understand. We eat, we digest, we have fuel. But we have learned that foods carry within them a vast array of healing agents about which we never were previously aware. We have finally become convinced that healthy, fresh food is perhaps the best preventive medicine a person can take and that carefully balancing our nutritional intakes is key to health and longevity.

Exercise. Research into the beneficial role of movement and strength began to emerge only in the late 1970s. Today, we understand that a lethargic life makes you prone to disease and saps you of the vitality necessary for assertive living. Moreover, we finally understand the physiology and chemistry of exercise as well as the right amounts and types for optimal living.

Anti-aging medicine. This branch of medicine looks at the human body from a cellular level. Stop thinking about, say, the stomach as a whole; it's the cells of the stomach that matter. What can we do to keep these cells replicating in a healthy, orderly way? What causes cells to mutate or stop reproducing? The belief is that by aiding your cellular structure through nutrition, vitamins, and such, you immeasurably extend your potential life span.

Mind-body medicine. If you've read health magazines lately, you know that the most widely predicted trend is the rise of mind-body healing techniques. Indeed, a staggering amount of research is confirming that optimism, faith, and a sense of purpose are among our most powerful healing agents. These notions were once dismissed as New Age-like and ridiculous. Today, major cancer clinics teach patients to meditate as part of their battle against the disease. And lots of studies confirm the healing power of prayer.

Together, these four areas of research are showing mankind that there is an extraordinary amount that we as individuals can do to lengthen our lives. To our delight, there is little conflict between the solutions arrived at by these different disciplines. Even better, the solutions are simple—in a nutshell, eat well, exercise often, and have a good attitude.

A Small Reality Check

Aging is a process that inevitably leads to one unavoidable, ultimate outcome. In this context, the goal of the *Men's Health* Longevity Program is to slow the deterioration as much as possible. This allows you to maintain youthful vigor beyond the usual time boundaries and then, at the end of your life, to die the old-fashioned way: of natural causes.

By this measure, things are already much better for men than they were in the past. A boy born in America in 1998 had a life expectancy of 73.4 years. At the start of the 20th century, the average guy punched out at the age of 46. Why, baseball star Nolan Ryan was still firing fastballs at 46. U.S. senator Strom Thurmond didn't sire the first of his four children until he hit the age of 68.

We can't assure you that you'll still be siring children at 68—and let's face it, do you really want to be planning weddings at age 90? But you will live a healthier, more satisfying life if you follow at least some of this program. You'll see immediate improvements in your health—mental as well as physical. You will look and feel better. And maybe, if you don't take up skydiving or collecting venomous snakes as a hobby, you will live much longer and stronger.

Getting with the Program

The *Men's Health* Longevity Program is a 12-week program that doesn't require you to undergo boot camp–like physical rigors or mental torture that only G. Gordon Liddy could endure (or enjoy). Each week has a unique theme, such as eating, aerobic exercise, or anti-stress techniques. Within that week are six daily tasks (on Sunday, you may rest). You will be asked to do unique things ranging from drinking a lot of water to spending an evening with your parents. You can perform most tasks at home. Some require some spending, some require appointments.

In total, there are 12 weeks of tasks with 6 tasks per week, meaning 72 tasks in all. In a perfect world, you would do the entire program. As you go along, some of the tasks will surprise you. Some will annoy you, some will amuse you. Most important, some should resonate with you. These you need to continue doing, particularly the eating-and-exercise ones, like having a good breakfast or taking a daily walk.

After 12 weeks, you will have sampled almost every possible thing you can do to improve and lengthen your life. You also will have figured out ways to integrate many of them into every day.

Throughout the book, but unrelated to the formal 12-week program, are prevention tips for men's 20 biggest health concerns about aging. The topics range from hair loss to back pain to heart disease. If you have a particular concern about aging or know that your family history makes you prone to a particular disease or health problem, you'll want to take this advice into consideration as well.

We know that you won't follow the program in every single detail. Maybe the prospect of calling your siblings or updating your wardrobe is more than you care to deal with immediately. Maybe you can't commune with your dog because you don't have a dog. Don't worry about it. Follow as much of the program as you can.

You already know this, but it bears repeating: In this life, talent counts for only so much. Dogged persistence—the will to keep on keeping on—is what separates the men from the boys, the wheat from the chaff, the quick from the dead.

Nowhere is that truer than in your endeavors to live a longer, healthier, more active life. We won't pretend that in 12 weeks alone, you will add a decade to your back end. We do hope that by the end of those 12 weeks, you will have made a commitment to live well and long by making lifelong habits of many of the tasks presented in the *Men's Health* Longevity Program.

As we've said, this program comprises 72 daily tasks. The idea is to do all of them at least once; the ideal is to integrate all of them into your future.

Think of this as a syllabus for the best course you'll ever take.

Appointments to Make, Money to Spend

Feeling good and living a long, fulfilling life comes with a price. Following this Longevity Program is going to cost you some time and money. That said, when you've finished reading what's expected of you, we think you'll agree that the price truly is a bargain. You can bet your life on that.

Depending on the task prescribed, the amount of time that you need to carve out of any given day can vary quite a bit. But on average, the program will take you 45 minutes a day. That's less time than many guys spend fiddling with the remote.

You may think you can't manage to find the time. Truth is, you can. Let us remind you of the great truism of time management: When you say, "I don't have the time to do that," what you are really saying is, "I choose to do something else rather than that." Scheduling your time is all about priorities.

We ask that for the next 12 weeks, you put your health, happiness, energy, and appearance at the top of your priority list. Now, most of the people putting this book together are fathers, so we understand that if you have a family, every single, possible, conceivable moment gets filled up with utterly meaningless but God-help-you-if-you-don't-do-them tasks, to the point that from the moment when you wake up at 6:30 A.M. until you crash at midnight, you've had about 37 seconds to yourself.

If you resemble that remark, we recommend the following: Get a babysitter and take your wife out to dinner. Explain to her that you want to make a serious investment into your health, your happiness, your future. Tell her that the guys at *Men's Health* Books have put together a brilliant 12-week plan that will get you eating better, exercising more, even looking better. But you need help. You're going to need an hour or so of solo time on most days. For her help, you'll do whatever it is that would please her immensely. Watch the kids every Sunday—or give her nightly back rubs. Trust us, everyone will win if you strike this deal.

Get Your Calendar Ready

As we've explained, this program is built of daily tasks. Most of them you can read the night before and have no trouble completing the following day, but not all. We ask you now to make some formal time commitments. If you want to get an A1 grade on your performance, you need to set up the following appointments prior to launching into the program. Before you can do even that, you need to target a Monday on which to start. Don't assume it should be next Monday. Launch the Longevity Program on a week when you can concentrate on it. Don't wait too long, though, or you'll never start.

Here are the daily tasks that will require a formal appointment or an unusually large chunk of time.

Week 1, Day 1. You will overhaul your kitchen. First, you'll clean out old and unhealthy food. Then, you'll stock up on the food of the future you. Doing this right could entail a full 6 hours of cleaning, shopping, and putting away food. With that in mind, you may want to start the program on a Sunday.

Week 3. This week, you will thoroughly explore the wide world of supplements. We ask you to go to a store every day, either to study the shelves or make purchases.

Week 4, Day 3. You'll get a professional massage. Do some homework on picking a good massage therapist (the chapter for this day provides some pointers), then make an appointment.

Week 5, Day 5. We ask that you take a day off from work for a personal vacation. Either set it up now with your boss or start working on your fake hoarse voice.

Week 6, Day 2. This day calls for a complete physical exam. If you have had one in the past 2 years, you can skip this. Otherwise, set up the appointment immediately, without hesitation or second-guessing.

Week 6, Day 3. Lucky you, you'll get your entire body inspected in just 2 days. This day is dentist day. If you haven't been to the dentist in 6 months or more, make an appointment now for a checkup.

Week 8, Day 1. This is the wardrobe version of what we put you through on Week 1, Day 1, with your refrigerator. Plan on taking at least 4 hours to do a thorough inventory of your closet.

Week 8, Day 2. Plan on a few hours of clothes shopping. If your to-buy list is long, you might wish to schedule a full day at the mall or outlet center to get it all done.

Week 8, Day 5. You'll get a haircut. We'll ask you to find a new, probably more expensive barber. You might need to make an appointment ahead of time.

Spend Money Like There Is a Tomorrow

Some guys dole out Trump-like sums for injections of yak liver cells or herbal enemas, hoping to feel and look better. Our plan costs a comparative pittance. Better still, it works. It's the best money you'll ever spend.

What will you buy? Will you spend $200 or $2000? That's up to you. You may not need to buy everything on our list. But no guy we know is so mentally and physically together that he doesn't need to change something. It depends on the current state of your mind and body as well as your commitment to improving yourself.

Food. If you subsist primarily on doughnuts and cheeseburgers, you will have to increase your daily food allowance to cover stuff such as oatmeal, brown rice, shrimp, pasta, fruits, and vegetables. These items aren't going to make you miss a rent or mortgage payment. But if your larder is currently a den of lard, the shopping we'll ask you to do on Week 1, Day 1 might set you back $150 or more.

Vitamins and herbal supplements. You may eat such a balanced diet and be in such hearty health that you will be satisfied to take our minimal recommendation: a multivitamin, a vitamin C supplement, and a vitamin E supplement each day. That would be a mere $20 or so for a few months' dosages. We'll also recommend that you stock six or so healing herbs. That could be another $50. We further recommend that you investigate other health supplements that might be appropriate for your unique needs.

One-day vacation. A day at the country club could set you back a C-note. A day in the country will cost you nothing. It's yours to decide. But treat yourself well.

Clothes. Upgrading your wardrobe may not have a direct impact on your health, but it will leave you looking better. And if you look good, you feel better about yourself. Once again, the cost will vary greatly from man to man. If you need to buy a new suit or if the last sport jacket you bought looked hip during the disco era, you may shell out some serious coin. Then again, your greatest sartorial needs may be no more serious than a couple of polo shirts and a pair of khakis. As with other aspects of this program, you can make changes incrementally.

Home gym. This is where you could spend the most—literally, thousands of dollars, depending on what you already own and your exercise preferences. At least initially, if you're content to purchase a very basic weight setup, you can invest as little as $200.

Health care. We hope you have health and dental insurance that covers checkups. If you don't, your physical and dentist visits could cost you $400, once you factor in the medical tests. A good massage might be $75 for a full hour, and a good haircut, at least $25. Finally, we recommend that you invest in some good-quality skin-care products. Spend a little more than would ordinarily make you comfortable; we'll wager that when the supply runs out, you'll have no problem convincing yourself to buy more.

A good calendar. One of the last tasks of the program is to start using a personal planner not just for work appointments but also for every scheduled event in your life, be it social, exercise, or personal. A good system may cost $25 to $50, but it should last a long, long time (paper inserts for subsequent years are relatively cheap).

Most of the rest of this program comes free. Doubling your water intake, taking a walk after dinner, improving your breathing, and spending extra time outdoors are just a few positive things you can do for health that cost you nada.

How to Keep Yourself on the Program

Okay, all the cards are on the table. You know what we're trying to do with this program. And you know you have everything to gain by following it. You may even be all fired up to take on the program, to really take your life in a new direction. We may be talking to the next Jack LaLanne.

But we also know you're only human. Some days, it's all too easy to let your eyes glaze over even though they may be on a prize that you consider eminently worthwhile. We've done everything humanly possible to make sure this 12-week plan gives you something new and fresh to try every day. Even so, we know you won't always follow through. Drift is a natural part of life. We just don't want you drifting so far that you go careening hopelessly off course.

That's why this chapter is going to address the issue of mindset—specifically, *yours*. We're going to help you lay down the law for yourself and establish goals, guidelines, and safety valves to make sure you stick with this program not for just 12 weeks but for the rest of your long life.

We hope that your specific goal at this moment is to get through this 12-week program. If it's not, give yourself an honest goal in its place, such as, "I will do at least 20 of the recommended tasks in this book during the next 2 months."

Once you've reached that goal, the harder work begins: creating lifelong ambitions, like a permanent exercise habit or a commitment to never again let work wring your emotions dry. To do this, you have to set up more specific goals, with specific time frames. We suggest you pick a fitness goal, a healthy-eating goal, and a few more goals geared toward your mental well-being.

Scoring Your Goals

Each year, when you sit down with the boss to review your work and haggle about how many percentage points over the cost of living you should get in your raise, you probably also spend a little time filling out a form in which you outline your goals for the coming year. Then you and your boss both sign the form, send a copy off to human resources, and promptly forget about it.

That isn't the kind of goal we want you to set here. No, we want you to set some meaningful goals, goals that aren't about posturing and satisfying the folks in HR but are completely, uniquely yours, answerable only to you. In other words, you can't cheat. Such goals must be honest and motivating and, unlike many work-related goals, achievable.

There is a science to goal making, but it's one in which you can earn a Ph.D. rather quickly. Here are some basics for setting goals and making them stick.

Commit it to paper. Writing down your goals for the coming year, the coming decade, and so on really isn't such a bad idea. Research shows that putting your goals in ink actually increases your level of commitment to those goals. But once you write them down, don't file them and forget them. Post them where you can see them—on the refrigerator door, say, or by your bed.

Be specific. Don't just jot down some feel-good generalities like, "I want to live longer." Make your goal specific and measurable. Write, "I want to cut my fat intake by 50 percent over the next month" or "I want to be able to bench-press 200 pounds within 6 months." As you follow the daily objectives laid out in this book, you'll start to get a better sense of how to set specific goals for yourself.

Be realistic. As you strive to make goals specific, you'll find that you have to make them achievable in the real world. "Your goal might be that you're going to exercise 5 days a week," says Robert Weinberg, Ph.D., a sports psychologist at Miami University in Oxford, Ohio. "But soon, you miss a day and you say to yourself, 'To heck with it. I guess I can't do it,' and then you drop it. But how realistic is it for anyone to exercise 5 days a week?" Don't set yourself up for failure.

Ditch the doubt. While part of our program encourages you to get more in touch with your inner self, don't overdo it. Too much analysis of yourself and your adherence to this program could put you on the slippery slope of self-doubt. Once you start to doubt yourself, it's easy to lose your motivation and give up. "Being aware is one thing; being self-conscious is another," says James E. Loehr, Ed.D., a sports psychologist with LGE Sport Science in Orlando, Florida. "Get outside your head and absorbed into the activity."

Keep it short. One of the reasons we designed this program as a system of daily assignments is because we know it's hard to stay motivated over a long period of time. You should follow that example and design your goals in similar short-range fashion. It's fine to have a long-term goal of living longer and better, but establish short-term goals whose sum will ultimately equal the big goal. That way, you get the reward and satisfaction of accomplishing goals on a regular basis.

Adopt the buddy system. Numerous studies have shown that you're more likely to meet goals and stay motivated if you have a partner whose goals are similar and who can goad and prod you when your will falters. That person may be your best friend, a coworker, or even your spouse. Elsewhere in this book, we tell you how important it is to be plugged into a support system of family and friends. Mutual motivation is just one of the reasons why it's important.

Review your progress regularly. Before your workweek gets underway, take some time every Sunday to review the goals of the previous week and to plan more upcoming, short-term goals. This regular review process helps you stay on track and can be very rewarding.

Know when to change. Trying to achieve even short-term goals can get boring sometimes, especially when those goals involve exercise and eating. If things start to feel routine, look at ways you can shake them up. If your exercise goals are getting blurry, try mixing up your workout routine. Maybe instead of a set schedule of weight training and aerobics, you could drop that for a while and take up cycling or running. Or maybe you could treat yourself to a kickboxing class. If you're struggling to come up with a new healthy meal that's tasty and satisfying, give yourself the okay to chow down on a burger and fries once in a while. Going off-course for a little while needn't be harmful. Just exercise a little self-control and know when to get yourself back on the program.

Build in reminders. As you plug away at your goals, take time to remind yourself of your big-picture goal of living a longer, better, healthier life. We're not talking about putting a reminder on the calendar. Remind yourself in a very concrete way. If you want a reminder with some shock value, pick up a newspaper and turn to the obituary page. Notice how many people your age or even younger have write-ups. For something a little more positive, play with your kids for an afternoon, and remind yourself that you will have an opportunity to do this with *their* kids, if you stick with the program.

Go with the flow. Life is a study in chaos. However much we may try to control our environment, every once in a while we have to take the curves that life throws us. Illness, job duties, or even fun stuff like vacations and activities with the kids can get in your way and sidetrack you from your goals. Our advice is to let it happen. Don't be so obsessive about hitting your short-term goals that you can't allow yourself the pleasure of the rest of your life. At the end of the week, when you review your goals, you can always tweak the next week's goals to make up for time lost.

The Habit of Life

As you go through the 12-week plan, you're going to have to go beyond setting goals. You're going to have to turn your goals into habits so automatic that you aren't even aware you're doing them. While you're building those habits, you're going to have to be ever on the alert for boredom and complacency, the two great adversaries that threaten to put you in the ground at an untimely age. Here are just a few guidelines to keep you on the right path.

Read ahead, plan ahead. Each day, we give you a task to perform. If at all possible, you should perform each task immediately upon reading it. But some tasks may require a few preparatory steps. Keep this book by your bedside, and each night, read ahead to see what your task will be the next day.

Pace yourself. If 12 weeks is too long or too short a time frame for you to work with, modify these plans as you see fit. We recognize that everyone works at his own pace. If you need 6 months to implement the strategies outlined here, that's fine. Conversely, if you want to cram this program into a concise 6-week regimen, you have our blessing.

Do a little something every day. We recognize that you probably have other things to do during your day besides prepare yourself to do the tasks we outline. You may not be able to do absolutely everything we suggest, exactly the way we suggest it. That's okay. But at the very least, try to do a little something from each of the daily assignments. You'll feel better and be more motivated to devote a little more time and energy to the next day's task.

Be kind to yourself. Some of what we suggest here isn't for sissies. It takes guts to commit to an exercise program, to take time to reach out to another person, to pitch out old, familiar stuff in favor of strange, new stuff. We know that. And we know that change can be hard, at least at first. So if, as you embark on the plan, it starts to feel like the going is getting a little too tough, you have our permission to cut yourself a break. If you need a day off from the plan to relax or deal with daily life, take it. Otherwise, you're going to end up being resentful of the program and even of yourself.

Stay open. Some of the tasks you will encounter in the next 3 months may seem strange or unconnected to the issue of longevity. For example, there are more tasks related to your mind and spirit than you may have expected from the guys at *Men's Health* Books. But they are here for a very good reason. If the *Men's Health* philosophy is about anything, it's about attitude—how to be your own man, without compromise, without apology. Moreover, some of the attitudinal work is one-time stuff. Improving your outlook doesn't require the ongoing time commitment that exercise and nutrition do.

Stay with the program. You have a chance, probably the best chance you've had in years, to truly lay the groundwork for a better, stronger, happier you. Don't let it slip through your fingers. Remember, it's a poor man who cheats himself.

WEEK 1

EAT FOR MAXIMUM ENERGY

Restock Your Refrigerator and Pantry

The Day's Task

Your health-and-longevity program begins the way any worthwhile work of monumental transformation does—with an act of wanton destruction.

Open your kitchen cabinets. All of them. Prop open your fridge and freezer doors. Pull your trash can alongside you. Not the wimpy, white kitchen can—get the mondo, super-size black one you keep in the garage for yard waste. Be sure to put a plastic bag in there; when you're done, you'll want to tie it up so wild animals don't come to feast.

Examine each item in your cabinets, fridge, and freezer. You have two questions to ask yourself: (1) Would I eat this? If yes, (2) should I eat this? If the answer to the first is no (hint: if the color of the food is different than it was when you bought it, answer no), throw it out. If the answer to the first is yes, look at the ingredients and the food itself and ask yourself, "Is this healthy?" If it's not, into the can it goes.

Unsure about what's healthy? Here are some hints. If it's high in fat—say, if more than one-third of the calories come from fat—get rid of it. If it's virtually without nutrients, chuck it. If it's highly processed, highly refined, or highly chemicalized, slam-dunk it into the barrel. When in doubt, throw it out.

So let that jar of high-fat mayonnaise shatter against the inside of the barrel. Smash that cream pie facedown. Revel in the splat it makes.

Now for the constructive part. Grab this chapter's grocery list and head for the store. Plan to be there a while. You have a lot of food to gather.

Keeping the right stuff in your kitchen is a proven way to be healthier and live longer.

- Experts say that diet contributes to 4 of the top 10 causes of death in the United States.
- Many of the common quality-of-life diseases (some potentially lethal) are related to poor diet. These include cataracts, memory loss, diabetes, obesity, high blood pressure, and impaired immune function.
- If death and quality of life aren't convincing arguments, perhaps money is. It's estimated that more than $23 billion a year in hospital costs would be saved if Americans ate a more healthy diet.

The max-health restocking plan we're about to give you is based on three really simple ideas about good eating.

1. Lots of plant-based foods. Grains, fruits, and vegetables are where the life-sustaining substances are found. The goal is to maximize the fiber, vitamins, minerals, and disease-preventing chemical powerhouses known as phytochemicals that are found only in plant-based foods.

2. Not much fat. Lowering the amount of fat you eat to 30 percent of your total calories significantly reduces your risk of serious disease, not to mention your waistline. That means that (if you're typical) nearly a third of the calories you consume can be fat and you'll still be better off than you are now. Your restocking assignment today will make it easy to cut down even more than that on artery-clogging, cholesterol-raising, heart disease–inducing, physique-ruining, life-shortening dietary fat.

3.Total satisfaction. Look at the shopping list that follows. Does it look like monk food? On the contrary, it's a supply line for 21st-century adventures in good eating. And that's our restocking philosophy at work: Always have the fixings for a delicious, healthy meal, and you'll always eat delicious, healthy meals.

Load Up the Fridge

With what should a man who is interested in eating well fill up his refrigerator? Here's a very full list. In recommending quantities of particular foods, we are assuming that you shop once a week for fresh food such as vegetables, fruits, milk, and meats and that you eat most breakfasts and dinners at home.

Keep in mind, though, that all this food that we're telling you to buy is for you alone. If you're going to be sharing with someone else, increase the quantities accordingly.

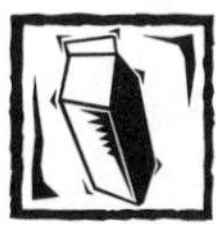

Beverages

Milk: One gallon of fat-free; you can do without the fat in whole milk
Orange juice: One gallon of real OJ
Other fruit juices: Like Concord grape juice and pineapple juice
Vegetable juice: V8, for example
Beer: You can keep a six-pack on hand—surprise, it has health benefits (better go fish it out of the trash can)
Water: A large pitcher of filtered water

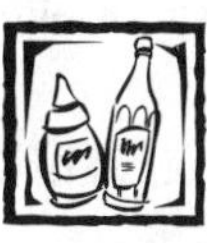

The Condiment Shelf

Load up on the traditional and the exotic. The idea is that no future meal, no matter how healthy, will ever be tasteless or dull.

Hot sauces: Two types: Tabasco and one crazy-named scorcher
Salsa: Healthier than you think
Mustard: Three types: golden, brown, and something fancy, like honey
Mayonnaise: It must be low-fat
Salad dressings: Two kinds: We suggest low-fat Italian and low-fat blue cheese
Garlic: The crushed kind in a jar
Maple syrup: Reduced-calorie
Chinese condiments: Chile-garlic paste, black bean sauce, hoisin sauce, oyster sauce, and plum sauce are staples of Chinese cooking; get them only if you are willing to wok
Italian condiments: Oil-packed sun-dried tomatoes, cured olives, and capers
Jalapeño peppers: Jarred or canned
Also: Ketchup, barbecue sauce, lemon juice, lime juice

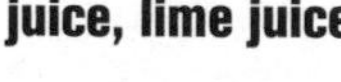

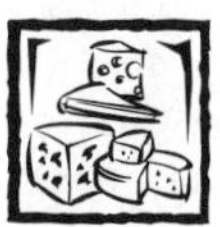

On the Shelves

Or some may fit better in the door. Point is, all you need is listed below. And what you don't need conspicuously isn't.

Butter or soft margarine: Butter freezes well, so a pound, which is four sticks, should last you at least a few months; avoid margarine with hydrogenated oils, as they contain the ill-reputed trans fatty acids
Cheddar cheese: The low-fat kind
Parmesan cheese: Grated
Cream cheese: Reduced-fat; once you open the container, cream cheese doesn't last that long, so buy small quantities unless you like green fuzz

Eggs: One dozen—that's for a few weeks, not one omelette
Yogurt: One quart of the plain, low-fat kind
Jelly: Two jars, two different flavors
Sour cream: One pint of the low-fat kind
Peanut butter: Natural reduced-fat
Pudding cups: Low-fat
Tortillas: Whole-wheat
Also: Flaxseed oil, applesauce, chocolate syrup

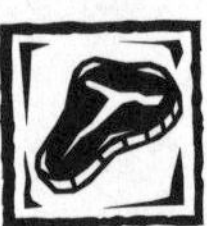

The Meat Drawer

Keep fresh meats for 2 days of meals. The rest should be frozen.

Turkey bacon: One pound; same taste as pig bacon, much less fat
Chicken breasts: Boneless and skinless; keep one or two in the fridge, put any extras in the freezer
Ground beef: Make sure it's extra-lean
Cooked shrimp: A small tub is enough for a meal—unless you love them, in which case get extra for salads or stir-frying with vegetables
Sliced ham or turkey: A half-pound of the lean stuff
Sliced cheese: A quarter-pound of any low-fat type, for sandwiches
Cheese block: A quarter-pound of any low-fat variety, to use for snacks

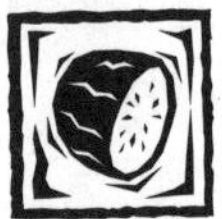

The Fruit Drawer

Start each week with at least 15 to 20 servings of fresh fruit on hand.

Apples: Six of your favorites
Oranges: A half-dozen; more if you squeeze your own orange juice
Summer fruit: As available; berries too
Melon: One cantaloupe or one-quarter of a watermelon

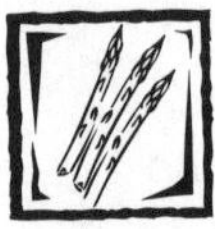

The Vegetable Drawer

Stock at least enough fresh vegetables for a salad and a cooked vegetable for each of the week's home-cooked dinners.

Lettuce: Not just iceberg but also a dark leafy lettuce or pre-mixed greens
Green onions: One bunch
Cooking vegetables: Four, like zucchini, broccoli, eggplant, or green beans
Ginger: A small hunk of the fresh root
Cucumbers: Two
Tomatoes: Three

Celery: Good for snacking as well as including in stir fries, soups, and salads
Carrots: Consider getting a pound for cooking and a 1-pound bag of baby carrots for snacks
Also: Green and red bell peppers, mushrooms

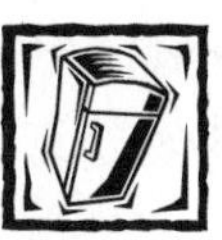

In the Freezer

The freezer is an underrated storage area where good foods last a long time. Keep frozen meats for four meals, prepared foods for two, and bags of fruits and vegetables. You should have room for the following.

Fish: Several fillets
Steaks: Extra lean and not bigger than 8 ounces each
Chicken: Skinless breasts
Dumplings: One pound, like wontons, ravioli, or pierogies
Vegetables: One-pound bags or boxes of varieties such as mixed vegetables, chopped broccoli, and spinach
Berries: A bag each of blueberries and strawberries
Soft pretzels: One box
Bagels: Six, preferably whole-grain; the small Lender's are fine
Bread: An extra loaf of whole-wheat
Ice cream: Low-fat vanilla or low-fat frozen yogurt
Waffles: One box of whole-grain

Stock the Pantry

Remember the obvious rule of space management: Keep the stuff you use a lot (cereals, cooking oils, pastas) close by, at a convenient height. Put the occasional-usage stuff low, high, or in the basement.

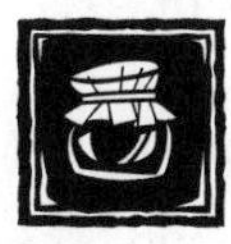

The Basics

Oils: You need these two: canola oil and olive oil
Vinegars: Again, two versions: red wine and apple cider
Dried herbs: Oregano, basil, thyme, Italian seasoning, parsley, and rosemary
Spices: Chili powder, ground cinnamon, ground cumin, and garlic powder
Flour: Or a flour mix, like Bisquick
Chicken broth: Stock both small and large cans
Pasta: Strand-type (such as linguini and spaghetti) and shape-type (fusilli, wagon wheels); whole-grain is best

Rice: Two large boxes of instant brown rice (instead of white rice); and 2 pounds of uncooked wild rice or a large box of instant rice

Noodles: Six packages of the ramen variety

Tomato products: Two cans each of whole tomatoes, tomato sauce, and tomato paste

Tea bags: Assorted herbal, plus green (which has the best health benefits) and English breakfast or Earl Grey

Refrigerator backups: Have these extras ready for when the refrigerate-after-opening items run out: salsa, ketchup, mustard, jelly, and peanut butter

Psyllium fiber: Like Metamucil or Konsyl

Also: Salt, pepper, soy sauce, cocoa, lemonade mix, coffee

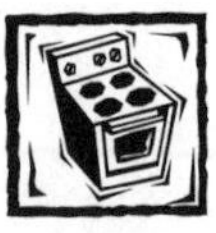

Ready to Eat or Heat

Cereals: Three boxes or bags, one very high fiber kind, like an all-bran cereal; one flake cereal, such as raisin bran; and either low-fat granola or wheat germ

Oatmeal: Packets are okay; a canister box is better (more fiber)

Breads: A loaf of whole-wheat bread, a whole-grain baguette, and a package of whole-grain muffins

Crackers: Two types, both whole-grain; try sesame rounds and wheat

Popcorn: A case of microwaveable, reduced-fat or fat-free

Tortilla chips: Make sure they're baked

Nuts: A pound or so of a raw and unsalted variety

Sunflower seeds: Go for shelled and unsalted; they're great for adding to salads

Canned fruits: Two each of pineapple chunks and pears in water

Canned vegetables: Two each of water chestnuts and bamboo shoots

Canned beans: Two each of black beans, chickpeas, baked beans, and chili beans

Canned tuna: Two or three small cans of the packed-in-water kind

Canned soups: Keep six cans of varieties such as minestrone and lentil, but no cream-based soups; also, keep plenty of instant soup packets on hand

Prepared side dishes: One box each of rice pilaf, black beans and rice, macaroni and cheese, and couscous blends

Also: Raisins, fruit bars, spaghetti sauce, red wine

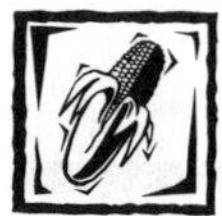

Fresh Foods

Onions: Two pounds
Potatoes: Four loose russets or reds and two sweet potatoes
Garlic: At least one large head
Bananas: One bunch
Tropical fruit: Like mangoes, kiwifruit, papayas, or pineapples; have at least one or two on hand

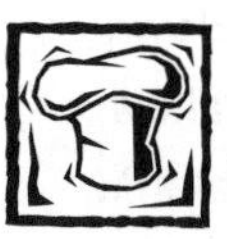

And If You Like to Cook

More nuts: One pound each of peanuts, walnuts, cashews, and pistachios
Specialty items: Such as hearts of palm, artichoke hearts, roasted peppers, and capers
Baking supplies: If you bake or have a bread machine, you'll need baking powder, wheat flour, bread flour, baking soda, cornstarch, and honey
Tofu: Buy brands that come in tightly sealed boxes, which store at room temperature for up to a year
Also: Sesame oil, red wine vinegar

Eat a Good Breakfast

The Day's Task

You're going to do just one thing different today. You're going to eat and enjoy breakfast.

Not only that, you're going to enjoy the kind of breakfast that will please your palate and energize your morning while it helps keep your weight down and your life span up. But you can't enjoy anything if you're rushing, so allow yourself plenty of time for a relaxed, unhurried meal. Use that time to eat in a seated position, not running out the door. And sit down at a real table, not in the driver's seat and not at your desk at work.

Comfortable? Okay. Here's how to eat breakfast.

Grab a bowl. Pour in a little of the high-fiber cereal you stocked up on yesterday, then fill it the rest of the way with the flake cereal. Pour in some fat-free milk. Top it off with a sliced banana or a generous pile of strawberries or blueberries or all three. Eat it accompanied by an 8-ounce (or larger) glass of orange juice.

Remain seated. Relax. Savor your coffee. (You didn't think we were going to deny you your coffee, did you? Just keep it to two cups.) Have a slice of toast from the whole-wheat loaf you bought yesterday. Spread on a little bit of low-fat cream cheese. Relax a few minutes more. Then, go to work.

Repeat every day for the rest of your life.

We're not suggesting that you always eat the same breakfast. But you should eat one that approaches this model breakfast in low fat content, fueling power, fiber, and nutritional goodness. And we suggest—no, we *insist*—that you do it daily. The reason for that is simple: Men who start their days with a meal tend to live longer, healthier lives.

Of course, if you're like a lot of guys, the whole business of eating breakfast at all is a radical proposition. If so, you've been paying a price for those mornings without meals. And you've been paying that price in the following currencies.

Your get-up-and-go. Ditching the most important meal of the day can leave you dragging and less efficient. "A lot of men skip breakfast, don't eat much for lunch, and wonder why they feel miserable by the time they get home," says Mack Ruffin IV, M.D., associate professor in the department of family medicine at the University of Michigan Medical Center in Ann Arbor.

Your weight control. Want to shed those extra pounds fast? Start eating breakfast regularly. Skipping a meal, especially breakfast, to "save" calories doesn't work. "Typically, men who skip breakfast eat more later, and then choose food higher in fat and calories," says Franca Alphin, R.D., a licensed dietitian at the Duke University Diet and Fitness Center in Durham, North Carolina.

Your longevity quest. You'll be reading a lot in upcoming chapters about how the vitamins, minerals, fiber, and disease-fighting antioxidants in fruits and vegetables are nearly miraculous in their anti-aging action. You're going to want a generous allotment of these life givers, and some of the top anti-aging foods known to man are classic breakfast fruits. Orange juice, for example, is the best source of the energy-essential, immune-boosting, eye-saving, and age-busting antioxidant vitamin C as well as of heart-helping folate, a B vitamin.

The strawberries and blueberries you add to your cereal are also first-rate anti-aging agents, but the best of the bunch may be the most familiar breakfast fruit of all. "The banana is probably the best form of food there is in the world," says Richard Honaker, M.D., a family physician in Carrolton, Texas. "It's the perfect mix of vitamins, antioxidants, fiber, and trace minerals."

So your humble task of the day, eating a good breakfast, just may be the cornerstone of your new Longevity Program. It lays the foundation for taking control of your meals so you can eat for health and vitality and enjoy yourself while you're doing it. It's hard to think of anything more important for living long and prospering.

"No matter what you've done the night before, have a normal breakfast," advises Paula Levine, Ph.D., of the Anorexia and Bulimia Resource Center in Coral Gables, Florida. "That way, you start the day off on the right foot instead of continuing the deprivation/binge cycle."

That's worth repeating: Always eat breakfast, no matter what. Pigged out at midnight? Eat breakfast. Overslept and have only 5 minutes to make it to a meeting across town? Eat breakfast. Girlfriend left you and you've already written your suicide note? Eat breakfast first.

The Best Kind of Breakfast

Making the commitment to eating breakfast every morning is a pretty fair piece of work for just the second day of your program. But you've actually done more than that. You've committed to eating a *good* breakfast every morning.

What's a good breakfast? Well, the one you're eating today is. We've already told you about the vitamins, minerals, and antioxidants it offers. Here are some other reasons why it's so good. Pay attention to them because they can be your guidelines for choosing other breakfast menus.

It has a good macronutrient balance. That means you're getting the right mix of carbohydrates (the majority), protein (a moderate amount), and fat (very little, but not zero). In the long run, that's the three-way ratio your body needs to function. In the short run—this morning, that is—it's the best combo for fueling up. The carbohydrates in the cereal, fruit, and toast bring on the energy, while the protein in the milk, cream cheese, and cereal, along with the fat (mostly in the cream cheese), help meter that energy so your head doesn't start nodding 5 minutes into that 10:00 A.M. meeting.

It has the right kind of carbohydrates. All those carbs in today's breakfast will provide you with energy to burn, literally. But not just any old carbohydrates will do the job right. Refined white flour and simple sugars fool you with a quick energy fix as they send your blood sugar soaring, but leave you lazy when your blood sugar levels plummet soon after.

That's one reason why we had you throw out those refined and sugary foods yesterday and replace them with the good stuff. It's not that a little jam or jelly on your whole-wheat toast is going to sabotage your breakfast, but if you go so far as to replace the whole-grain cereal with sugared cereals named after cartoon characters or video games, you exchange nutrients, fiber, and energy for a lot of empty calories and a mid-morning slump. Who needs it?

It has loads of fiber. Before your 12 weeks are up, you're going to consider fiber one of your best friends, and there's no better time to get a generous healthy dose of it than at breakfast. Fiber helps prevent heart disease, reduces your risk of certain kinds of cancer, helps keep your weight down, and slows the processing of energy from the carbohydrates so your vim and vigor last longer.

That's a big reason why you're eating bran cereal today instead of eggs, lots of fruit instead of bacon, and whole-wheat toast instead of white toast. These foods are fiber-packed, especially the cereal. A good rule of thumb is to read the cereal box to make sure your choice has at least 7 grams of fiber per serving. Your best bet for that, of course, is those super-fiber cereals. But if you tend to balk at breakfasting on what look like rat pellets and taste like nothing, take a tip from today's breakfast: mix in the hard-core stuff with a cereal you do like, such as a better-tasting (but still pretty darn high in fiber) bran cereal like raisin bran.

Brave New Breakfast Worlds

We called this chapter Eat a Good Breakfast, not Suffer through a Good Breakfast. Fruit and cereal are great, but not every day. How about some variety?

No problem. The trick is breaking out of that boring breakfast box. No internationally recognized law requires cereal or eggs for breakfast. Let your imagination or palate run wild. Just remember what we said about low fat, high fiber, macronutrient balance, and vitamins and minerals. Here are some ideas, all with at least 7 grams of fiber and not too much fat or too many calories.

Have a bowl of oatmeal topped with fruit and ground cinnamon. Add a piece of whole-wheat toast covered with fruit jam. Also have a few slices of melon. Drink your orange juice.

Okay, this one is relatively tried-and-true. But oatmeal is so great for breakfast that we feel duty-bound to mention it. Rolled oats are a whole grain that's nutrient- and fiber-rich. And they're a get-up-and-go food, delivering lots of nicely metered carbohydrate energy.

Whip up a stack of whole-grain pancakes topped with bananas or berries. Don't forget the orange juice. Do forget the butter and maple syrup. Your typical pancake-and-syrup breakfast is a feast of fiber-poor and nutrient-challenged refined white flour with a lot of sugar poured over it. But, of course, you have to have pancakes occasionally. So make them with a whole-grain mix or with a half-cup of wheat germ added to the batter.

Try a baked potato. Top it with a cup of broccoli, 2 tablespoons of fat-free sour cream, 2 tablespoons of salsa, and ¼ cup of cheese—with orange juice, of course. Plenty of dinner foods make good breakfasts.

Eat a sandwich for breakfast. Make it with fat-free turkey on light whole-wheat bread with fat-free mayonnaise and tomato. Have a banana on the side and orange juice to wash it down.

Make a bean burrito. Fill a whole-wheat tortilla with fat-free refried beans (not meat), 2 tablespoons of salsa, and ⅛ cup of grated cheese. Later, tell your friends that you had a burrito for breakfast and that it was probably a heck of a lot healthier than what they had. Did we mention the orange juice?

Eat a Good Dinner

The Day's Task

Tonight, we present you with the perfect weekday dinner: a tossed salad, sautéed vegetables and shrimp on brown rice, a whole-wheat baguette with Italian cheese, and a dessert of mango and yogurt. You'll need to do the cooking at home. Don't let this frighten you.

Making a salad isn't rocket science. Throw about one fistful of loose green lettuce leaves or salad greens into a wide soup bowl. Cut six slices of cucumber and about half of a tomato and place on top the greens. Take a bottle of olive oil, put your thumb over the top, and shake just enough oil on top of the salad so that when mixed, all the ingredients will have the slightest amount of oil on the surface. If there's oil pooled at the bottom of the bowl, you've used too much. Sop it up with a paper towel. Put your thumb over the top of a bottle of red wine vinegar, and shake on about half as much as the amount of oil you used. Add a light sprinkling of salt and pepper.

Make the entrée. Slice up half of a small zucchini, half of a red bell pepper, a quarter of a medium onion, and three or four mushrooms. Pour about a tablespoon of olive oil into a skillet, heat it up, and add one clove of chopped garlic or ½ teaspoon of garlic powder. Throw in the zucchini, pepper, and mushrooms, and sauté for a few minutes. Next, toss in about six large shrimp (large shrimp are about 25 shrimp to the pound, so you need approximately ¼ pound). Continue cooking for another 3 to 4 minutes, or until the shrimp turns pink. Meanwhile, cook about ½ cup of instant brown rice according to the package directions. When the shrimp and vegetables are almost done, throw on healthy pinches of pepper, dried thyme, and dried oregano, and mix. Put the brown rice on a dinner plate. Pour the vegetables and shrimp right onto the rice.

Prep the bread. Good grocery stores make French baguettes using whole-grain wheat. If you can find one of these, great. (If not, use two slices of whole-wheat bread.) Toast about a 3-inch hunk that's been sliced open lengthwise. Put it on a small plate, and add two slices of reduced-fat provolone or mozzarella cheese. These cheeses taste good straight from the refrigerator, but if you like, you can melt them on the bread in a toaster oven.

Pre-make the dessert. Use a mango if you have one, or you can substitute a generous helping of strawberries or blueberries. Grab a good peeler and remove the skin from the mango. It's a bit of a challenge, but it only takes a minute. Carefully slice the meat off the mango. Give yourself a reward and take the mango pit to the kitchen sink, lean over the sink, and suck the remaining juice and meat off the pit—it's one of life's simple, messy pleasures. Wash your hands and face and get back to the dessert. Place about half of the mango slices on a plate. Plop a small scoop of low-fat vanilla frozen yogurt on top. Throw it in the freezer until you are ready to eat it, but not longer than 30 minutes.

Next, pour yourself a glass of red wine.

Finally, pour yourself a large tumbler of water.

Bon appétit!

Dinner is not the time to get heavy. Notice a few things about this dinner right away? For one, it's relatively light, though far from skimpy. For another, it includes lots of different foods. And finally, it's probably much better eats than you're used to. None of this is coincidence.

"Most Americans make dinner their heaviest meal of the day, which is a mistake," says John Amberge, an exercise physiologist at the Sports Training Institute in New York City. What's the point of fueling up at the end of the day? Research has shown that food eaten shortly before bed not only tends to keep you awake but also has a greater tendency to be stored as fat.

Dinner is a chance to get pro-longevity nutrients. A week ago, you may have eaten in the evening for pleasure and to satisfy your hunger. As of today, you eat dinner for pleasure, for satisfaction, and to provide yourself with a generous portion of the very best nutrients, the kind that help you live a long life and feel good enough to want to. Variety is the way to get those nutrients. And tonight's dinner has lots of variety. Here's a partial rundown of the benefits you're getting.

- The brown rice delivers fiber, as do the vegetables, the whole-grain bread, and the mango. So do certain kinds of pasta made from whole grains, which you can use instead of the rice.

- The shrimp is your main protein source in this dinner, and it's rich in vitamin B_{12}, which is good for immunity and helps prevent age-related memory loss.
- The vegetables and fruit—from the salad at the beginning of your dinner to the mango at the end—are loaded with those phytochemicals we talked about.
- Olive oil is high in monounsaturated fat and low in saturated fat, which is just what you want in an oil. Aside from keeping your cholesterol levels down, olive oil provides vitamin E, the antioxidant superstar that helps save your heart, your eyesight, your memory, maybe even your gums.
- The herbs you used to wake up those vegetables deliver super health benefits as well as zing for your tastebuds. For example, rosemary is rich in antioxidants, thyme is heart-healthy, and oregano may block the carcinogens in cooked meat.
- Red wine is brimming with a family of phytochemicals called phenolic compounds, antioxidants that protect you from heart disease. Red wine contains phenolics that have the ability to neutralize free radicals, unstable oxygen molecules that create "bad" cholesterol, which clogs arteries. There's good evidence that the alcohol itself, in moderation, is protective as well. Experts advise that you limit your intake of wine to one 5-ounce glass daily, or you could be throwing the health benefits out the window. Cheers.
- The low-fat frozen yogurt in your dessert gives you calcium for strong bones.

A healthy dinner is a taste treat. When we tell you to eat a good dinner, we mean good tasting just as much as we mean good for you. Tonight's model dinner should convince you of a welcome fact about the eating aspect of your Longevity Program: nutrient-rich meals are pleasurable.

Sure, some of the foods that you like are decidedly unhealthy, like a fat-marbled cut of prime rib the size of a catcher's mitt. But more often, it's the dinners you don't enjoy that do more harm than good—like when you open a can of mystery meat because nobody wants to cook or when you settle for fast food and regret it because afterward you feel like you ate the paper bag that contained the food.

So keep a sense of pleasure in mind when you think about dinner. You won't miss the bad stuff if you concentrate on the good stuff. Tonight's dinner is the kind that will make you feel great while you're eating it *and* afterward.

How to Eat Dinner

You're going to be eating a lot more dinners over the coming decades. And, much as we'd like to, we can't be there to suggest a meal for you every night. But we can tell you, right now, the thinking behind tonight's model dinner. With the following general guidelines, you can eat for longevity every night, whether you do the cooking or somebody does it for you.

Focus on carbohydrates. The brown rice and vegetables in the model dinner are a fine example of a carbohydrate focus. So is the pasta that you might choose to substitute for rice, and so are the potatoes of the great American meat-and-potatoes tradition.

It's the meat half of the meat-and-potatoes combination that you need to deemphasize at dinner. Fact is, you don't need all the protein (we'll talk about that in a minute) and you certainly don't need all the saturated fat that comes with red meat. So it makes good sense to focus instead on what you do need—the fiber, vitamins, minerals, and other nutrients that come with grains and vegetables.

If you're a meat-and-potatoes kind of guy, you're probably wondering, "If I can't have the steak I deserve at dinner, when can I have it?" You're better off eating a piece of meat like that at lunch. A noon meal that's too carb heavy can lead to the so-called afternoon slump that turns you into a clock-watching zombie instead of the productive human being you really are. So while carbohydrates are going to be in the majority of your meals, have them at dinner—not lunch.

Stay lean and mean with the protein. We're not prohibiting nighttime protein outright. The trick is to keep it secondary and keep it light. Whether it's the sautéed shrimp we recommended for tonight or something like salmon, tuna, crab, clams, or mussels, seafood is an excellent evening protein that combines well with carbohydrates such as rice or pasta.

And nowhere will we ever say that meat should be permanently banned from the dinner table. But it should be lean meat, like skinless chicken or turkey. If you want red meat occasionally, choose the leanest cut you can find and keep the serving down to about the size of a deck of cards. There will be plenty else on your plate to fill you up.

Speaking of light, that goes for the pasta too. Or the potatoes. Or the rice. Or any of the carbohydrates, for that matter. It's not so much the pasta or potato itself that's light or heavy, it's what you put on it. For example, lasagna should be in small servings because the cheese and meat add extra protein and fat. For the same reason, stay away from heavy cream sauces or lots of butter. A better option is marinara, a meat-free sauce with basil, a bit of olive oil, and a shake or two of Parmesan cheese. Or add a package of mixed frozen vegetables to whole-wheat pasta and cover it with tomato sauce, which, incidentally, helps prevent prostate cancer. Kick up the flavor a notch or two with plenty of garlic and fresh parsley.

Pick some vegetables, any vegetables. You can't really go wrong with vegetables unless you load them up with butter, cheese, or cream sauces or deep-fry them. Instead, stir-fry or steam your vegetables, and zing them with spices. That way, you'll get the fiber and beneficial phytochemicals without the cholesterol-raising saturated fats.

Same goes for salads. Adding fresh vegetables like tomatoes, spinach, broccoli, and beans turns that dull pile of lettuce into a nutrient-rich and much tastier opening course. But drowning it in one of those glutinous dressings only adds calories and fat. Stick with a little bit of heart-healthy olive oil, vinegar, and spices.

The same thing applies to soups. Avoid the heavy, cream-based or cheese-based soups. With all the healthy vegetable soups, bean soups, tomato-based soups, and broth-based soups to choose from, you'll never miss those creamy cholesterol raisers.

To be sure, these guidelines for eating a good dinner every night probably call for a few habit shifts on your part. But they're really not all that drastic, considering that they make the difference between killing yourself a meal at a time and eating for a longer, healthier life.

Eat Smart throughout the Day

The Day's Task

This morning, try to eat breakfast at around 7:00 or 7:30. After breakfast but before you go to work, you need to prepare some food for the day, as follows:

1. **Rinse and polish an apple, and put it in a plastic bag or container with about an ounce of low-fat cheese.**
2. **Take out six whole-wheat crackers and dab a little natural peanut butter on each. (Take it easy; this is a high-fat food in any form). Make three little cracker sandwiches and put them in another bag.**
3. **Throw a few carrots in yet another baggie.**
4. **Pour about 6 ounces of grape juice into some kind of plastic container with a top that won't leak, or take a juice box of the stuff.**

Stick all this into your briefcase, your lunch pail, your coat pocket, your gym bag, wherever you can get your hands on it easily during the day. Then, at 10:00 or 10:30 A.M., 2 to 3 hours after breakfast and 2 to 3 hours before lunch, give yourself a 10-minute break to enjoy the apple and cheese with a big glass of cool, clean water.

Eat lunch as usual at noon to 1:00. Later, at 3:00 to 4:00 in the afternoon, take another break to munch away on the peanut butter crackers and the carrots, washing them down with the grape juice.

Then, don't think about eating again until dinnertime.

No big deal, right? A couple of much-needed breaks and pleasant snacks during the day aren't what you'd call a major personal sacrifice in the cause of good health. In fact, you may wonder, just what do they have to do with feeling better and living longer?

Plenty. Each snack offers a lot more than 10 minutes of pleasure. Snacks can help you feel more alive throughout the day by delivering the right kind of energy just when you need it. They make it easier to eat good lunches and dinners by keeping you away from the famine-then-feast rhythm that leads you to overindulge on harmful foods. And the kind of snacks we're talking about give you two more chances to ingest the life-enhancing, longevity-stretching nutrients that good food provides.

That's a far cry from what most folks call a snack. A snack, the thinking goes, is eating any old thing any old time. That usually means cookies, candy, chips, doughnuts, nachos, and so on. These snacks have nothing to do with reenergizing other than a short-lived burst of energy from the sugar or refined white flour. They're not a way of controlling appetite or maximizing meal quality—quite the opposite. And helpful nutrients? Forget it. With that kind of snacking, they're not even on the radar screen.

The snacks suggested here are completely different, though ultimately just as satisfying. What you're doing today is taking control of your snacks, turning the perfectly natural desire for between-meal eating into your health-and-longevity ally. A lot of it has to do with what you actually put in your mouth, of course. But a lot of it also has to do with timing.

Spreading It Out

Simply put, the 4 to 6 hours between breakfast and lunch is too long to go without eating. Ditto the period between lunch and dinner, which might be even longer. The most obvious drawback is energy supply. When you're running on empty, you're going to drag.

So an energy boost is benefit number one of your well-timed snacking. That mid-morning nosh will make those 10:30 meetings seem a little less interminable. And that mid-afternoon food break means you can finish the day strong, with your mind on your work instead of on dinner.

There's more to it than that, though. By actually planning your snacks in advance, determining what they'll be and when you'll eat them, you take more control of your eating patterns. That obviously makes for healthier snacking, the kind that delivers nutrients and long-lasting energy instead of empty calories and cholesterol-raising fats.

It gives you more control over your actual meals as well. Those timely snacks take the desperation out of your mealtime hunger, allowing you to concentrate on quality at lunch and dinner instead of on inhaling food to placate your growling stomach.

What your snacking today really accomplishes, then, is to more evenly spread out your daily calories, not just over breakfast, lunch, and dinner as we suggested in the last chapter but over *five* meals spaced evenly throughout the day. The 300 to 350 calories in each of your snacks should be subtracted from your lunch and dinner totals.

Dietitians and nutritionists have a name for this: *mini-meals*, or even more colloquially, *grazing*. The idea is to eat smaller meals, and more of them, throughout the day. And there are even more health benefits to this than those we've already mentioned.

For one thing, it's been shown that you burn more calories if you eat smaller meals more frequently. There's also an anti-aging benefit of smaller meals. At least one key study indicates that lower-calorie meals may keep blood sugar and insulin levels steadier. High blood sugar levels set off by bigger meals may set the stage for damage to collagen and DNA and accelerate signs of aging such as wrinkles and cataracts. High insulin is a known risk factor for heart disease.

All that is in addition to what you've surely noticed on your own—that big meals can make you lazy afterward. Eating a big meal diverts blood to your digestive system and away from your brain, making you sleepy. So now you know why a too-big lunch, especially one that's almost all carbohydrates, can lead to the dreaded afternoon slump when you return to work.

Hard-core mini-mealers take the concept to its logical extreme by eating as many as seven snack-size meals 2 to 3 hours apart. They toss the whole concept of breakfast, lunch, dinner, and snacks out the window. We're not asking you to do that. But if you plan and time your snacks the way we've suggested, you're on your way to eating smart all day long.

Anatomy of a Snack

Planning your snacks means you have to make a few more food choices during the day than you may be used to making. And when you're eating for longevity, you usually can't make those choices by tossing some quarters into the junk food machine and selecting a knob to pull. Here are some ideas to start you thinking.

- The best overall plan is to design your snacks so they include foods you tend to skip—fruits and vegetables, perhaps, or yogurt.
- Remember the "mini" in mini-meal. Carry your snack foods in single-serving

sizes so you won't overeat. Divvy up big bags of crackers into snack-size plastic bags.

- Fill your desk drawer with instant soups. "Noodle soups sound like they're a snack for kids, but they're a great snack for everybody," says Neal Barnard, M.D., of the Physicians Committee for Responsible Medicine in Washington, D.C. Make sure some are vegetable soups with fiber-rich lentils.
- A bagel topped with a piece of low-fat cheese is a complete snack on its own.
- Stash nonperishable goodies such as mini-boxes of raisins, cans of vegetable juice cocktail, and whole-wheat pretzels in your desk or car or briefcase.
- Another desk drawer idea is packets of instant oatmeal.
- If there's a lunchroom fridge at your job, stock things like low-fat yogurt, baby carrots, or juices that you'd prefer to drink cold.
- Eating out for lunch? Take the opportunity to order your afternoon snack to go. If there's an appetizer on the menu, it can become a mini-meal. Or get half of an entrée in a doggie bag.
- For home snacks, make sure your kitchen is stocked with fixings for a few mini-meals that you can make in seconds, such as whole-grain cereal with 1% or 2% milk or low-fat vanilla yogurt with frozen blueberries.
- It's okay to expand upon the usual snack concept as long as you keep the calorie count to no more than half of that of your regular meals. For example, a tuna sandwich made with whole-grain bread is a fine, balanced snack choice. Aim for healthy snacks in the 300- to 350-calorie range.

Double Your Water Intake

The Day's Task

Today, you'll learn where all the bathrooms at work are and where each urinal is in those bathrooms and maybe even which gas stations on your way home offer the cleanest rest room facilities.

That's because today you're going to start drinking water. Lots of water. Probably at least twice as much water as you usually drink in a day. Your ultimate goal is to guzzle down so much water that you'll need to visit a bathroom every 2 to 4 hours where, not to put too fine a point on it, your urine will run nearly clear and in appreciable volume.

Your task is actually quite straightforward: Make sure you drink at least eight 8-ounce glasses of water.

A minimum of that much water a day is good for more health benefits than you ever thought possible from such an innocent-looking liquid.

Some 60 to 70 percent of you is water. Your body uses water for every metabolic reaction, for building tissue, for regulating body temperature, for lubricating your joints. Without water, those and every other bodily function would simply stop. In just a few days.

But unless you're planning to get lost in the desert, immediate survival is not what your new, increased water quota is all about. It's about feeling a lot better and living a lot longer. Inadequate fluid intake can aggravate problems all over your body. And chances are, your intake is indeed inadequate—at least it was until today.

"Most people are in a dehydrated phase," says Chris D. Meletis, N.D., professor of nutrition at the National College of Naturopathic Medicine in Portland, Oregon. "They should be feeling like a grape; instead, they feel like a raisin." Here are some reasons why it's so much better to feel like a grape.

Water prevents kidney stones. Drinking plenty of fluids dilutes the concentration of calcium and magnesium salts in urine that can otherwise cause kidney stones, one of the most painful conditions ever to curse man.

Water helps keep your weight down. When water mixes with food, you feel more full more quickly and for longer, so you're less likely to overeat.

Water keeps you regular. Fluids aid elimination, and when you combine high water intake with regular exercise and lots of fiber in your diet, constipation problems tend to disappear.

Water lowers your risk of bladder and colon cancers. We men run a higher risk of bladder cancer than women do. But in a 10-year study of nearly 48,000 men, those who drank six 8-ounce glasses of water daily were half as likely to develop that cancer as those who drank just a glass a day.

Another study shows that men who drank 32 ounces or more of water per day—only four glasses—had 92 percent lower risks of colorectal cancer than those who drank 10 ounces or less. It seems that drinking more water dilutes cancer-causing toxins and speeds them through your digestive system.

Water battles a cold. Drinking those eight 8-ounce glasses of water a day also can help you beat a cold. Antibodies in your throat can kill cold viruses, but dehydration can deactivate them by drying up the mucous membranes where they hang out. Water also works as an expectorant for productive coughs. And, of course, it replenishes lost fluids when a fever is burning you out.

Water fights fatigue. Your cells must be hydrated no matter what, so if there's not enough water available, they take water right out of your bloodstream. Your body adapts to the resulting lower blood volume by slowing down. That spells fatigue. Conversely, however, extra water increases your endurance during exercise.

Water saves your memory. Your brain is 75 percent water by weight and is the first organ to be affected by dehydration. Hence, low fluid levels in your body may result in memory loss and confused thinking, especially in older folks.

Priming the Water Works

Once you're convinced that water can do a lot more for you than slake your thirst on a sunny day, you're on your way to meeting that eight-glass daily requirement. But you may find that after this first day in your new water world those eight glassfuls won't always find their way down your throat. It's not that you don't want to drink water every 2 hours. It's just that you forget.

Furthermore, you can't rely on thirst alone to drive you to drink. By the time you're thirsty, you're already in the beginning stages of dehydration. Strive for the eight-glass minimum whether you feel parched or not. What you need, then, is a water strategy. We have some ideas for you.

First of all, keep in mind that a lot of drinkable liquids are mostly water and can count toward your eight glasses. Pure, no-calorie water is best, but if you really would prefer a glass of, say, apple juice instead of one of those eight glasses of water, go for it.

There are two important cautions, though. First, while beer, soft drinks, coffee, and nonherbal tea are indeed fluids, drinking eight glasses of any of them is obviously not a healthy alternative because of the alcohol, the caffeine, and the calories. What's more, alcoholic beverages and any fluids with caffeine in them act as diuretics and actually cause you to lose fluid. To keep on the plus side, then, a good rule of thumb is to count each caffeinated drink as a half-glass and each alcoholic drink as minus one glass, meaning that you need to drink an extra glass of water for each shot of booze.

Here are some tricks of the water trade to help you reach your goal.

The pre-meal gulp-down. Mealtime is a great time to drink your water, for lots of reasons. If you get in the habit of drinking two glasses before each meal, you take care of three-quarters of your quota right there. Have a glass before your midmorning and mid-afternoon snacks, and you cross the finish line.

But you do even more than that. By drinking just before meals, you maximize your water benefits because the sodium in your food helps you retain the fluid better. Furthermore, a Dutch study showed that those two pre-meal glasses of water can make you feel less hungry, so you may eat less, helping to keep your weight down.

The constant companion. One way to remember your water is to carry it with you, especially at work. There's nothing unusual these days about toting around a 32-ounce plastic bottle of good-tasting water. A nice advantage is you can sip those 32 ounces at your leisure, not necessarily 8 ounces at a time. Once you emptied it, you're halfway to your daily water goal.

The gourmet touch. You'll be much more likely to drink water if you really like it. A squeeze or two of fruit juice can turn that humdrum glass of water into something you look forward to. And for lots of guys, colder is better. Fill a half-gallon (64-ounce) bottle halfway with water and stick it in the freezer overnight. The next morning, fill it the rest of the way for cold water all day long.

Now go find the rest room.

Have a Fruit-and-Vegetable Jamboree

The Day's Task

Today, you're going to eat an amazing, astonishing nine servings of fruits and vegetables. And it's going to be easy. Trust us.

- **Have a 6-ounce glass of orange juice at breakfast and a banana with the meal, perhaps cut into your cereal. Or, instead of the banana, have a half-cup of frozen blueberries.**
- **Eat a medium-size apple during your mid-morning snack.**
- **Have a half-cup of cooked or raw chopped vegetables with lunch—your choice of veggie.**
- **Have some carrot sticks with your mid-afternoon snack.**
- **Down a 6-ounce glass of grape juice when you first get home from work.**
- **With dinner, have a salad and a serving of steamed or sautéed vegetables.**
- **Finally, end your day with a piece of fruit for dessert.**

Not so bad, was it?

Vegetables and fruits do so much for your longevity quest in so many different ways that we'd tell you to eat more than nine servings if we thought you'd do it. Unlike the deprivation so often associated with healthy eating—cut down on this or don't eat that—the goal with fruits and vegetables is to eat a lot. Except in the case of certain medical conditions, it's pretty hard to overdose on fruits and vegetables.

You may not have thought of them this way, but fruits and vegetables are energy foods. For the most part, they're fiber-rich carbohydrates, ideal for optimal energy flow. Fruit, in particular, may be the perfect workout food.

While other sugars give you a quick burst of energy, fruit sugars deliver a steady stream of carbohydrate energy over a few hours.

All those vegetables and fruits help you keep your weight down too. With some notable exceptions like coconuts and avocados, most fruits and vegetables have little or no fat and not much in the way of protein either. They still have calories, of course, but filling up on their fiber will push fat and excess calories out of your system.

It's a scientific fact that fruits and vegetables protect you from top killers like cancer and heart disease. For example, European researchers who investigated the dietary habits of 2,112 men in Wales over a 13-year period found evidence that regularly eating fruits and vegetables slashes the risk of dying from cancer. A study of 976 people in California showed that those who ate the most fruits, vegetables, and grains were less likely to develop precancerous colon polyps than were those who ate the least number of these foods.

By eating lots of fruits and vegetables, you reduce your cancer risk in at least two ways. The fiber they provide pushes digested food through your gut faster, giving potential carcinogens less time to damage cells in your digestive tract. But also, the antioxidants that are so abundant in fruits and vegetables destroy cell-damaging free radicals. They also may actually reverse existing cell damage before it leads to cancer.

Here's another encouraging statistic from the medical literature. If you increase your intake of fruits and vegetables from the four daily servings that most Americans eat to the nine we're recommending, you can reduce your risk of heart disease by 15 percent and your risk of stroke by 27 percent. That assumes you also cut back on dietary fat, but as we just said, eating lots of fruits and vegetables helps you do just that.

The most exciting news about the magic of produce has to do with the thousands of phytochemicals that are still being discovered within them. It's in this class of chemical compounds found only in plant-based food where a lot of life-sustaining antioxidant action is found.

That's a big reason why eating lots of fruits and vegetables at any age has been shown to slow down, brake, or even reverse many of the unpleasant developments associated with the aging process. Heart disease and cancer are just two such problems that antioxidants combat. They also help keep your mind sharp, your bones strong, your eyesight keen, and your immune system powerful enough to fight off infections and other illnesses.

There's even some promising evidence that the phytochemicals and other good things in fruits and vegetables retard the aging process itself at the cellular level. In other words, if your antioxidant intake is high from eating lots of fruits and vegetables, you may be biologically "younger" than others your age who have low antioxidant intakes.

You may live longer as a result. Researchers studied 22 healthy Italian centenarians, average age 103, and found one of the things that set them apart from younger folks: They ate more than twice as many vegetables.

All-Star Produce

Science is just beginning to uncover all the good things that phytochemicals can do for you. And there's still a lot to be learned about how different phytochemicals work together. But one thing that researchers are already pretty sure about is that no one fruit or vegetable contains all of the different phytochemicals. That's one of the reasons we've asked you to shoot for nine servings today. Eating a lot of different fruits and vegetables is key to getting maximum health benefits.

So no fair chomping down nine bananas today and congratulating yourself on a job well done. Go for variety. That said, however, we're going to give you a lineup of some of the top fruits and vegetables that research indicates pack an awesome wallop of health and anti-aging benefits. Don't limit yourself to these, but let them inspire you and perhaps help you make some choices to get the nine-a-day ball rolling.

Berries. Who doesn't like strawberries and blueberries? These are precisely the two berries that animal studies indicate help reverse the effects of aging on your mental functioning. It seems that these berries contain a lot more antioxidant phytochemicals than most other fruits or vegetables.

Spinach. Okay, it's a cliché to talk about how healthy spinach is for you. But there's just too much great stuff in it to ignore. For example, if you never thought of spinach as good for your eyesight, think again. It's rich in lutein and zeaxanthan, two phytochemicals that have been shown to slow or reverse age-related vision problems.

Furthermore, spinach is one of the best food sources of vitamin E, an antioxidant that works as an immunity booster. Vitamin E also helps prevent memory decline, as does another vitamin found in abundance in spinach—folate. One more thing: Spinach helps keep your bones strong well into older age.

That's because it's rich in potassium and magnesium. In a 40-year study of 600 men, researchers found that men with the lowest intakes of those two minerals lost roughly four times more bone density in their hips than men with the highest intakes.

Orange juice. You're probably already well aware that orange juice is a first-rate source of vitamin C. Well, it turns out that vitamin C is good for your eyes. One study found that the subjects who took vitamin C supplements had 75 percent lower risks of cataracts over time than those who didn't supplement. Not only does orange juice offer plenty of that vitamin C but it's also a source of lutein and zeaxanthan, the two eyesight-saving antioxidant phytochemicals also found in spinach. And like spinach, orange juice is a rich source of folate, the B-vitamin that's essential for maintaining memory.

Don't underrate orange juice as an energy food. Its role in replenishing your vitamin C supply is important for your vim and vigor since research has shown that low vitamin C levels can interfere with your body's energy processing.

Tomatoes. Tomatoes should hold a special place in the hearts and prostates of men. One study showed that men who ate two or more servings of tomato products a week significantly reduced their risks of prostate cancer. The phytochemical hero here seems to be an antioxidant called lycopene. And, in a case where fresh is good but high concentration is better, tomato sauce apparently gives the greatest protective benefit.

Broccoli. Broccoli is another all-around player in the anti-aging game, and one study provides yet another reason to eat lots of this nutrient-rich life sustainer. Researchers who followed almost 50,000 men for 10 years found that those who ate just two half-cup servings of broccoli a week got bladder cancer only half as often as those who rarely ate any broccoli. That matters because bladder cancer is three times more common in men than in women.

Grape juice and grapes. A few days ago, we told you that red wine contains antioxidants from the family of phytochemicals called flavonoids that help ward off cancer and heart disease. Well, grape juice is the nondrinker's red wine. In fact, a cup of Concord grape juice packs more antioxidant power than 20 raw carrots.

Grape seeds are also antioxidant gold mines, studies show. Are we really suggesting you eat grape seeds? No way. But the grapes themselves are certainly worth eating. And even seedless grapes seem to include most of the antioxidants found in the seeds.

ADVENTURE IN GROCERY LAND

You're a man, and you do not readily admit to fear. So we're asking you to be brave and to try some new fruits and vegetables. Several business shifts and food trends have transpired to fill your local produce section with unusual and unusually good selections. Try these. They taste great, they're easy to prepare, and they are all enormously healthy for you.

Tropical fruits. Pineapple. Mango. Papaya. Star fruit. Kiwifruit. These fruits taste outstanding. The main challenge with tropical fruit is getting the skin off without mangling the inside. With a little practice, you'll figure it out. Get past the peeling issue, and you're in sweet, juicy heaven.

Asian greens. The vegetables of China, Japan, and southeastern Asia have become widely available in America over the past few years. Many are quite easy to cook: a fast sauté in oil, plus some garlic or ginger, and they're done. Items to try include bok choy, napa cabbage, Chinese broccoli, and Japanese eggplant.

Leafy greens. Cheap, packed with nutrients, pungent, and ready for hot spices, Southern-style greens like kale, mustards, collards, chard, and even dandelion greens are great for preparing in bulk and eating throughout the week. Boil them in broth with a touch of vinegar or hot sauce until wilted and tender, and you have a classic American dish.

Salad greens. Forget iceberg lettuce. Myriad salad greens are available with far greater taste and health benefits. For a start, try red leaf lettuce: It looks great and tastes sweet and crunchy. Move on to baby spinach, arugula, romaine, or the mesclun (or "spring") mixes now available. These tend to taste more bitter than iceberg, but they also have much more snap, flavor, and personality.

Enjoy the Jamboree

Recognizing the health-and-longevity power of fruits and vegetables is one thing. But making a habit out of nine daily servings of them is another, isn't it? Once you decide to do it, however, you'll see how easy and enjoyable it is. Here are some hints to bear in mind.

Know your servings. When you need to figure out what a single serving is, the rule of thumb is that it's usually equal to a half-cup. That's about the size of a tennis ball. If it's a raw leafy vegetable, make it a full cup. One piece of raw fruit also constitutes a serving—one medium apple or banana, for example. But if the fruit is chopped, cooked, or canned, a half-cup is a serving.

Count juice as a serving. Three-quarters of a cup of fruit juice or vegetable juice is a serving. Just make sure that what you're drinking is 100 percent juice and not some juicelike liquid consisting mostly of sugar, water, dye, and preservatives. Fruit punch is not juice. A "fruit drink" is not juice either. Neither is anything with "ade" in its name. If you don't squeeze it or juice it yourself, look for the freshest juice you can find, noting the purchase-by date.

Split meals down the middle. One thing that will really help you load up on vegetables, especially at dinner, is to remember the 50-50 rule. Simply make sure you fill half your plate with produce, and divide the other half among everything else.

Go for variety. Put as many different fruits and veggies on your plate as you can. That will not only get you a better array of anti-aging and pro-health plant nutrients but also keep your appetite for vegetables permanently whetted. International fare is a mother lode of new and great-tasting plant-based entrées. For starters, just check out the vegetable stir-fry dishes at a Chinese takeout.

Study menus. When you eat out, remember that just about any menu has to have some vegetable dishes prepared in a way you might never have considered. Steal some ideas and give them a try at home.

Have a little fat. You don't have to be totally gun-shy about adding butter or cheese sauce to your vegetables. Yes, we warned you against smothering veggies with these fats or deep-frying them. But if the taste and texture of a little bit of butter or cheese or olive oil will make you want to eat more servings, go for it.

In fact, a small amount of added fat actually jacks up the benefits of certain vegetables. Broccoli, for example, is a rich source of beta-carotene, one of the major antioxidants. But beta-carotene is fat soluble, which means it has to hitch a ride on fat molecules to make the trip through your intestinal wall. Without a little fat in the mix, your body won't absorb nearly as much beta-carotene.

Eat it all. Fruit and vegetable skins usually house the majority of the food's fiber. By peeling an apple or discarding a potato skin, you lose a vital part of the benefits. If the skin is edible, eat it.

If it's not, as in the case of oranges and grapefruit, don't cut them into pieces—just peel the skin off. That way, you'll eat more of the white, stringy, fiber-filled and flavonoid-rich membrane of the fruit.

10 Ways to Prevent Digestive Problems

1 **Eat several small meals spread through the day rather than two or three big meals.** Many nutrition experts now recommend eating six times a day: the usual meals cut substantially in size, plus three healthy, fairly sizeable snacks in mid-morning, mid-afternoon, and a few hours before you go to sleep. The benefits are many, including less strain on your digestive system (and hence less gas, bloating, and acid problems), an even flow of nutrients into your bloodstream, and a greater diversity of nutrients.

2 **Keep it clean, clean, clean.** Stomach pain and diarrhea are symptoms, not the end problem. And most often, they indicate that something foul has gotten into your digestive tract. Minor cases of food poisoning happen all the time. So don't get lax about the basic rules of kitchen hygiene: clean your produce well, use only the freshest of meats and seafood, quickly scrub surfaces and utensils that touch raw food, cook everything thoroughly enough to kill the cooties, and don't leave exposed food sitting around on the counter or the table any longer than necessary.

3 **Eat lots of fiber to keep waste smoothly and happily moving through your system.** Insoluble fiber, like that in vegetables and wheat bran, absorbs water as it heads through your colon. Soluble fiber, found in fruits, some beans, and grains, dissolves in water to form a gel in your digestive system that helps soften stool. The American Dietetic Association recommends you eat 20 to 35 grams of dietary fiber daily. If you're going to bump up your intake, do it gradually to minimize gas. Some good high-fiber foods are bananas, apples, prunes, figs, sweet potatoes, black beans, black-eyed peas, broccoli, sunflower seeds, wheat germ, and whole-grain cereals like All-Bran and Fiber One.

4 **Run plenty of water through yourself.** Drink at least six to eight 8-ounce glasses of water to help keep your stool soft and on the go, says William B. Ruderman, M.D., of Gastroenterology Associates of Central Florida in Clearwater. Be extra vigilant about drinking your water when you're eating all the fiber you're supposed to or increasing your fiber intake, as fiber needs water to work properly.

5 **Get moving to get moving.** Aerobic exercise, particularly running and rowing, are good for speeding up the flow of food through the digestive process. Exercise may speed up bowel transit time by creating changes in bloodflow or nerve activity to the bowels. And the more intense the exercise,

the faster you'll move out the waste, says Benjamin Krevsky, M.D., a gastroenterologist at Temple University School of Medicine in Philadelphia.

6 **Say no to sorbitol.** Your small intestine can't absorb this artificial sweetener, commonly found in sugar-free gum and candies, very well. Sorbitol heads to your colon, where resident bacteria ferment it, leading to gas and diarrhea. The compound is also found in strawberries, cherries, plums, prunes, and peaches, according to Seymour Katz, M.D., clinical professor of medicine at New York University School of Medicine in New York City. If you're having gas and diarrhea, cut way back on these sorbitol-containing foods.

7 **Go sparingly on the dairy.** If you're dancing the bathroom quickstep and don't know why, avoid dairy products for a while. Your gas and diarrhea may cease to be a problem. Many people, particularly African-Americans and people of Asian and Mediterranean descent, don't produce the enzyme lactase that digests a sugar in milk called lactose. The result is lactose intolerance. Aside from the obvious foods, like ice cream and cheese, look for the words milk products, casein, and whey on the labels of processed foods, Dr. Katz says.

If you just can't say no to dairy, take supplements containing lactase before you eat dairy, or buy dairy products already treated with lactase. Look for these in health food stores and supermarkets.

8 **Deflate your vegetables.** If beans or other foods make you puff up like the Hindenburg, use some Beano before you eat them. This product, which comes in a liquid that you sprinkle on the food or a tablet that you take beforehand, contains an enzyme that helps you digest a troublesome complex carbohydrate in the food. Follow the dosage information on the label. "Use it once, and you may have no gas at all after that particular meal," says Eugene Oliveri, D.O., a gastroenterologist in East Lansing, Michigan.

9 **Start the morning with a hot drink.** If you can't get things moving along, have a hot drink in the morning, says Harris Clearfield, M.D., section chief of gastroenterology at the MCP Hahnemann School of Medicine in Philadelphia. It doesn't matter whether you choose tea, coffee, or even hot water; they can all stimulate the reflex that triggers a bowel movement, he says.

10 **Don't hold it.** When your body tells you it's ready to have a seat and do its thing, don't make it wait. If you wait too long, your gut will start to reabsorb water from the stool it's holding, making the substance harder, drier, and more difficult to push out.

10 Ways to Prevent Weight Gain

1 **Make a commitment to your health.** Losing weight is about much more than vanity. Far more serious is that if you are more than 20 pounds over your ideal weight, you are at serious risk for many potentially deadly conditions, including diabetes, high blood pressure, and heart disease.

Life is all about choices, and since most of us tend to put on weight as we age, you need to choose wisely. An excellent way to keep your weight under control is to make a small, steady commitment at the start of every day. A quick 10-minute walk when you wake up, followed by 10 pushups and 10 crunches, will burn just a modest number of calories, enough to lose 3 pounds in a year. But doing these things will let you make a powerful statement to yourself about how you want to live and will make weight loss far easier to achieve overall.

2 **Don't diet.** Diets are the exact opposite of a healthy lifestyle because they make you look at your ideal weight as a destination point. A healthy life is a process, not a destination. Plus, when you eat less than you should, you become obsessed with food, which is exactly want you do not want. Instead of beginning and quitting diets all your life, choose meals based on the Food Guide Pyramid, which you'll find on pretty much any box of food on your supermarket shelf. You already know the highlights: Enjoy generous helpings of fruits, vegetables, and whole-grain breads; choose lean meats and fish and low-fat dairy products; and go easy on the fats, oils, and sweets.

3 **Heed the power of the calorie.** It's this simple: If you eat more calories than you burn, you store them as fat. Eat 3,500 more calories than you burn (and it won't take long), and you'll gain a pound. Certainly, don't count every calorie you put in your mouth. But do spend some time reading the labels on foods. This will help you gain a general awareness of calories and make better choices. A lightly active man who weighs 160 pounds should eat 2,866 calories each day.

One of the first things you'll notice about food labels is that the portion you're supposed to eat is a lot smaller than the portion you want to eat. Here are some handy guides: one serving of meat is the size of a deck of cards, a serving of cheese is the size of a golf ball, and a serving of pasta is the size of a tennis ball. Minimize temptations by putting the correct serving size right on your plate rather than serving meals family-style, with heaping serving bowls on the table.

4 **Make every calorie count.** Foods that are higher in fiber, like fruits, vegetables, and whole grains, make you feel fuller longer and help you eat less throughout the day. To work fiber into every meal, have whole-grain cereal for breakfast, sandwiches on whole-grain bread for lunch, and black bean soup or chili for supper. Remember to count the calories you drink too. Beer, sodas, juices, and sports drinks are all high in calories. Stick with calorie-free water, seltzer, plain iced tea, or diet soda.

5 **Really enjoy your food.** If you eat in front of the TV or over the stove, you probably shovel in food without thinking, So, gather your loved ones and eat together as a family at the table. This will help you to eat more slowly and mindfully. Since it takes 15 to 20 minutes for your brain to get the message that your stomach is full, this will keep you from eating more than you need to.

6 **Ride out cravings with a call.** Cravings kill many weight-management efforts because too many people give in to them too easily. Studies indicate that the average craving passes in 4 to 12 minutes. So before you give in, distract yourself for a few minutes. Call a friend, walk around the block, do whatever it takes to get you away from the fridge.

7 **Become restaurant savvy.** Restaurants are designed to make you stay longer and eat more. Here are some ways to fight back: Grab a snack before you go out. That way, you'll eat less when you stop for a meal. If you really are hungry when you get to a restaurant, quickly drink a carbonated beverage or tomato juice

Avoid the tempting descriptions and pictures on the menu. Tell the waitress what you want in broader terms: grilled fish or chicken, say, with steamed vegetables. Any restaurant can make that.

8 **Exercise for at least 30 minutes, 5 days a week.** The easiest exercise plan of all is to walk, building up to at least 30 minutes of brisk walking five times a week. When scientists compared nearly 350 middle-aged twins, they discovered that the twin who was more active was slimmer than the other despite the shared genetic makeup.

9 **Forge new relationships.** Social gatherings = food. We meet for lunch, go out for dinner, break for coffee. Plan some new social events around motion, not meals. Play golf with friends, bowl with your kids, work out with your wife. To make commitments to exercise, you need cooperation and support.

10 **Stop working late.** According to a study of Japanese office workers, employees who worked late into the night put on the most weight. Working overtime can lead to skipped workouts and later dinners, usually ordered from fattening fast food places. Try to put in extra hours it at home, or go into work early.

WEEK 2

EXERCISE TO GET LEAN AND HEALTHY

Do a Morning Stretching Routine

The Day's Task

Set your alarm clock to wake you up 15 minutes earlier than usual. Then, get a good night's sleep.

Good morning. Don't argue with the clock; just get out of bed. Don't change out of your sleep clothes. Proceed directly to a room with some nice light and space, but no other people, and stand in the middle of it. Take three deep breaths, each for a count of four in through your nose and a count of four out through your mouth.

For the next 10 minutes, do the basic stretching routine described in this chapter, six stretches done slowly and pleasurably. When done, jump around a little, shaking your arms and getting loose.

Then, proceed with your day. (And remember: eat breakfast.)

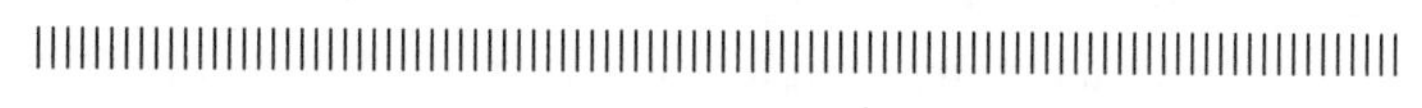

The benefits of a morning stretching routine are far greater than you might expect. There are the physical benefits: stretching jump-starts your body, sending blood to every corner and putting your muscles into action. Nagging morning body aches melt away. You'll be more flexible and supple, and therefore less prone to the minor muscle hurts that can occur in a day. Best of all, consistent stretching improves your chances of preventing or reversing the loss of range of motion that occurs as you age.

Then there are the mental benefits. Stretching helps release brain chemicals that give you a feeling of well-being. Moreover, the quiet calm of a private morning stretching routine is just plain good for your head, relieving stress and giving you time to sort out and strategize your upcoming day. In fact, this day's task would fit perfectly in the week dedicated to anti-stress tactics.

Guys usually consider stretching as the last part of a workout, something you do after a long run or a weight-training session. The morning routine we are prescribing has many of the same benefits, but is different. The morning routine is for starting the day—getting your blood flowing, stretching your joints, getting your whole body limber and primed. It is a whole-body program. A workout stretch is often targeted to the muscles you just worked out and is done to lengthen them out after intense usage, with a key goal being the prevention of cramping and soreness.

Stretching Techniques

Along with walking and running, stretching is among the most natural, intuitive forms of exercise. But no matter how organic the movements are, doing any of them improperly can hurt you. Here are several bits of advice for integrating smart stretching into your life.

Do it slow and easy. Stretching should be a gentle, fluid motion. Don't bounce or jerk; you could tear a muscle. The muscle tightness you feel may be mildly uncomfortable but should never be painful. If you experience pain, ease up a bit or try another stretching routine that extends the same muscles.

Hold it. When you're in a stretch position, hold it for 20 to 30 seconds. In order to sufficiently extend the muscle cells, you need to maintain a stretch for more than the few seconds that many people do. When possible, repeat stretches two or three times.

Breathe deeply. You may be tempted to hold your breath while holding a stretch. Don't. You may tighten up and feel pain if you don't breathe as you are stretching.

Customize your stretches. Think about which areas of your body are tightest or least flexible and how they limit your activities. You can't sit on the floor cross-legged with your kids or grandkids? You feel older than Neanderthal man every time you bend over? Then concentrate your stretching routines on the areas where you most need more flexibility. There are plenty of good books on stretching and even more books on yoga that offer hundreds of effective stretches.

Incorporate stretches throughout your day for both the physical and mental benefits. If in the morning you catch a little of CNN, the *Today* show, or ESPN highlights of the previous night's games, stretch while you watch TV. Need a break from the computer screen? Do a few stretches. If stretching bores you, at least you can do it concurrent with something you enjoy.

The Core Stretching Routine

Even if you're gung-ho about stretching, you probably can't commit a lot of time to it in the morning. You have to get ready for work and eat breakfast, maybe do your regular workout too. No need to worry. Here is a stretching routine you can complete in less time than it takes to read the morning paper, while still getting your entire body loosened up.

Lying overhead arm stretch. (1) Lie on your back with your knees bent at a 45-degree angle, feet flat on the floor. The small of your back should be pressed firmly against the floor. Extend your arms straight up over your chest, with your palms facing your knees.

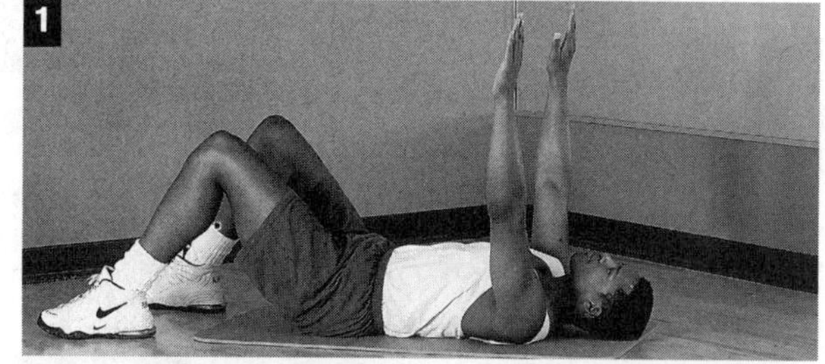

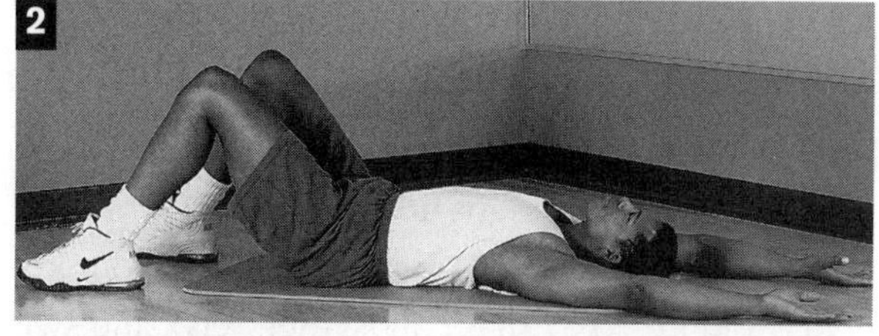

(2) Slowly lower your arms straight back over your head. Try to press the backs of your hands and arms flat on the floor. Hold for 20 to 30 seconds, then relax. Slowly bring your arms back to the starting position before repeating the stretch.

Bowing shoulder stretch. (3) Get down on all fours with your hands and knees about shoulder-width apart. Keep your back flat, your neck straight, and your eyes on the floor.

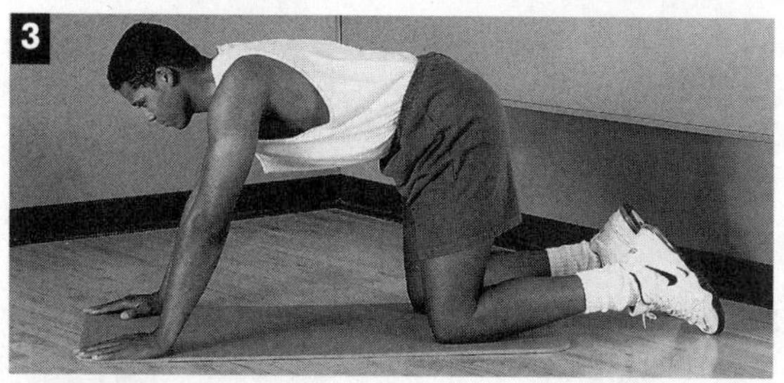

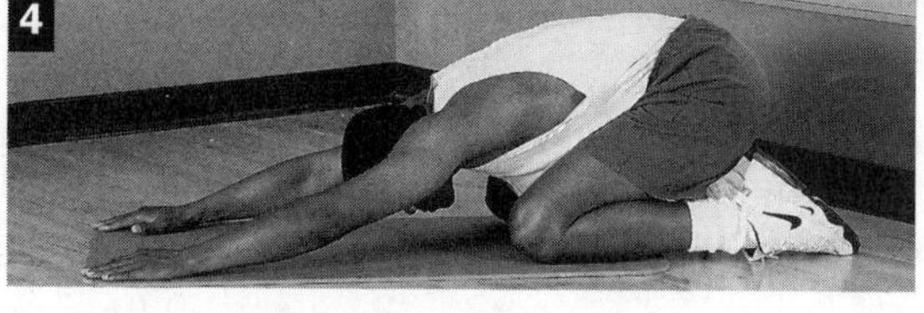

(4) Without moving your hands, sit back on your heels, letting your arms extend in front of you. Slightly push down with your palms until you feel a stretch in your arms and hips. Hold for 20 to 30 seconds. Relax, then repeat.

Bending chest stretch. (5) Stand a few feet away from a table, feet shoulder-width apart. Extend your arms and lean your hands on the table, bending forward at the waist. Don't round your back or hunch your shoulders forward.

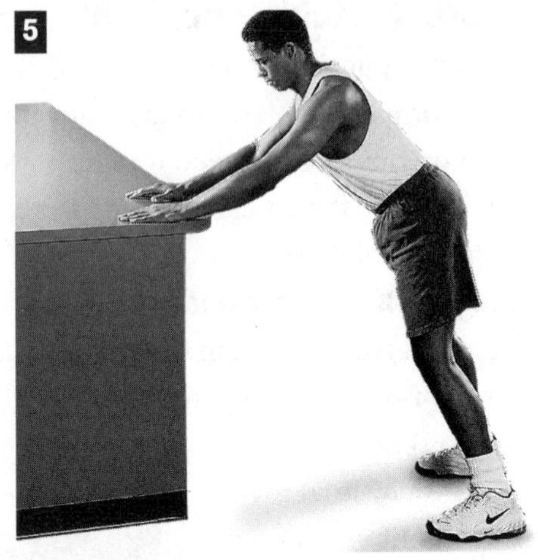

(6) Continue bending forward until your arms and back are parallel to the floor, keeping your knees slightly bent. Push your chest and head toward the floor until you feel slight tension. Hold for 20 to 30 seconds.

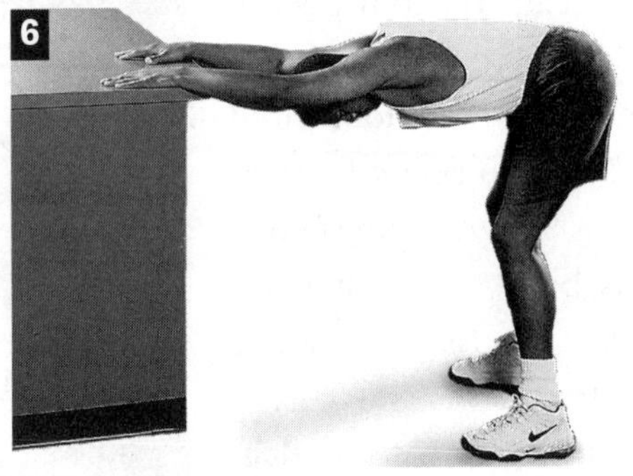

Kneeling calf stretch. (7) Kneel on your left knee, resting your right forearm on your right thigh. Slightly lean forward at the waist, keeping your back straight.

(8) Shift your weight to your right knee, bending it as far as you comfortably can. Keep your right heel on the floor. Shift your left leg so that the inside of your knee and lower leg are flat on the floor. Hold for 20 to 30 seconds, then relax and switch legs.

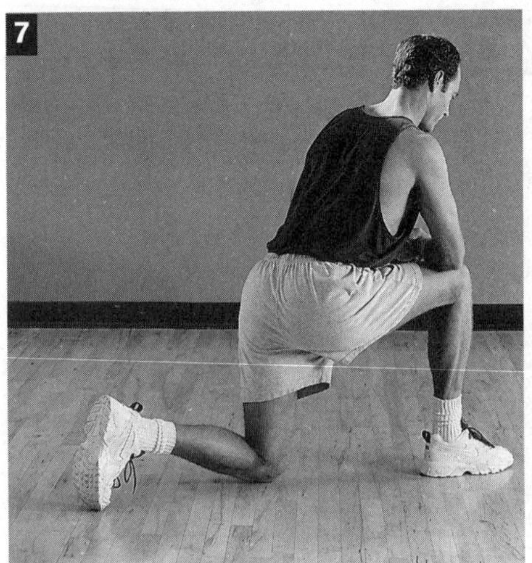

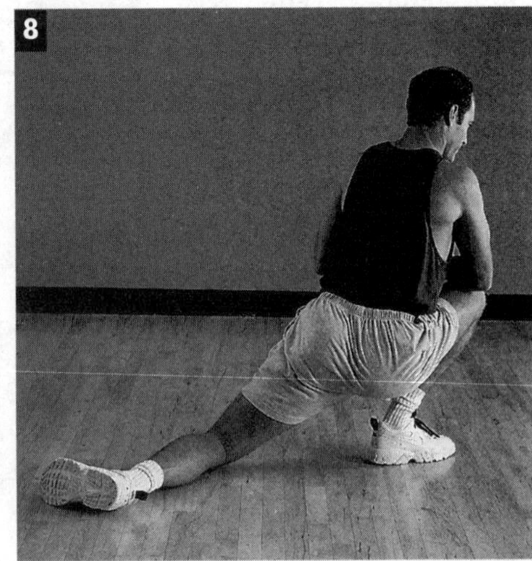

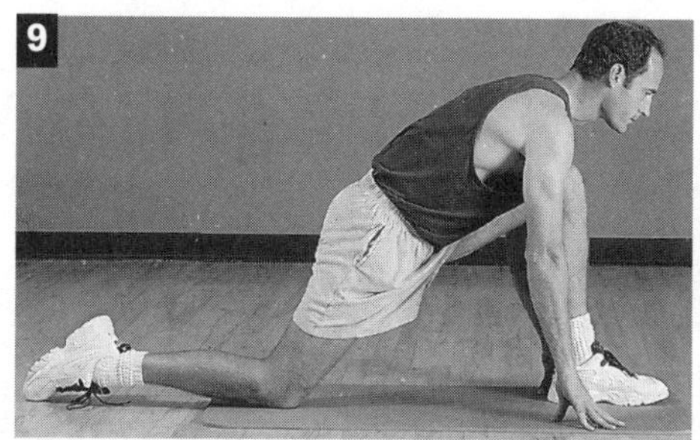

Kneeling quad stretch. (9) Get down on all fours. Move your left leg in front of your body and bend it at a 90-degree angle. Extend your right leg behind you so that your knee, your shin, and the top of your foot are on the floor to help support your body.

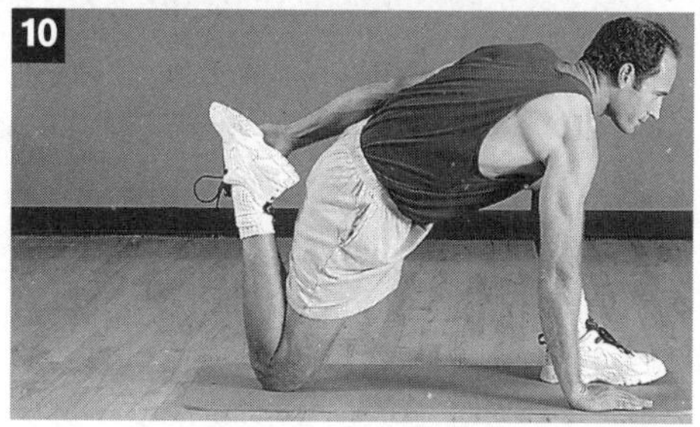

(10) Keeping your right hand flat on the floor, use your left hand to reach behind your back to grab the top of your right foot. Pull your heel toward your butt as far as you comfortably can. Keep your back flat and your head in line with your torso. Hold for 20 to 30 seconds, then relax and switch legs.

Standing hamstring-and-butt stretch. (11) Extend your left leg and place the back of your heel on a table or stair at about waist height. Your right foot should be flat on the floor and your right knee slightly bent. Keep your torso straight and your head in line with your spine.

(12) Slowly bend at the waist while keeping your back flat. Grab your left shin with both hands and pull your upper body toward your leg, going as far down as you comfortably can while maintaining a flat back. Hold for 20 to 30 seconds, then relax and switch legs.

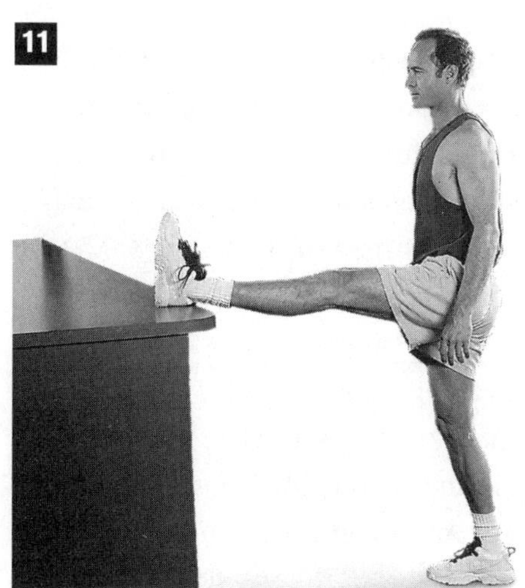

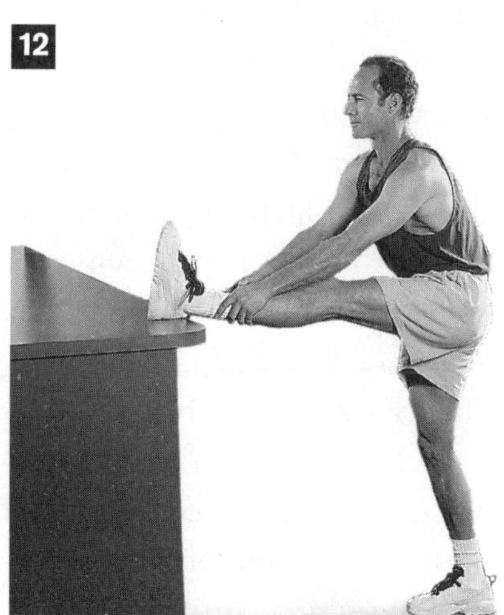

Develop a Walking Habit

The Day's Task

An hour after finishing dinner, head outside and walk at least 30 minutes, covering at least 2 miles. Weather is not an issue unless it is downright dangerous out there.

If you wish, drag your wife or kid or buddy with you; walking is a great time for talking.

It doesn't have the bold intensity of martial arts or pumping iron, but the simple act of walking will help you live a healthier and longer life. Skeptical? A Finnish study that followed 16,000 twins for an average of 19 years found that those who took brisk 30-minute walks at least six times a month were 44 percent less likely to die than their less active twins.

A second study tracking men ages 35 to 60 concluded that those who walked 11 to 20 minutes a day were less likely to develop high blood pressure than those who didn't walk. And men who walked 21 minutes or more reduced their odds by 30 percent.

Thirty minutes of brisk walking most nights keeps your body's engine running smoothly by increasing your heart rate and boosting lung capacity. This, in turn, moves oxygen and other nutrients throughout your body more efficiently. Your metabolism speeds up, which helps melt that layer of lard around your middle that's been expanding like bread in the oven. A 170-pound man who walks 2 miles in a half-hour burns 309 calories. If he does that five times a week, he burns more than 1,500 calories.

There are secondary benefits to these evening walks as well. The biggest is stress relief. A walk is a great time to think or to talk—or better yet, to not think or talk. It's pure decompression time in the great ol' outdoors. Evening walks also get you out of that quintessential American postdinner habit of watching television. This is a good thing.

Consider coaxing your honey into joining you; she'll share the same health benefits as you. One study tracked 84,000 female nurses for 8 years and found that women who walked 3 to 4 miles per hour at least 3 hours a week had a 54 percent lower risk of heart attack and stroke than those who were sedentary. Even those women who walked at a slower pace had a 32 percent lower risk.

An added benefit if your favorite woman joins you is time alone to talk without distractions. You'll come to really like this. And for sure, she will. Trust us on this.

Plus, you'll see things in your neighborhood you never noticed while zipping by in your car. Pleasant people. Animals. Kids laughing. The sound and feel of wind. Strange fauna. Nubile neighbors. Who knows?

Walking makes you feel better in so many other ways. Various research has shown that walking burns calories, reduces blood pressure, raises high-density lipoprotein or "good" cholesterol, and relieves stress.

Like any other aerobic activity, walking is going to do you the most good when you reach between 60 and 80 percent of your maximum heart rate. See Day 6 of this week to find how you determine these percentages.

The nifty thing about walking is that you needn't have any special skills to do it. You don't have to be in great shape. And you don't need to buy special gear, except perhaps shoes. More on shoes later.

Stride Right

Sure, walking is easy, but to get the most from your meanderings, there are some steps you should take.

Don't overstride. Long strides may seem like the way to cover more ground faster. But in fact, your real goal is to take more steps per minute than you normally would. The idea is to walk briskly; that is, fast enough to get your heart pumping but not so fast that you can't hold a conversation.

Keep your body loose. Don't walk stiffly with your arms at your sides. Instead, bend your arms at roughly 90-degree angles. Swing your arms close to your body, from your lower breastbone to the backs of your hips, to generate speed and balance.

For maximum efficiency and speed, walk in a straight line. Imagine a line drawn on the route you walk. Your right foot and left foot should be stepping on that line.

Speed up when going down hills. You need not walk as fast up a hill to get your heart pounding and have a good workout. But most guys walk down that hill at the same pace or slower. That makes it hard to keep your heart rate up. Instead,

SEVEN WAYS TO GET MORE FOOT MOTION INTO YOUR LIFE

1. **Always take the stairs.** Skip escalators and elevators, particularly when you are going up or down just one or two stories.
2. **Lock up your remote control and change television channels manually.** For the typical adult male television watcher, that means standing up and sitting down about 20 times per minute. Yes, we're serious.
3. **Park your car far from the door.** Stop circling around parking lots like a four-wheeled vulture. Take a spot some distance away and walk in.
4. **When you golf, never, ever take a cart unless the course mandates it.** If you believe in the expression that golf is "a good walk spoiled," you want to at least guarantee yourself the "good walk" part.
5. **Walk during your lunch hour.** It doesn't take 60 minutes to eat. Walk outside for 20 minutes and then grab your chow.
6. **Never sit when on the phone.** Get a hands-free phone for the office. That will better allow you to stand up, move about, pace.
7. **Launch a weekend hiking routine.** A nice little routine that works as well for families as individuals is to drive to a remote spot every Saturday or Sunday morning, take a rugged nature walk for an hour or two, then go home. It's kind of like church, but personal and outdoors. Be sure to leave the cell phone at home. Hang a water bottle from your belt instead.

go as fast as you can. This isn't a problem, of course, on a treadmill. You can set the degree of incline and keep it there.

Do not carry hand weights or wear ankle weights. Neither will improve your workout. In fact, they can throw your body out of kilter, slow you down, and put you at risk for injuries, which are otherwise a walking rarity.

Shoe News

Since walking is a relatively low-impact activity, you don't have to agonize over what shoes to buy as if deciding what stocks to invest in for your 401(k). That said, don't just wear sandals or your work shoes. You can do a number on your toes, Achilles tendons, knees, and arches if you stride hard in the wrong shoes.

The bottom line is if you walk regularly, invest in walking shoes. Here's what to do.

- Try on shoes at midday or later. Feet can swell by up to a half-size over the course of a day.
- When you try on shoes, wear the same type of socks that you will wear when you go walking.
- Look for shoes that provide stability, that is, ones that keep your feet from rolling inward too much when you walk.
- Walking shoes should feel sturdy and hug your entire foot, providing solid support all around.
- A good shoe will provide shock absorption, minimizing the jarring impact of your feet hitting the ground.
- Good shoes are not only solid and stable, but flexible. Try bending each shoe at the angle to which your foot naturally bends. If it doesn't bend easily, it may resist your foot when you try to walk briskly. Bear in mind, too, that shoes will become more flexible as you break them in and that hiking shoes will be—and should be—more rigid than walking shoes.
- Test-walk shoes on a hard surface. If the area where you try on shoes is carpeted, walk to a part of the store that isn't. Then, go at a fast pace, just like you will after dinner.
- Don't buy the cheapest model you see. The old adage that you get what you pay for is true of walking shoes too.

Aerobic Session Number 1 (Outdoors)

The Day's Task

Take 60 minutes of personal time for outdoor exercise. Early morning, prior to getting ready for work, is particularly good. Put on some comfortable clothing appropriate for the weather: T-shirt, shorts, and athletic shoes if warm, sweats in colder temperatures. Do a 5-minute warmup of walking, jogging in place, and shaking your arms. Then, for the next 30 minutes, take up an activity that keeps you moving without a break and accelerates your heartbeat to the point that you are working and breathing hard but can still converse without gasping. You choose the activity: a run or fast walk, a bike ride, some aggressive hoops shooting and rebounding, whatever. Follow up with 5 minutes of walking and light stretching to cool down. Allow yourself 20 minutes to clean up with a tepid shower and get dressed.

Let us clear up whatever confusion still exists here. Aerobics and aerobic exercise are not the same thing. Aerobic exercise is anything that accelerates your heartbeat for a sustained period, generally 20 minutes or longer. That's why it's also called cardio exercise. Running, bicycling, skiing, shadow boxing—it's guy stuff.

Aerobics is a small subset of that. It's basically group aerobic exercise in which an instructor leads a class through a formal program of movement. Completely forget about aerobics for now. Rightly or wrongly, its reputation has become tarnished for many guys. Most grown men don't want to work out in a co-ed class to thumping, loud dance music. If you're among them, be proud of that.

But if you want to feel good and live longer, you have to have a regular routine of aerobic activity. You'll get an amazingly wide array of benefits from exercising your most vital muscle, your heart.

Lifesavers

Here is what you can achieve by engaging in aerobic exercise regularly.

Longevity. Your ticker will tick longer if you exercise it. Researchers tracked more than 21,000 men of varying levels of fitness for as long as 24 years and found that the guys who jogged, played tennis, and the like almost every day reduced their death rate by 57 percent over their least-fit peers. The most diligently aerobic among us figure to live nearly 9 years longer than our neighbor who spends weekends in his backyard hammock, scientists speculate. Those of us who stay moderately fit have a 6-year edge.

A lean body. Aerobic exercise continues burning calories even after you stop. Researchers at the University of Missouri found that seven active men who bicycled for an hour each burned 600 calories during a workout and another 120 calories in the 9 hours afterwards.

A healthier heart. Aerobic activity may bring reductions of up to 25 percent in your resting heart rate. Why should you care? Because fewer beats per minute means your heart is stronger, pumping more blood with each contraction.

Cleaner blood. Cardio workouts reduce total cholesterol and heart-damaging blood fats called triglycerides while increasing high-density lipoprotein (HDL), or "good," cholesterol. When you exercise has a lot to do with how well this works. When a group of 21 men exercised 12 hours before a high-fat meal, they reduced their triglycerides by half. The figure was 40 percent when they exercised an hour before the meal. But when they worked out after a high-fat meal, they reduced the fat in their blood by only 5 percent.

Protection against colon cancer. Men who exercise regularly have half the risk of colon cancer of those who are more sedentary, concluded researchers at Harvard University and Brigham and Women's Hospital in Boston. Exercise accelerates digestion, so potential carcinogens spend less time in the intestinal tract.

Protection against diabetes. Aerobic activity improves insulin sensitivity and reduces your overall insulin level, reducing your odds of getting diabetes.

Lower blood pressure. Aerobic exercise stymies the increase in blood pressure that's common as we grow older.

A better attitude. Studies show that cardio exercise can be an effective antidote to mild to moderate depression.

Mental sharpness. Researchers at the University of Illinois split 124 subjects into two groups. One group walked up to 45 minutes a day, three times a week. The other group stretched for an hour, three times a week. After 6 months, the walkers scored 15 percent higher on tests measuring their ability to focus and perform multiple tasks. It's believed that aerobic exercise may improve bloodflow to the area of the brain that controls the ability to sort and process information.

Better sex. Aerobic exercise appears to boost men's levels of testosterone, the hormone that fuels so much of our sex drive. Exercise also enhances bloodflow throughout the body, and adequate bloodflow is critical to long-lasting erections. It even produces those feel-good brain chemicals called endorphins that can increase your arousal and possibly the intensity of your orgasms.

Better sleep. Depending on when you do it, a cardio workout can help you sleep. If you exercise 5 to 6 hours before bedtime, your metabolism will slowly drop at the same time that your body is naturally winding down for sleep. But if you exercise too late at night, you may get too hyped up to sleep.

Start Me Up

So many activities are aerobic that you're almost guaranteed to find one or several that you enjoy. And that's a key to sticking with it: find an activity that's fun. This chapter focuses on those exercises you can do outdoors. On Day 5 of this week, we'll discuss in more detail those that you can do indoors.

Keep in mind, though, that lower-body exercises such as running and bicycling build aerobic fitness faster than upper-body exertions such as rock climbing and swimming. A study of 16 people who ran on treadmills or climbed for 20 minutes found that the two groups posted similar heart rates, but the runners used 14 percent more oxygen, getting the better aerobic workout.

Before you start an energetic aerobic program, however, consult with a doctor first if you answer yes to more than one of the following questions.

- Are you over the age of 45?
- Has any male family member died of a heart attack before age 55? Or has any woman in your family died of a heart attack before age 65? Do you have at least one family member who has had bypass surgery?
- Do you smoke cigarettes?

- Has your doctor ever told you that you have high blood pressure? Or has your blood pressure been measured more than once at greater than 140 over 90? Or do you take high blood pressure medicine?
- Has your doctor ever told you that you have high cholesterol? Or do you know if your total cholesterol is greater than 200? Or is your HDL cholesterol less than 35?
- Do you consider yourself physically inactive at work and during your leisure time?

Outdoor Man

Here are some cardio sports and activities you can do outdoors.

Cross-country skiing. If you live in a winter climate that permits it, cross-country skiing is one of the best calorie-burning workouts you can get because it's one of the few sports that works both upper- and lower-body muscles. In an hour, a 155-pound man will burn between 1,000 and 1,500 calories.

Cross-country skiing doesn't jar your joints or muscles the way running, basketball, and soccer do. But as with other sports, you can surely get injured if you attempt to do too much too soon. A few weeks before hitting the snow, start hiking and speed walking on the same sort of hilly terrain that you will be traversing on your skis. To get your upper body primed, take along your ski poles. Take long strides and kick off with your feet while planting and pushing off the ground with your poles. Consider using old poles in order to protect your equipment.

Inline skating. For a good workout of your legs, hips, and butt, this is the ticket. You'll burn about 550 calories an hour—more if you tackle some hills.

While gliding on skates is easy on the joints, some guys inevitably get hurt in falls. Take a few precautions, though, and you'll get a terrific cardio workout and live to tell about it. Go only as fast as feels comfortable. Wear a helmet, wrist guards, and knee and elbow pads. Take lessons, if you need them.

To get the best aerobic workout possible while inline skating, figure on averaging 8 to 12 miles an hour for at least 20 minutes. Continually move your arms for more momentum and a better calorie burn. Skate low in long, powerful strides.

Mountain biking. Cycling of any sort, including on a stationery bike, can give you a good aerobic workout. But mountain biking is especially intense. Unlike in traditional cycling, you use your upper body as well as your lower body in mountain biking, jerking over logs and other trail impediments. By using more muscles, you burn more calories. And you exert more energy traversing rugged terrain than you do on a smooth road. Still more calories burned.

CAMP CARDIO

Okay, tough guy. Think you have the cardio exercises whipped? Then you might want to sign up for a cardio boot camp course at a health club or buy a video of the same.

The drills vary, but you can expect to be put through a variety of heart-pounding exercises adopted from martial arts, calisthenics, and sports ranging from boxing to bicycling. Boot camp backers say the variety not only prevents boredom but also makes it less likely you will strain a particular muscle group.

And unlike in the military, you won't have a drill instructor with a gargoyle face and cesspool breath barking in your face like a rabid dog. Cardio boot camp is tough, but civilized.

As with inline skating, you should take a few safety precautions when mountain biking. Wear a helmet. Before you go out the first time, get instruction so you'll know how to ride over and around obstacles and how to brake and shift properly. Go easy on downhills until you've become a whiz on the bike. Have the seat adjusted to a level that best enables you to handle the bike.

Running. This is good fat-burning exercise, but can be a literal pain if you don't approach it smartly. First, the benefits. Running at a leisurely 12-minute-mile pace burns about 10 calories a minute. If you run an 8-minute mile, you'll burn around 15 calories a minute, or 600 calories over the course of a 40-minute run.

Running is hard on your feet and joints, however. Each time your foot pounds the ground, it hits with a force equal to three to four times your body weight.

You can minimize the chance of injuries by easing up a bit if you feel sore. Don't increase the distance of your runs by more than 10 percent a week. Begin and end each run with a 10-minute jog to warm up and cool down. Don't buy cheap shoes. Run on soft surfaces such as dirt or grass; or run on a high school track, which may have a spongy, rubber surface that's easy on the feet. Avoid running on cement and concrete, when possible.

Running can be tedious, but it doesn't have to be. Run with friends or join a running club, and seek new routes to roam.

Swimming. This sport doesn't melt calories to the extent of some others on our list, but it will give you a fine total-body workout. Your legs, hips, abdominals, chest, shoulders, and upper back all come into play.

Slicing through the water is gentle on the body, but swimming isn't without injury risks. It's a physically demanding sport, and shoulder injuries are common among overzealous newcomers. Start by warming up with a 400-yard swim: 200 yards of freestyle, 100 yards of backstroke, and 100 yards of breaststroke.

While you can get a perfectly good workout by doing the same stroke at the same pace for a half-hour or so, you'll burn considerably more calories by completing an interval workout. This consists of a series of swims separated by a specific amount of rest, the interval. A typical workout includes several sets of swims with a 10- to 30-second interval after each swim, then several minutes' rest after each set. You could do 10 repetitions of 50-yard freestyle swims, for example. Or try 5 reps of 100-yard freestyle swims, giving yourself a short rest after each swim.

Another way to maximize your workout is to perform a variety of strokes, not just freestyle. Doing so enables you to hit more muscles and improves your flexibility by bringing different motions into play.

Alternatives

Even if you're sometimes too busy to engage in formal aerobic exercise, there are ways to give your heart a good workout. Here are a few suggestions.

- Rake leaves the old-fashioned way, with a rake. Leaf blowers don't count.
- If you use a power lawn mower, switch to a push mower.
- If you live near an ocean, lake, or river, use it. Kayaking, canoeing, or rowboating are all bold and tough upper-body aerobic workouts.
- Try some extreme yard work. Digging holes, cutting down trees, splitting logs, and spreading a few hundred pounds of mulch can all provide a good mix of strengthening and aerobic exercise.
- Play with your kids. Not computer games, but physical activity. Go one-on-one against your son on the basketball court. Play soccer with your daughter. Take both of them on a hike in the woods, on the beach, or in a park. Not only will you get an aerobic benefit, you'll be instilling healthy habits in your children too.
- Climb. It could be trees, rocks, building facades, mountain paths, ropes. All are tough and real workouts. Just remember that to make it aerobic exercise, you need to sustain the intensity for at least 20 minutes. Short bursts of exertion build muscles but don't strengthen your cardiovascular system.

Get Active at Work

The Day's Task

We assume you will be dedicating 8 hours to work today. If not, consider yourself on the clock from 9:00 A.M. to 5:00 P.M. Your task today is to do all of the following during your work hours:

- **Go up or down a minimum of 12 flights of stairs.**
- **Do at least eight 30-second stretches (we outline several good office stretches in this chapter).**
- **Take at least four brisk walks of 5 minutes each.**

You can do these at any time. Even if you already do some of these, you need to do all of the rest. Obviously, scattering the movements throughout your day makes the most sense. In fact, that is the healthiest thing to do. It's what we want you to do.

To make sure you get to everything, write down on a clean sheet of paper "Stairs" and the numbers 1 through 12, "Stretches" and the numbers 1 through 8, and "Walks" and the numbers 1 through 4. Fold up the paper and place in your shirt pocket with a pen. Check things off as you go.

Truth is, filling your day with small bursts of movement will not burn a whole lot of calories or give you taut muscles. But it will do more for you than you could possibly guess.

If you learn one thing from this chapter, it should be this: Fitness is not about 30 minutes of exercise done three or four times a week. Fitness is an attitude, a lifestyle, a personality. Your goal in life is to be active and vital at all times. That is the key to longevity.

There are physiological reasons why moving throughout the day is good for you. Research confirms that you can get almost the same health benefits by doing several short spurts of exercise during the day as you would if you did one 30-minute workout.

Just as important are the psychological benefits. Energized people feel young, act young, and are just plain happier.

So are you an active person? The answer can be found in the hundreds of small choices you make every day. Do you smack the snooze button on the alarm clock, or do you get up in time to eat a healthy breakfast and do a few stretches? Do you climb trees with your kids, or do you watch videos with them? Do you hire the neighbor's kid to cut the lawn while you watch the ball game, or do you do mow the grass yourself? Is your hobby bicycling, or is it the surfing the Internet?

Extend that to work. When you arrive at the office, do you park as close to the building as you can, or do you park where there are plenty of spaces and enjoy the brisk walk in? If your office is on the third floor, do you take the stairs or the elevator?

Our message here is that even at work, you need to be active. It's the attitude of long life. It is also, by the way, the attitude of success. In other words, it's good for your career. Trust us. Your energy and good attitude will be noticed.

Office Max

It's easy to discreetly fit in more vigorous exercise at work and to do it without getting so sweaty that you drive colleagues screaming from a staff meeting. Here are a few ways, some of which amplify today's assignment.

Walk around the perimeter of the floor on which your office is located. Then, take the stairs up to the next floor—or down to a lower floor if you're at the top—and walk the circumference of that floor. When you finish that floor, hit the stairs again and do another floor before returning to your office via the stairs.

If much of your time is spent driving, be sure to get out of the car at least every 2 hours. Once out, stretch, walk, jump, shake, do some calisthenics. Don't just go into the doughnut shop and plop down on a stool. Use as much of your break time as you can for movement.

Find a lonely stairwell and walk up and down. In just 10 minutes, you can burn 91 calories going up and 34 coming down. Descending stairs can be tough on your knees. If you feel any knee discomfort, take the elevator down.

A variation that's guaranteed to tax your calves is to step up on a stair with your right foot, slowly raise your right heel off the ground, then step up with your

The Fidget Factor

Even if you're enduring one of those 10-hour, no-time-for-lunch (or exercise) days at work, you can burn some calories without ever leaving your desk.

Mayo Clinic researchers fed 16 women and men of average weight food containing 1,000 more calories per day than required to maintain their weights and limited them to low levels of exercise. Then, they measured which participants stored the most and the least amounts of the additional calories as fat. The study volunteers gained an average of 10 pounds in 2 months. But those who were most active without actually exercising—who fidgeted, shifted in their seats, adjusted their posture, and so forth—gained the least weight. One volunteer burned up an average of 692 calories per day through such seemingly meaningless movements. Conversely, those participants who moved around the least gained the most weight.

So the next time you feel yourself squirming in your seat when the boss asks you a question you can't answer, take solace. At least he's helping you manage your weight.

left foot and raise your left heel. Since you'll be walking on the balls of your feet, hold on to the railing for balance.

Buy an indoor basketball setup and, once a day, take a few minutes to practice your layup. Do that thing you used to do back when you played at your driveway hoop: pretend it's the last 5 minutes of the NBA championship and you are the hero ("The crowd roars!"). Better yet, get a workplace pal to join you for a fast game of Horse or 21.

Do as many pushups and crunches as you can, or do lunges and squats. Or take two chairs (without wheels), position one on either side of you, put your hands on the seats and your legs straight out on the floor in front of you, and do dips. It is not at all ridiculous to do some no-gear exercises at work.

Load your car trunk with water bottles. Every 2 hours, walk to it for a new one. This achieves several things. It guarantees that you take breaks. It works in a brisk walk several times a day. It keeps you drinking water, which is extremely healthy. And it saves you money because water by the case is far cheaper than all that soda and coffee from the cafeteria.

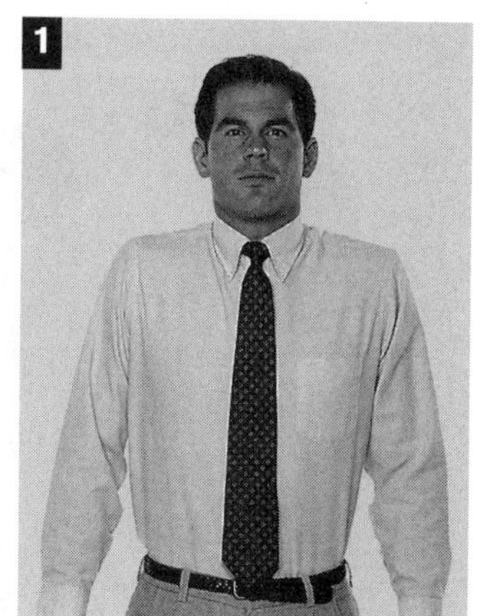

Every time you get a phone call, stand up. If the call is longer than 30 seconds, pace while you talk. Anything that gets you out of your chair more often is a good thing. Plus, standing will give you a mental and physical boost that could very well help you be more alert and clever on the phone.

Office Stretches

It's another pressure cooker day at work, and your body is rebelling. Your neck, your shoulders, your back, your entire body feels like a taut rubber band ready to snap. Here are a few stretches and exercises you can quickly do in your office to help you unwind, Rubber Band Man. Find an empty conference or stock room, or merely go to an empty office. Then, all you need is a chair and a wall.

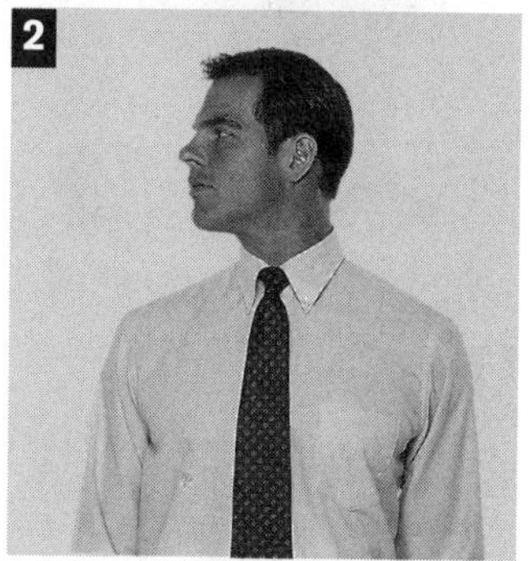

Shoulder shrug (1). Sit or stand with your arms hanging loosely at your sides. Shrug your shoulders up. Hold for 5 seconds. Relax your shoulders downward. Repeat one or two times.

Neck rotation (2). Sit or stand with your arms hanging loosely at your sides. Turn your head to one side, then the other. Hold for 5 seconds on each side. Repeat one to three times.

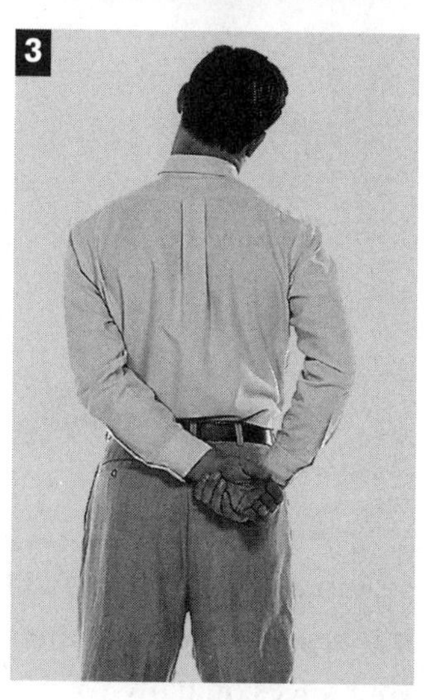

Arm and shoulder stretch (3). Lean your head sideways toward your right shoulder. With your right hand, gently pull your left arm down and across behind your back. Hold for 10 seconds, then relax and repeat with your head to the left, your left hand pulling your right arm.

Shoulder and wrist stretch (see photo 4 on page 72). Interlace your fingers above your head, palms up. Push your arms slightly back and up. Hold for 10 to 20 seconds. Repeat. Don't hold your breath.

Trunk rotation (see photo 5 on page 72). Stand with your hands on your waist. Gently twist your torso to the right until you feel a stretch. Hold for 10 to 15 sec-

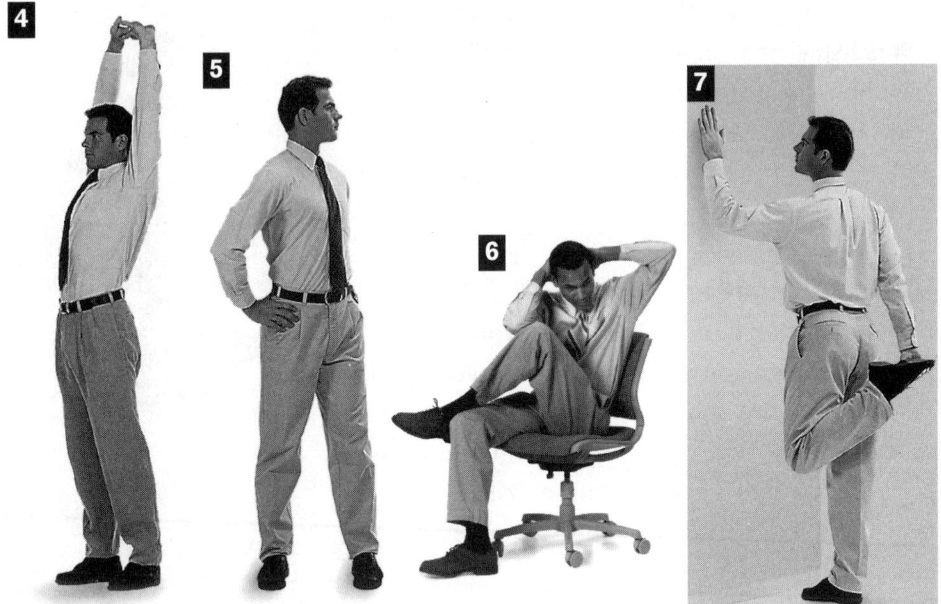

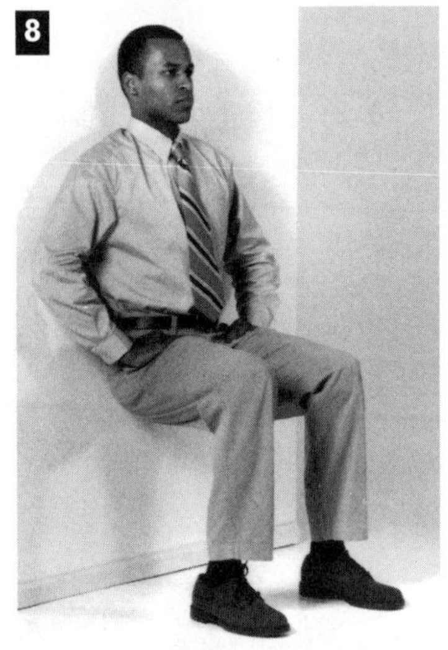

onds. Repeat to the left. Keep your knees slightly flexed. Don't hold your breath.

Seated ab builder (6). Sitting upright, interlace your fingers behind your head. Lift your left knee, and bend to touch it with your right elbow. Return your foot to the floor. Repeat with your right knee and left elbow. Do at least five on each side.

Quad stretch (7). Stand two steps from a wall and place your left hand on the wall for support. Standing straight, grab the top of your left foot with your right hand. Pull your heel toward your butt as far as you comfortably can. Hold for 10 to 20 seconds. Repeat with your right leg.

Extended wall-sit (8). Stand with your back against a wall, feet hip-width apart. Slowly slide down and walk your feet out until it is almost as if you were sitting in a chair. Don't go below a 90-degree angle at your knees or allow your knees to pass your feet. Your back will be supported by the wall, and your quads, hamstrings, and glutes will support your body weight. Hold for 5 to 10 seconds, then slide back up. Repeat five times.

Aerobic Session Number 2 (Indoors)

The Day's Task

Just like on Day 3 of this week, we need you to set aside 60 minutes of your day for a full aerobic workout. You'll follow the same format: 5 minutes of warmup, 30 minutes of aerobic exertion, and 5 minutes of cooldown and stretching, with the rest of the time allotted to changing clothes, showering, and getting dressed again. There is just one big difference today: we want you to work out inside your house.

We've already explained the benefits of aerobic exercise. And we've made clear that you need to do it frequently. All you need from us now are some ideas for working out indoors on those all-too-frequent days when circumstances do not permit an outdoor excursion.

Roughly half of American households already own indoor exercise equipment, such as stationary bikes or treadmills. Most of them are covered in cobwebs. So get out the vacuum, remember the money and hassle involved in getting this equipment purchased and carried into the house, and use it with gusto.

Or don't. In this chapter we list several indoor aerobic workouts that require little to no special gear. Give these a try, or, better yet, do a little of each to fill your 30 minutes.

Jumping Rope

As boxers will attest, skipping rope works your entire body—legs, abs, chest, shoulders, back, and arms—and will have you puffing in no time. A 165-pound man jumping rope can burn more than 400 calories in a half-hour, exceeding jogging or cycling. Regardless of where you jump rope, make sure you have plenty of space so you don't get snagged on a pipe in the basement or on another guy's head at the gym.

Jumping rope is an impact sport, so don't jump high and land hard. Instead, lift your feet off the floor just high enough for the rope to pass quickly beneath you. Land on the padded balls of your feet to avoid knee injuries.

Make sure your rope is long enough. When you stand in the middle, the ends of the handles should reach your armpits. Your wrists and forearms, not your shoulders, should turn the rope. Keep your arms at your sides, with your elbows tucked in. Wear well-padded cross-trainers or aerobics shoes.

Calisthenics

Calisthenics can be another way to get a full-body workout while improving your heart health. The key to burning calories and getting your heart pumping is to push yourself hard and take minimal rest between exercises. In fact, one approach would be to run in place for a few minutes, do one of the exercises below, resume running for a couple of minutes, move on to the next exercise, and so on. Stay in nonstop motion for 30 minutes. It's a tough workout.

Jumping jack. This is the classic guy calisthenic. Start with your arms at your sides, your feet together, and your back straight. Jump a few inches off the floor, bringing your arms in a wide circular path over your head and clapping lightly, if you wish. As you raise your arms, spread your legs until your feet are a little wider than shoulder-width apart; that's the position you want to land in from your first jump. Repeat over and over until you approach the point where you can't speak because you're breathing too heavily.

Stepup. Stand in front of a sturdy chair or bench. Step up then down, alternating feet. Do two or three sets of 12 to 15 repetitions per foot.

Crunch. Lie on your back with your knees bent and your feet flat on the floor. Rest your fingertips lightly on the sides of your head and put your elbows out to the sides. Tilt your pelvis so that your lower back stays flat on the floor, then curl your body up so that your head and shoulders come off the floor. Take 3 seconds to lift your head and shoulders, pause for a second, then take 3 seconds to lower your head to the floor. Do 15 to 20.

Lower-back extension. Lie facedown on the floor, with your arms against your sides. Raise your head so that your shoulders are 6 inches off the floor, then lower.

RAGE AGAINST THE MACHINE

If you are going to invest in an expensive piece of aerobic equipment, be sure to buy something you think you'll use. Here's a list of some popular machines and the percentages of buyers still using them within 5 years after purchase, according to a *Consumer Reports* survey.

Motorized treadmill	53%
Strength-training machine	44%
Air walker, strider, glider	39%
Cross-country ski machine	39%
Stationary bike	36%
Nonmotorized treadmill	27%
Stairclimber	27%

Do 12 to 15 repetitions. If this is too easy, lie facedown and place your arms in front of you. Then, lift your chest, arms, and legs off the floor simultaneously.

Pushup. You know the drill. Just your hands about 2 feet apart. Do 12 to 15 repetitions.

Pullup. Use an underhand grip on the bar and pull yourself up until your chin is over the bar. Keep your back and arms straight. Do 12 to 15 repetitions.

As you get better at calisthenics, you can make them harder. Place a 5-pound weight plate across your chest while doing crunches, for example, and hold it in place by crossing your arms. Take 5 seconds going down and 5 seconds going up when doing pushups and pullups. It's important to continually make small changes in the order of your exercises and the way you do them in order to maximize the benefit you receive from them.

Boxing

Whether you punch a heavy bag or a speed bag or just the air, boxing is an intense workout. A 150-pound palooka who keeps at it for a half-hour can burn about 200 calories. If you're a heavyweight, the figure will be higher.

Even if you have no plans to step into the ring with anybody, consider hiring an instructor or picking up a video or book on how to correctly throw jabs, crosses, hooks, and uppercuts. You can injure a shoulder or break a wrist if you don't use the proper form.

Professional boxers fight 3-minute rounds with a minute of rest in between. Strive for this in your workouts, but don't expect to do it immediately. Work up to it; boxing is grueling exercise. Once you're able to last 3 minutes, try to increase the number of punches you throw or decrease the amount of time you rest. This will help keep things interesting.

Trampoline

If you have kids, chances are pretty good that you already have a mini-trampoline around. If not, they're cheap and readily available. Use them for jumping, running in place, and random hopping about. Trampolines provide a nice way to integrate fresh movements into a calisthenics regimen.

Aerobics

Let us acknowledge that workout videos for men do exist, that not every aerobics video is cheesy and feminine, that possibly, remotely, conceivably, there's a tape that you'd enjoy working out to. You don't know until you try. At least you're going to get a well-rounded workout featuring some visual candy to keep you entertained.

Juggling

Okay, this won't leave you panting like boxing or rope jumping will. But a 150-pound man can quicken his heartbeat and burn 135 calories in 30 minutes of tossing objects in the air.

Unless you're flipping flaming torches or chainsaws, there is little danger that you'll hurt yourself juggling. Nor do you need fancy gear or equipment. But you ought to check out a video, book, or Web site to learn how to get started. Here are a few hints.

Start practicing with beanbags, not balls; and stand at a table that is between knee and waist height, such as a kitchen table. You can make beanbags by putting beans or coins in socks, knotting them, turning them inside out, knotting them again, and turning them inside out once again.

Then, you are ready to start playing catch with yourself using one beanbag, then two, then three. When you drop one, it will hit the table, not the floor, and because it's a beanbag, it won't bounce or roll away.

Discover Your Heartbeat

The Day's Task

Today's exercise is mental, not physical. Grab a paper and a pencil.

1. **Let's say that you are 40 years old. Subtract your age from 220. The difference, 180, is a rough estimate of your maximum heart rate, or the maximum number of times your heart can safely beat in 1 minute.**
2. **Multiply your maximum heart rate by 0.6. Continuing with our example, multiplying 180 by 0.6 yields 108. This is your minimum target heart rate for your aerobic workouts. Below that level of heart activity, you really aren't getting much health benefit.**
3. **Multiply your maximum heart rate by 0.8. In our example, that gets you 144. That's the maximum target heart rate you should have in a workout. Move above that, and you significantly overexert yourself and put your body in jeopardy.**
4. **Memorize those two numbers, 108 and 144 in this case. They are the range in which you want your heart to beat while doing aerobic exercise.**

In the previous chapters, we told you that an aerobic workout is any activity that keeps your heart beating at an elevated rate for 20 minutes or more. That raised the question of how hard you need to do aerobic exercise in order for it to pay off. Today's task teaches you how to determine the absolute optimal level of exertion for your unique body and age. The numbers you just calculated are a big part of this.

Admittedly, your two numbers provide you with a very broad range. Exactly where you should be within that range depends mostly on your level of fitness. Here's an easy scale: If you are out of shape, sustain 60 percent of your maximum heart rate during your aerobic workouts. If you are in adequate shape, sustain 70 percent. If you are seeking a very high level of fitness, are already very healthy, and have high stamina, you can move up to 80 percent.

Even if you are fit, limit your high-intensity, "80 percent" workouts to once a week. Going at a fast and furious clip more often can result in injuries to muscles, ligaments, and tendons, setting back your fitness program. And going all-out too often may also leave you burned out and finding excuses not to exercise.

If you last exercised regularly when athletic shoes were called sneakers, you need to start out slow and easy. Don't even consider trying to reach the 80 percent range until you've been working out for at least 3 months. Stay at 60 percent of your maximum heart rate. Your heart is a muscle; it needs to get in shape too.

Time is your heart's friend. If you have plenty to spare, you can embark on a more leisurely but also more beneficial workout. If you're willing to spend 60 to 90 minutes at it, exercising at only 40 to 60 percent of your maximum heart rate will give you a quality cardio workout and will ease your muscles into the program as well. But if you're in good enough shape to do so, increase the effort to higher than 60 percent of your max, and reap weight loss and heart benefits in less time.

A Different Method

Want a more precise method for determining your target heart rate? This method is more complicated but takes in two variables, your age and your resting heart rate. The latter is a good indication of your current fitness level. The higher it is, the less in shape you are, and thus the lower your target heart rate for exercise. Here goes.

1. Find your resting heart rate by taking your pulse before getting out of bed in the morning. It'll probably be between 50 and 80 beats per minute. Let's say you're a 40-year-old man with a resting heart rate of 70, and you want to exercise at 60 percent of your maximum heart rate.
2. Subtract your age from 220. Then, subtract your resting heart rate. You'd take 40 away from 220, then 70, leaving you with 110.
3. Find 60 percent of that difference. In our example, you'd multiply 110 times by 0.6, which yields 66.
4. Add back your resting heart rate. The sum is your target heart rate. In our example, that would be 66 plus 70, or 136 beats per minute.

Determining the Beat

All of this number crunching is useless if you don't know how many times your heart beats in a minute. The crucial skill is taking your pulse. Here's how to do it.

Place two fingers, but not your thumb, on your wrist near the base of your

COUCH POTATO BLUES

So, wise guy, you're wondering if you could elevate your heart rate without getting winded or breaking a sweat. What if you could induce a rapid heartbeat by placing yourself in a stressful situation, say, listening to Mötley Crüe perform polka music every night? Could you lose weight and otherwise improve your health as if you were exercising?

No. If it were that easy, high-strung, nervous people would be among the most physically fit folks in the world. A couch potato could become buff by watching thrillers on television.

It's a rise in oxygen intake and energy expenditure that does the trick. The increase in heart rate is merely a marker for these changes.

thumb and feel the pulsations. Count how many times your heart beats in 10 seconds and multiply this number by six. If you find it easier to do, substitute your neck for your wrist. Find the beat on either side of your Adam's apple.

If you're uncomfortable groping for a pulse, consider investing in a heart rate monitor. The monitor straps around your chest and transmits heart rate readings to a receiver that is similar to a wristwatch. This gizmo gives you a second-by-second account of your heart rate. So if your target rate is between 108 and 144 and your monitor shows you at 130 while you exercise, you know you are in your heart-training target range.

A heart rate monitor is more accurate than taking a 10-second pulse, and it's more convenient. Instead of stopping periodically during a workout to measure your pulse, you simply glance at your wrist receiver without missing a beat.

Heart rate monitors vary in the number of bells and whistles they feature. For about $100, you can buy a basic model, which displays your heartbeats per minute, period. Or you can spend more for a monitor that can be programmed for specific target zones and that beeps when you fall out of your range. Other models include a memory function and can provide additional data, such as average heart rate and time spent in, above, and below a target zone. Some units even calculate calories burned and transfer data to a personal computer, where the information can be analyzed and stored. You can even buy a heart rate monitor with headphones that allows you to play music and has a humanlike voice interpret your data.

10 Ways to Prevent Arthritis and Arthritis Pain

1 **Stay within your weight limits.** If you need another reason to lose weight, here it is: Extra weight puts extra strain on your joints and puts you at greater risk for osteoarthritis, says Alan Lichtbroun, M.D., assistant professor of rheumatology at the University of Medicine and Dentistry of New Jersey Robert Wood Johnson Medical School in New Brunswick. This wears out your cartilage and allows the bones in your joints to rub together. Ouch.

2 **Get up and move.** Even if you don't need to lose weight, you do need to keep the muscles and ligaments that support your joints strong and flexible. Be sure to work out regularly, combining aerobic exercise and strength training, to help reduce your chances of osteoarthritis, says Howard R. Smith, M.D., chief of rheumatology at Meridia Huron Hospital in Cleveland.

3 **Practice safe stretching.** Add stretching to your exercise routine to help keep your muscles strong, which in turn will protect your joints from wear and tear. Stretching will also help keep your joints flexible. Before you start your exercise, begin with about 10 minutes of warmup, just enough exertion to start a light sweat, followed by stretching. Try to hold each stretch for 15 to 20 seconds, then relax and repeat. Never bounce while you're stretching, says Emil Pascarelli, M.D., professor of clinical medicine at Columbia-Presbyterian Medical Center in New York City.

4 **Be gentle with your joints.** Treat your joints like you do your kids: lovingly. You want them to be good to you when you're older. When you carelessly slam into walls at the racquetball court, get tackled on the Sunday-afternoon gridiron, or rough yourself up in extreme sports, you risk joint injury, increasing your chances for arthritis.

By all means, get plenty of exercise, but make sure it's not too jolting on your system, says David Pisetsky, M.D., Ph.D., of the Duke University Arthritis Center in Durham, North Carolina.

5 **Set your thermostat wisely.** Both heat and cold can ease arthritis pain if you use them the right way. The trick is to know which one to pick and when to pick it. If you feel sore and achy, apply heat to the troublesome area. Wrap a heating pad or hot pack in a towel and apply it to your painful joint for 20 minutes. Repeat three times a day, suggests the Arthritis Foundation in Atlanta.

But if you feel a sudden flare-up of pain, take the opposite approach. Wrap a plastic bag filled with ice cubes or a bag of frozen vegetables in a pillowcase since you don't want to hold ice directly on your bare skin. Then, apply it to the trouble spot for about 20 minutes. Wait at least 45 minutes before you put it on again.

6 **Stand up straight.** If your car's front end is poorly aligned, your tires can wear out unevenly. If your body is poorly aligned—we're talking about bad posture—you can put too much pressure on certain joints, causing bone and cartilage to wear away. Sit and stand so that your bones are evenly balanced. While you're sitting, hold your head and upper back straight, your knees level with your hips, and your feet flat on the floor, Dr. Lichtbroun advises. Stand so your shoulders are vertically in line with your hips and your hips are vertically in line with your knees and feet.

7 **Vary your exercise pattern.** To keep from adding wear to the same points in your joints, walk or jog different routes so you don't stress your knees and hips the exact same way day after day, says Dale L. Anderson, M.D., author of *Muscle Pain Relief in 90 Seconds*. Seek out a mixture of terrains from day to day, such as hills, fields, pathways, and flat areas.

8 **Eat plenty of fish.** Oils in certain fish contain omega-3 fatty acids. Get enough of these in your diet, and you can actually lower the level of inflammatory substances in your body and reduce pain from rheumatoid arthritis, which is caused by inflammation in your joints, says John Thompson, M.D., professor of medicine at the University of Western Ontario Faculty of Medicine and Dentistry in London. Herring, salmon, mackerel, and tuna are the ultimate omega fish.

9 **Antioxidize yourself.** Be sure to get plenty of vitamin C, both as a daily supplement and from foods like green leafy vegetables, citrus fruits, and potatoes. In a Boston University study of 640 people with and without osteoarthritis in the knees, those who got the most vitamin C had three times less disease progression than the people who got the least. On its own, this antioxidant may not help you completely avoid arthritis, but it may prevent it from becoming severe.

10 **Pass on the purines.** Go easy on the red meat, aged cheeses, and alcohol. These foods are particularly rich in a chemical called purine that raises levels of uric acid in the body. Uric acid settles into joints and gives you gout, an agonizing form of arthritis, says Doyt Conn, M.D., of the Arthritis Foundation.

10 Ways to Prevent Back Pain

1 **Take frequent walks, using good form.** Walking is the best way to prevent back problems, says Jerome F. McAndrews, D.C., of the American Chiropractic Association. It strengthens and warms the large muscle groups that hold your back in its proper position. As you walk, check out your reflection in bright, shiny objects and make sure your form is good. Don't lean forward; bring your weight back on to the heels of your feet and feel the ground solidly beneath you. While you move, think about lengthening your spine, standing up very straight. Imagine your spine is an arrow pointing up, away from the ground.

2 **Choose a work chair that is firm and supportive.** Sitting may sound like an easy job, but nothing is simple when 200 muscles and 33 bones are folded into an unnatural position, particularly when they are held there for hours at a time. Here's the anatomy of a perfect chair: Look for a high-end office chair with a seat height and seat pan (the forward-back tilt of your seat) that can be adjusted to meet your needs. The chair should have a firm cushion on the seat and armrests on the sides. Position the seat so that your knees are just slightly lower than your hips and your feet are flat on the floor. The back support should just touch the small of your back.

3 **Improve your sleeping arrangements.** You spend roughly a third of your life in your bed (more if you're lucky). Choose a firm mattress with good support. Rest your head on a medium-size pillow that keeps your head, neck, and spine in a straight line; you don't want your head angling up as it would with big or multiple pillows. Invest in several other pillows so you can sleep on your back with pillows under your knees, or on your side with your knees curled up and a pillow between your legs. Whatever you do, don't sleep on your stomach, which twists your neck and back, says John E. Thomassy, D.C., a chiropractor in Virginia Beach, Virginia.

4 **Learn proper lifting techniques.** Any time you lift a heavy object off the floor, you put your back muscles at risk. Here's the proper technique to minimize that risk. Get close to the object you're lifting. Plant your feet shoulder-width apart. Squat down, bending your knees and keeping your back straight. Firmly grab the object, surrounding it with your arms, then tighten your abs and lift with your legs. As you stand, keep your back and neck straight, as if you had a broomstick attached to your spine. If you can't keep your back straight, the object is too heavy, advises Dr. McAndrews.

5 **Stretch your back muscles three or four times a day.** The following stretch takes about 90 seconds. Do it every 4 to 6 hours during the day, says Dr. McAndrews.

Stand up and lean forward with your hands on your thighs and your legs straight. Arch your back until you feel a gentle pull on the muscles down your back. Hold for 30 seconds, then stand up straight.

Reach straight up with your right arm and lean to the left until you feel the muscles stretch along your right hip and waist. Hold for 30 seconds. Repeat on the other side, raising your left arm and leaning right.

6 **Strengthen your abdominal muscles.** Strong abs lighten the load on your spine and back muscles, helping to protect you from back pain or injury. The gold-standard abs exercise remains the crunch. Every day, do crunches until exhaustion or for 10 minutes, whichever comes first, according to Kenneth Light, M.D., of the San Francisco Spine Center.

7 **Give yourself occasional back rubs.** With either your palms or the backs of your hands, rub your lower back until you generate heat. "The friction will warm the area and increase circulation," says Michael Reed Gach, Ph.D., of the Acupressure Institute in Berkeley, California.

8 **Practice a single yoga pose called the cobra.** This common posture helps strengthen your spine and back, says Mara Carrico, a yoga instructor in Encinitas, California. Do it two or three times a day. Here's how.

Lie on your stomach. Bend your elbows and place your hands underneath your shoulders. Keep your legs hip-distance apart. Tighten your buttocks. As you inhale, straighten your arms to raise your chest up, and look forward while keeping your lower body on the floor. Hold this position for 10 to 20 seconds, then release and lower your chest back to the floor.

9 **Lose extra weight, particularly if it shows up around your belly.** If you are overweight, you are putting strain on your spine and fatiguing your back muscles. If the muscles are already fatigued and you go to lift something too heavy, the muscles are going to give.

10 **Adopt back-friendly habits.** Everyday activities like shaving and talking on the phone are so mundane that it's easy to forget how you're contorting your body while doing them. For example, when you shave, leaning toward the bathroom mirror puts stress on your neck and lower back, which can create disk and muscle problems. Instead, shave standing up in the shower with a shower-safe mirror or no mirror at all (you get a better shave in the shower anyhow, and you get to skip the lather).

Similarly, cradling a phone between your head and shoulder sets you up for spasms in the large, flat muscles of your upper back. Instead, hold the phone in your hand or use a headset.

WEEK 3

THE SAVE-YOUR-BODY SUPPLEMENT PLAN

Day 1

Browse a Supplement Shelf

Day 2

Take a Multivitamin

Day 3

Take a Vitamin C Supplement

Day 4

Take a Vitamin E Supplement

Day 5

Stock Your Herbal Shelf

Day 6

Decide on Other Supplements

Browse a Supplement Shelf

The Day's Task

You have an easy job today. All you have to do is a little browsing.

Take this book and walk into a big store like Wal-Mart or one of the larger drugstores or a well-stocked health food store. Head straight to the supplement aisles. Your eyes will be assaulted with a bewildering array of vitamins, minerals, and various other sundries to swallow. The purpose of your browsing today is to de-bewilder this array.

Do this by relating what you read in the rest of this chapter to what you're looking at in the real world. Pick up the merchandise. Read the labels. Rattle the bottles. The store manager doesn't know you have no intention of buying.

Don't try to memorize anything. You'll only drive yourself crazy, and going crazy is not good for your Longevity Program. Just poke around, compare, and let yourself get used to this brave new world of health in a bottle.

Americans flock to these same shelves, spending more than $3.1 billion a year on supplements. Indeed, it's estimated that even more M.D.'s (one in two) take supplements than other adults (one in three).

That speaks well of the efficacy of supplements. But what is a supplement? Try this on for size: A dietary supplement is a pill, capsule, tablet, or liquid that contains at least one of the following: a vitamin, a mineral, an amino acid, an herb, or a similar substance such as fish oil or psyllium.

Note that the word is *supplement*, not *replacement*. Food is always your best source of vitamins, minerals, and other nutrients. You take supplements for one of two reasons: (1) to make sure you're getting enough of the natural chemicals your body needs for basic, everyday functioning or (2) to get a medical benefit that goes beyond your body's basic need for the substance.

In the case of vitamins and minerals, the minimum amount you need, as assessed by scientists hired by the federal government, is given as a Daily Value (DV). On supplement labels, the Daily Values and any other amounts are usually given as weights, using grams, not ounces. Since the weight is almost always less than a gram, you'll usually see it in thousandths of a gram, or milligrams, abbreviated mg. Sometimes, the weight is so small that it appears in micrograms (mcg), which are millionths of a gram. A few vitamins (A, D, and E) are measured in international units, or IU. Some labels don't tell you the actual amount of a vitamin or mineral, but rather what percentage of the Daily Value the supplement provides.

But even though the Daily Value is an accepted standard, many experts recommend getting more of certain nutrients. For example, the DV for vitamin C is just 60 milligrams for adult men, meaning that is the minimum amount your body needs each day to function. However, many doctors believe that vitamin C in daily doses as high as 1,000 or even 2,000 milligrams provides a host of medical benefits (you'll hear more about this later in this chapter and again in 2 days).

But just because supplements are natural doesn't mean you can take them without restraint. At minimum, too much of any one vitamin or mineral is a waste of money. At worst, it can cause health problems. If you're on prescription drugs or have a chronic health condition, it's a good idea, too, to check with your doctor before taking any supplement.

As you poke around the vitamin area, you'll notice that some products are "natural" and others are synthetic, or formulated in a lab. Truth is, your body usually doesn't notice the difference, but your wallet does because the synthetics are cheaper. So are generics as opposed to brand names. What's important is to find the letters *USP* on the label. They stand for United States Pharmacopeia, and they constitute a promise that the vitamins in the bottle contain the indicated amount of nutrient and will dissolve properly inside you.

One more task during your label investigations is to check for an expiration or sell-by date. This date matters because if you take the supplement after it, there's no guarantee of potency.

Seek out the bottles of multiple vitamins, also called multivitamins or multis. Actually, all three of those terms are misnomers since most of the good products include minerals as well as vitamins, often but not always at the Daily Value amount. A better term is *multivitamin with minerals*. Whatever you call them, they're a darn convenient way of getting pretty much all the vitamins and minerals you need in one little pill.

What All Those Vitamins Are

To a lot of guys, vitamins are either a confusing jumble of letters and Greek words or little Flintstones characters that you chew. But vitamins are actually just chemicals that your body needs in varying amounts. The exciting stories of vitamins are the more recent discoveries. At first, vitamins were considered important only for preventing deficiency diseases, like scurvy from a lack of vitamin C. But it turns out that vitamins are key for keeping at bay killers like heart disease, cancer, and diabetes. What's more, they improve your eyesight, strengthen your bones, increase your energy, and keep your mind sharp.

Vitamins, then, are worth getting to know. So let's go down the list.

Vitamin A. This compound is critical for healthy eyes and skin. It's measured in international units, of which you need 5,000 daily. One interesting thing you may notice on some labels is that a lot of those 5,000 IU might come from a chemical called beta-carotene. Beta-carotene is not vitamin A but rather a precursor of it. That means it converts to vitamin A once it's in your body.

Vitamin B. B is more complex than other vitamins because it's, well, a complex. There are lots of related vitamins in the B family.

- *Biotin* and *pantothenic acid* are two energy producers that are so common in American diets that you're unlikely to need supplements to ensure reaching the Daily Values, which are 300 micrograms and 10 milligrams, respectively.
- *Choline* is the most recent vitamin knighted as "essential" by the National Academy of Sciences, so it has begun to appear in multis even though your diet almost surely provides enough in the natural form called lecithin. Pronounced KO-leen, it helps protect your heart and liver. You need 550 milligrams daily.
- *Folic acid* is a real big shot in the B family since it's known to fight heart disease, boost immunity, aid brain function, and perhaps even discourage prostate and colon cancers. You might see this on some labels as *folate* or *folacin*, but all supplements actually contain the more potent form, folic acid. Folate is what you get in food like beans, orange juice, and spinach. But this may be one case where supplementing is more effective than relying on food sources. You'd need to eat twice as much folate to get the Daily Value of 400 micrograms of folic acid.
- *Niacin*, or nicotinic acid, helps your body use sugars and fatty acids for energy. You need 20 milligrams daily. Super-high doses are sometimes used to reduce cholesterol under a doctor's care but, unless buffered, can cause a temporary uncomfortable, hot, itching sensation accompanied by a rash or redness.

- *Riboflavin* is another energy producer. The DV is 1.7 milligrams. You can get some of that from white bread since by law it must be enriched with riboflavin and several other B vitamins.
- *Thiamin* helps turn carbohydrates into energy. The DV is 1.5 milligrams.
- *Vitamin B_6*, also called pyridoxine, is an immune-boosting vitamin that helps produce antibodies that fight infection. Like many of the B vitamins, it's important for your heart. One study found that people deficient in vitamin B_6 were twice as likely to develop heart disease. It has also been linked with memory function. You need 2 milligrams a day.
- *Vitamin B_{12}* is also important for immunity and brain functioning. Also known as cobalamin, B_{12} (along with B_6 and folic acid) is associated with lower levels homocysteine, an amino acid that's linked with heart disease when there's too much of it circulating. The Daily Value is only 6 micrograms, but the older you get, the more important that amount becomes.

Vitamin C. Also called ascorbic acid, C is the most popular vitamin supplement on American shelves, and for good reason. Besides its immune-enhancing and energy-processing properties, it's an antioxidant, meaning it can slow down or prevent all kinds of age-related problems. As mentioned, the DV is 60 milligrams, but you can probably benefit from more, as you'll see the day after tomorrow.

Vitamin D. This vitamin makes it possible for you to absorb the calcium you need for strong bones, which is why you'll see it in a lot of calcium supplements. It may also keep arthritis in check. The Daily Value is 400 IU, but you may have to double that when you hit 50.

Vitamin E. Thanks mainly to its antioxidant properties, vitamin E has gone from a fringe vitamin to a vitamin superstar. The DV is 30 IU, but that appears to be woefully low. We'll tell you more about that in Day 4 of this week.

Vitamin K. If you didn't know about this one, you're not alone. But you need 80 micrograms of K for adequate blood clotting. Very few people need to supplement this vitamin, and you shouldn't either without doctor's orders.

What All Those Minerals Are

There are 56 different minerals floating around in the average man's body, but don't expect to find all 56 as you investigate the supplement shelves. More than half (29, including gold and silver) aren't inside you for any particular reason, as far as anybody has been able to figure out.

The rest, though, have biological purposes, and 16 of them are considered essential. How essential? "The essential ones are the ones that if you don't get them, you'll eventually drop dead," says John N. Hathcock, Ph.D., of the Council for Responsible Nutrition in Washington, D.C.

As long as you eat, you're not likely to drop dead from mineral deprivation. Still, take note of the following ones, either within multivitamin/mineral supplements or on their own.

Calcium. Essential for strong bones, calcium also helps fight high blood pressure and colon cancer. You need 1,000 milligrams (more when you're older) that can come from milk or milk products, a supplement, or even antacids like Tums.

Copper. This assists the heart, immune system, connective tissues, brain chemistry, and absorption of other minerals, like iron. You need 2 milligrams.

Iron. Iron is essential for energy processing, but for men the more important issue is the problem of excess. Too much iron may raise your risk of heart disease, some cancers, and liver damage. You almost surely get more than you need in your diet, so your goal with iron supplements is usually to avoid them.

Magnesium. It's crucial for muscle activity and nerve-impulse conduction, but magnesium also may protect you from heart disease, diabetes, and even migraine headaches. The Daily Value is 400 milligrams.

Selenium. This one works as an antioxidant and shows promise as a cancer fighter and a preventer of gum disease, among many other benefits. You may notice that it's included in some but not all multivitamin/mineral supplements. As its own supplement, look for selenium as selenomethionine, which is the least toxic and most absorbable form. The DV is 70 micrograms.

Zinc. "When we look at zinc deficiency, it tends to affect males more than females," says Forrest H. Nielsen, Ph.D., of the Human Nutrition Research Center of the USDA. What it affects is your sperm count and sex drive, pretty good reasons to make sure you get enough. But zinc also provides a good illustration of the dangers of overdoing it with mineral supplements. Too much zinc actually depletes your copper supply, suppressing your immune system. So stick to the Daily Value of 15 milligrams, which is usually what you'll find in a multivitamin/mineral supplement.

What All Those Herbs Are

The new kids on the shelves you're browsing just happen to be the oldest of the lot. Plant-based medicine has been around for millennia, but now it's a staple along the supplement aisle.

The herbs are there for a good reason: People buy them. Researchers working for a supplement company recently concluded that 23 percent of the population uses herbal remedies, 11 percent on a regular basis and 12 percent for specific conditions. Not coincidentally, pharmaceutical giants such as SmithKline Beecham and Warner-Lambert have jumped into the herbal supplement market.

People buy herbs for just as good a reason: they work. And they're mostly safe. They can help prevent many diseases and heal just as many, without help from prescription drugs. "They're what Mother Nature gave us," says Eve Campanelli, Ph.D., a holistic family practitioner in Beverly Hills, California. "Herbs work, and they don't have all the side effects."

We'll take a look at some of the individual herbs on Day 5 of this week. Today, it's enough work to just figure out what's going on with all that stuff on the shelves. First off, you'll notice that many herbs are presented in combination, often with some sort of formula name. Ignore those as you would background static; look for single herbs.

You'll find them in several different forms. In those neat-looking little 1- or 2-ounce dark bottles are *tinctures*. The plant has been processed in an alcohol base that absorbs the active ingredients, yielding a long-lasting and potent liquid that lets you take your herbs by the drop or spoonful. The label might indicate the potency of the tincture as a ratio of herb-to-alcohol. For example, a 1:5 is much stronger than a 1:10.

You'll also see herbs in *tea* form, as either prepackaged tea bags or loose tea leaves. If you're in a natural food store, you'll find bulk herbs in large containers, from which you help yourself.

Some more exotic presentations might be in the containers or on nearby shelves. They include *solid extracts*, highly concentrated herbal goos that you eat or dissolve in water; *essential oils* that are usually for topical use or steam treatments; and *juices*. But most of the shelf space will probably be taken up by bottles of herb *capsules* or tablets.

These last forms provide the easiest way to buy and use herbs. But there are capsules and there are capsules. See if you can tell by the label whether the capsule has been filled simply with a ground-up, powdered herb (not the best choice) or by a freeze-dried extract (usually more potent and stable).

Then see if the label promises a certain amount of one or more chemical constituents of the herb. This *standardization*, as it's called, may be expressed as a percentage or as a milligram count, and it's the only way to make sure that the cap-

HOW MANY PILLS CAN YOU TAKE?

Put aside any lingering negative notions you have about pill takers. Forget your mother's taking a green, a purple, three white, and a striped tablet each day when you were a kid and your vow never to do that. Forget as well any notion that pills are for women or hypochondriacs or girly men.

"Accept the fact that for good health and a longer life, it is common to take three to six supplements a day," says Kenneth A. Goldberg, M.D., founder and director of the Male Health Center in Dallas. Just for perspective, be aware that many prominent anti-aging and weight-loss doctors advise their patients to take 20 or more supplements a day and that a surprising number of Americans do just that (you needn't get close to that number). If you need more convincing, understand that athletes are among the biggest consumers of natural supplements, says Dr. Goldberg.

So get into a routine. You might wish to get yourself a daily pill dispenser. Each Sunday, you can divvy up the week's take. Start each morning with a bowl of cereal with fruit, a big glass of water, and your morning supplements. No one will see you but the dog. After a while, it becomes second nature.

sule will deliver the real goods. It works because for many herbs, scientists have been able to single out chemicals that they believe are the active ingredients or that serve as markers indicating that the active ingredients are there. If there's enough of that chemical there, the herb is probably potent.

For example, ginseng products are so popular that they're all over the shelves. But see if you can find one with a label promising that each capsule contains 4 percent total ginsenosides, the main active ingredients. Such a product meets the accepted standard.

What All Those Other Things Are

If vitamins, minerals, and herbs had the supplement shelves to themselves, browsing would be less confusing. But as you learned during Week 1, there are plenty of other substances in nature that help your health. And even though good food is the best way to get them, lots have found their way onto the supplement shelves, for better (sometimes) or for worse (usually). Do a search for supplements that might fall into the following casual categories.

Hormones. Your body's own hormones taper off with the years, so by supplementing with hormones, you'll supposedly live longer and feel younger. DHEA (dehydroepiandrosterone) and melatonin are two that are in vogue, with the latter proven effective for preventing jet lag.

Phytochemicals. These plant substances that often act as anti-aging antioxidants are the reason you've been eating so many fruits and vegetables since Week 1. Some have been put into capsules, including lycopene (which puts the red in tomatoes and is thought to reduce your risk of prostate cancer) and quercetin (an anti-allergy phytochemical found in grapes, green tea, tomatoes, and onions).

Protein supplements. These are often sold as powdered drinks that promise to deliver enough of the essential amino acids (protein building blocks that your body doesn't make itself) to ensure that all those weights you lift translate into real muscle. But supplements of individual amino acids are also sold, such as creatine for bulking, L-glutamine for preventing exercise-induced immune suppression, and erection-friendly L-arginine.

Other nutrient supplements. Such products offer beneficial nutrients found in certain foods, without the foods. For example, the heart-helping essential fatty acids found in flaxseed and fatty fishes can be swallowed as salmon oil or flaxseed oil supplements.

Enzymes. Proteins such as the antioxidant coenzyme Q_{10} are found in your body, in food, and in supplements.

Targeted combos. These are just what the term implies: combinations of every imaginable kind of supplement that addresses a specific problem. For example, male virility combinations might combine herbs (such as ginkgo, yohimbine, and ginseng) with minerals (like zinc and selenium) and B vitamins.

Take a Multivitamin

The Day's Task

Take $10 back to the store you visited yesterday. Once again, head straight for the supplement shelves. This time, ignore everything except for the multivitamins.

Look for a multivitamin that lists minerals as well as vitamins on the label. Try to find one without iron or with very little. Two good candidates are One A Day for Men, which costs about $9 for 60 tablets, and Centrum Silver, which costs about $9 for 100 tablets. Make sure you check the expiration date.

Take the bottle to the checkout counter and pay for it. Go home, and at your next meal, swallow one of the multivitamin/mineral tablets.

You've just taken out some health insurance. Not the kind you have to write a check for every month but the kind that makes sure you get the vitamins and minerals you need even if you have an off day from good eating. As long as you don't fall into the trap of thinking that a multivitamin is a substitute for eating well, your daily dose is going to give you an extra edge.

Multis boost your immunity. They ensure that you get the immune-enhancing vitamins and minerals that you need most.

Multis reduce your risk of cancer. In a study, nurses who took multis for 15 years had 75 percent less colon cancer than those who didn't take them.

Multis help your heart. Research suggests that those who take daily multivitamin supplements have significantly lower homocysteine concentrations in their blood, a reduction linked to healthier hearts.

Multis keep your gums healthy. When researchers at the State University of New York at Buffalo evaluated blood samples from 9,862 subjects, they found that those with the highest vitamin A and C levels had half the rate of gum disease of those with the lowest levels. And high selenium levels were linked to a 13-fold reduction in cases of gum disease.

The Very Model of a Major Multivitamin

The main thing here is just to make sure that enough of the vitamins and minerals you need are in the multi you choose. You've probably noticed that most multivitamin labels offer a pretty long list of nutrients. Here are the key ones.

Folic acid. Aim for 100 percent of the Daily Value of 400 micrograms. If the label says "folate" instead of "folic acid," that's okay.

Niacin. Aim for 100 percent of the DV of 20 milligrams.

Riboflavin. Aim for 100 percent of the DV of 1.7 milligrams.

Vitamin A. Aim for 100 percent of the DV of 5,000 IU.

Vitamin B_6. Aim for 100 percent of the DV of 2 milligrams.

Vitamin B_{12}. Aim for 100 percent of the DV of 6 micrograms.

Vitamin C. Aim for 100 percent of the DV of 60 milligrams. That's still not enough, but you usually won't find much more in a multi.

Vitamin D. Aim for 100 percent of the DV of 400 IU.

Vitamin E. Aim for 100 percent of the DV of 30 IU. Again, that's too low, but it will have to do in your multi.

Thiamin. Aim for 100 percent of the DV of 1.5 milligrams.

Calcium. Get as close as possible to the DV of 1,000 milligrams.

Chromium. Aim for the DV of 120 micrograms. Some multis have more.

Copper. Aim for 100 percent of the DV of 2 milligrams, assuming the same multi also offers 100 percent of the DV for zinc.

Magnesium. You'll probably find 100 milligrams in your multi.

Selenium. Not all multis include it. The DV is 70 micrograms.

Zinc. Aim for the DV of 15 milligrams. Make sure that the percentage of DV for zinc is close to the percentage of the DV offered for copper.

(Iron, by the way, may only increase your risk of heart disease and cancer. Some multis include all 18 milligrams of the DV. Stay away from those.)

A dosage should be indicated on the label. It's usually one tablet, but sometimes it calls for two or more to get the percentages the label indicates.

Once you're in the habit, the nutrients are absorbed best if you down your tablet with some water at a meal. That meal should include about 5 grams of fat (1 tablespoon of margarine) to help with the absorption of the fat-soluble vitamins, A, D, E, and K.

Take a Vitamin C Supplement

The Day's Task

This morning, it's back to the supplement shelves again. (Sure, you could have saved time and gas by taking care of this yesterday, but we're focusing on one thing at a time here.) Say hi to your good buddies, the store employees, and take a look at some vitamin C supplements.

Choose a large bottle with tablets containing 100 milligrams of vitamin C each. You've probably already had your breakfast, so take three of those tablets with your mid-morning snack today. (Starting tomorrow, take those 300 milligrams with breakfast.) At night, with dinner, take two more.

Any questions? Here's one that's probably on your mind: "Why do I need to take more vitamin C? I'm already drinking a glass of orange juice every morning. I get even more C with my multivitamin. I'm actually getting more than the Daily Value. What gives?"

What gives is that you can really jack up the health benefits of vitamin C by taking considerably more than the DV of 60 milligrams. There's a long list of good things that vitamin C can do for you, and all those good things are backed up by scientific research. As a rule, that research involves vitamin C doses considerably higher than the DV of 60 milligrams.

So C is one vitamin (E is another) where you're going to leave the DV behind. In fact, there's a movement afoot to raise the DV of C to 200 milligrams. Even now, a typical recommended daily vitamin C dosage for a typical guy like you will range from 200 to 1,000 milligrams. We suggest that you supplement with 500 milligrams a day (in addition to the 60 milligrams in your multi) to take maximum advantage of vitamin C's age-blocking, disease-preventing antioxidant properties.

The question that remains is a good one: Can't you get that much through food? After all, we've been ranting since Week 1, Day 1 about how food is the best way to get any nutrient, including vitamin C. Well, food *is* the best way to get vitamin C and you *can* get enough from eating and drinking. The question is, will you?

Let's look at the arithmetic. Orange juice is far and away the best readily available food source of vitamin C, at about 60 milligrams per 6-ounce glass. Unless you're ordering fresh-squeezed juice at one of those froufrou brunch joints that hit you up for $3.50 for a glass the size of a bottle cap, you'll probably drink more than 6 ounces. So let's call it 100 milligrams. You'll get some more vitamin C from certain fruits and vegetables, notably other citrus fruits, cantaloupe, strawberries, broccoli, cauliflower, and peppers. And then there's the 60 milligrams from your multi.

That might add up to 200 to 300 milligrams of C, which is enough for some pretty good health benefits. But it's not 500 milligrams. You'd have to drink even more orange juice and really go to town on those vitamin C–rich vegetables to get to 500 milligrams.

What's more, it's important that you consistently get your vitamin C quota every day, not just most of the time. No matter how diligent you try to be, it's not so easy to do that through food and multis alone, especially since most fruits and vegetables are not really all that rich in vitamin C.

That's where C supplements come in. Again, we're talking about insurance. Swallow those 500 milligrams daily, split into morning and evening doses to keep your blood levels of C high throughout the day, and you know you're getting enough no matter what.

By getting enough, you're doing yourself a big favor. The health and longevity benefits of vitamin C are legion.

What C Can Do for You

Getting straight to the point, vitamin C helps you live longer. Research from the UCLA School of Public Health indicates that a 35-year-old man who takes in 300 milligrams or more of C a day has a life expectancy 5.5 years longer than a man whose daily intake is less than 50 milligrams.

Researchers point out that the increased life expectancy might have as much to do with the overall healthy habits of typical vitamin C–takers as with the vitamin C itself. That should be fine with you. Being nearly one-quarter of the way through a 12-week health-and-longevity program, you have nothing to be ashamed of in the healthy-habits department. Meanwhile, it's a smart move to get your daily quota of vitamin C.

Among other things, vitamin C is an antioxidant, meaning it scavenges for cell-destroying and disease-inducing free radicals. By neutralizing those unstable oxygen molecules, vitamin C may slow down the aging process while protecting you from a whole array of health problems. To wit:

Vitamin C enhances your immunity and strengthens your resistance to infections. "Vitamin C is a factor in normal immune cells," says Dennis D. Taub, Ph.D., of the National Institute on Aging. Numerous studies have confirmed that vitamin C is needed for a healthy immune system.

Vitamin C saves your eyesight. The nutrient decreases your risk of cataracts. It is concentrated in the lens of your eye up to 50 times more than in your blood, which is a pretty good hint that it plays a major role in eye health. Research has confirmed that suspicion, with one study revealing 75 percent lower risks of cataracts in those subjects who supplemented with C over a 10-year period.

Vitamin C improves your skin quality. It plays a role in forming collagen, which is needed for healthy bones, joints, and especially skin. Collagen also fortifies your blood vessel walls and forms scar tissue.

Vitamin C gets the lead out. Researchers have discovered that if your vitamin C levels are low, your body may be more likely to absorb and retain lead from sources such as drinking water and lead-based paints. Study coauthor Howard Hu, M.D., of Harvard, evaluated 747 men and found that those who took in a daily total of less than 109 milligrams of C had the most lead in their blood and bones. That can cause serious problems. "Even low levels of lead have been linked to elevated blood pressure, kidney dysfunction, and anemia," says Dr. Hu.

Vitamin C increases muscle strength. In a study at California State University at Fullerton, 37 students in a strength-training program took either 1,000 milligrams of vitamin C or a placebo every day. After 8 weeks, the vitamin C group had a 15 percent increase in the strength of their knee muscles. The other group posted a 3 percent gain. "Vitamin C helps muscles recover after intense exercise," says William Beam, Ph.D., the study coauthor.

Vitamin C protects against heart disease. In a Boston University study of 129 patients with arterial blockages, the patients who had recently suffered heart attacks also had the lowest levels of vitamin C. It may be that vitamin C prevents fatty acids in the arteries from rupturing and causing heart attacks, says lead researcher Joseph Vita, M.D.

Vitamin C reduces your cancer risk. That conclusion can be drawn from population studies that simply show that people with diets high in vitamin C have lower rates of cancer.

Vitamin C helps ease sunburn. It slows the oxidation damage that causes sunburn, says Richard Wagner, M.D., a dermatologist at the University of Texas at Galveston. A German study determined that taking high doses of vitamins C and E for several days before sun exposure can help lessen the severity of sunburn. For 8 days, 20 subjects took either 2,000 milligrams of C and 1,000 IU of E or placebo tablets. After exposure to ultraviolet rays, the C-and-E group developed milder burns.

Vitamin C is good for your gums. When researchers at the Buffalo campus of the State University of New York evaluated blood samples from 9,862 subjects, they found that those with the highest vitamins C and A levels had half the rate of gum disease of those with the lowest levels.

Vitamin C helps you handle stress. It assists your adrenal glands in the production of epinephrine and norepinephrine. Those are the hormones responsible for mobilizing energy so you can respond appropriately to stressful situations. "It is well-known that you need more vitamin C when you're under physical stress—for instance, when you have a cold," says Robert Jacob, Ph.D., of the USDA Western Human Nutrition Center. "But psychological stress also makes the adrenal glands crank up production, so it makes sense that you would need more vitamin C then too."

Vitamin C boosts your energy levels. You probably don't think of vitamin C as an energy pill, but one of the first symptoms of vitamin C deficiency is fatigue, notes Balz Frie, Ph.D., of the Linus Pauling Institute at Oregon State University in Corvallis. "Vitamin C is required for the synthesis of carnitine, which transports fatty acids into the mitochondria, the tiny powerhouses that generate energy inside cells," he says. "If you don't have enough vitamin C, you can't synthesize carnitine, so you can't convert all the fatty acids into usable energy."

Studies have borne this out. At Arizona State University, researcher Carol Johnston, Ph.D., found that people did much better on treadmill tests when they took 500 milligrams of vitamin C daily.

Take a Vitamin E Supplement

The Day's Task

One guess where you're going today. Yep, back to the supplement shelves. This time, look for the E vitamins, the ones that usually come in those easy-to-swallow gel capsules.

Check the labels (as you're now used to doing) and find a bottle that gives you 400 IU of vitamin E in each capsule. That way, you'll need to swallow only one a day. Also, make sure that the label promises that the capsules contain d-alpha tocopherol.

Take one at your next meal.

Vitamin E is the big Exception. No, that's not the reason they call it vitamin E, but it is the reason it joins the multivitamin/mineral and vitamin C on your supplement list. E is an exception to at least three rules of nutrient intake: the Daily Value standard, the get-it-in-food commandment, and the notion that it doesn't much matter whether a supplement is "natural" or not.

With E, the Daily Value (DV) is, by majority consensus of our experts, so low as to be virtually irrelevant. That's why you're taking more than 13 times the DV of 30 IU.

Also, you can't get nearly enough E from food, no matter how hard you try. In fact, it can be unhealthy to make the attempt. That's why you're taking supplements instead of sending your fat intake through the roof by over-loading on E-rich foods.

And natural is definitely preferable when you supplement with E. That's why you're taking the natural d-alpha tocopherol instead of the synthetic dl.

Let's look at those issues one at a time because they make up a pretty good object lesson of why supplements can be godsends for your health and longevity.

First, let's talk about the dosage. Like vitamin C, vitamin E has a DV that's way below what studies show can help you. For example, in one key study linking vitamin E to heart protection, the subjects were given up to 800 IU of vitamin E. In a more extreme example, German study volunteers were given a cool 1,000 IU before sun exposure to show E's ability to reduce sunburn symptoms.

We're not recommending anything like 1,000 daily IU of vitamin E. As with any other vitamin or mineral, you can overdo it. In E's case, the issue is slowed blood clotting, so it's a good idea to talk to your doctor before taking high amounts of E (say, more than 400 IU) or before supplementing with any amount if you are already taking blood-thinning drugs or have a bleeding disorder.

But you don't need to take megadoses to reap E's benefits. You just need to take a lot more than the DV. A minimum helpful dose would be at least 100 IU a day and more likely 400 IU. Those amounts are quite safe, says Iswarlal Jialal, M.D., professor of clinical nutrition at the University of Texas Southwestern Medical Center at Dallas Southwestern Medical School. If you're like most Americans, you probably weren't getting anywhere near that much until today.

What about food? While it's always best to eat your nutrients in their natural food form, no matter how dedicated a healthy eater you may be, the only way to get protective amounts of E is by supplementing.

Here's why: Olive oil is one of the best sources of vitamin E there is and probably the healthiest vegetable oil you could choose. But you'd have to drink 3½ cups of olive oil a day just to hit the lowball E recommendation of 100 IU. Or you could go for corn oil, drink 8 cups of it, and get your full 400 IU. Nuts and seeds are other E-rich foods. Figure out a way to eat 2½ pounds of almonds, and you're all the way up to 50 IU with only another 17½ pounds to go before you make it to 400 IU.

As we hope is obvious, that kind of eating is absurd in theory and would be downright suicidal in practice. Though there are some less fat-filled natural E sources (like spinach and whole grains), most are pretty darn fatty: vegetable and seed oils, peanut butter, sunflower seeds, and nuts. And fatty or not, there's no way you can eat enough of them to get the levels of E you need.

The final issue is natural versus synthetic. While it's not a major concern with most other nutrients, natural is better with E because of absorption. One study showed that your body absorbs vitamin E from natural supplements twice as well as from the synthetic stuff. So confirm that you're buying vitamin E from natural sources by looking for the word *d-alpha tocopherol* on the label. The synthetics will say *dl*.

By the way, E is a fat-soluble vitamin, which means you should take it with a meal or snack that includes a little fat, just as you do your multi. And since E comes in gel capsules, you have the advantage of being able to break an extra one open and rub it into wrinkled areas of your skin once a day. That softens wrinkles and crow's-feet.

Taking the E Train

There's just no other way to put it: Vitamin E is one hell of a great vitamin. Since the odds are pretty good that you've only been getting piddling amounts of it until now, your new 400-IU-per-day routine will very likely make a huge difference in how you feel now and how you feel decades from now.

And since you're taking it along with vitamin C, that difference may be even huger. The two work well together. During one period of study, a pool of subjects who took both C and E supplements had 42 percent fewer deaths from all causes than those who took neither or just one of the two.

But vitamin E brings its own benefits to the longevity party. First and foremost, it's a star-quality antioxidant, which means it actually fights the aging process and the problems that go with it. Vitamin E literally saves your cells.

By now, you just might be convinced that antioxidants—whether they're vitamins, minerals, phytochemicals, or whatever—are among your most powerful health-and-longevity allies. But if you're still a tad hazy on what exactly these guys are, don't sweat it. That puts you in the same category as about 99 percent of the world's population. So let's run through the antioxidant thing from the top.

When you use oxygen to burn food into energy, that oxidation creates as a byproduct highly reactive altered oxygen molecules called free radicals. These unstable molecules do some needed cleanup work, but excess free radicals damage cells and tissue. These free radicals are one electron short, so they flit about seeking to steal electrons from your body's healthy molecules. That not only damages your cells but also creates more aging-inducing free radicals.

Antioxidants stop this molecular chain of destruction (called oxidative stress) by offering their own electrons to the free radicals instead. Your body makes some of its own antioxidants, but you need more from outside sources. Vitamin E is one of the best of those sources.

As a strong antioxidant, vitamin E retards the aging process as a matter of course. But its specific heroic deeds are even more impressive. Here's a list of them.

- Studies are pretty clear that vitamin E protects your immune system, helping your body fight off disease now and on into old age, when immune function usually begins to weaken. It may even protect you from colds and flu.
- Where vitamin E really shines is in preventing heart disease, including heart attacks. One big reason is that free radical damage ups the danger of high cholesterol counts. And, as we've seen, vitamin E is a first-rate destroyer of free radicals. The heart study we alluded to earlier found that people with heart disease who were given 400 to 800 IU of vitamin E daily had 75 percent lower risks of heart attack that those who didn't get E.
- Vitamin E also protects you from certain cancers, including two top man killers, colon cancer and prostate cancer. To cite just one of many studies, Finnish researchers found that men who took just 50 milligrams (about 75 IU) of E a day had a 32 percent lower incidence of prostate cancer than the nonsupplementing study subjects.
- Diabetes may also be on the pro-E list. Again in Finland, researchers who studied 944 men found that those with the lowest levels of vitamin E in their blood were four times more likely to have diabetes than those with higher levels.
- While a weakened memory is one of the more unwelcome age-related possibilities, vitamin E may help you stay sharp as you age. In fact, vitamin E has been shown to delay the progression of severe dementia in people with Alzheimer's disease.
- A number of antioxidants are thought to protect your eyesight, vitamin E among them. Along with C, E can significantly cut your risk of cataracts.
- Yes, vitamin E really can reduce sunburn severity, though it's certainly no substitute for a topical sunscreen. Some subjects in the German study we mentioned earlier took high doses of C for 8 days, others took high doses of E, and others took placebos. Then, the lot of them were exposed to ultraviolet rays. The E takers developed milder burns. So did the C takers. Again, it's because those two vitamins slow the oxidative damage that causes sunburn.
- If none of that converts you, this will: Vitamin E may perk up your sex life. That's because it prevents testosterone from breaking down. And when testosterone doesn't break down, your libido stays up.

Stock Your Herbal Shelf

The Day's Task

It's herb-buying day. If the supplement shelves you've been frequenting for the past 4 days are a little weak in the herb department, take your business to a health food store with a generous selection of herbs in all forms.

Out of the hundreds of herbal products you see there, pick out about a half-dozen herbal supplements. That's a modest introduction to the world of herbs but a promising one for your health.

Pay for the herbs, noticing that many of them are far from cheap. Take them home and put them on your herbal shelf.

We know just what you're thinking. You don't *have* an herbal shelf.

That doesn't matter. The actual shelf part is unimportant. These guys don't take up a lot of space.

What matters is that you start to dip into the herbal pool, even if you only get your toes wet at first. The reason that this matters is the same reason that vitamins matter, the same reason that minerals matter, the same reason that all that good eating you learned during the first week of the program matters. After all, a big chunk of your Longevity Program is as simple as putting things into your body that will make it feel better, work more efficiently, and last longer. The herbs you buy today will do that, safely and naturally.

Science has begun to put its seal of approval on many age-old herbal remedies for treating or preventing common problems. Hard-core herbalists, citing thousands of years of results, promote many more herbs—far beyond what science recognizes. You, however, are going to limit yourself to the herbs we recommend here, the value and safety of which have been well-established.

Don't forget that a few days ago we gave you a brief primer on herbal supplements as you browsed the shelves for the first time. Take another look at that section before you hit the shelves again for some actual herb purchases.

One other thing: The herbs you'll see on the shelves are usually quite safe, but don't assume that you can take huge doses just because herbs are natural. Stick to the recommended doses on the labels, unless a professional has indicated otherwise. And if you're going to use herbs to self-treat a specific condition, consult with your doctor first. Some can have side effects and can interact with prescription medicine.

Herbs That Heal

Okay, you're going to stock up on a few herbs. Which ones? Not to dodge the question, but that often depends on what you want to accomplish. The best way to reduce the mind-boggling number of herb choices down to something manageable is to ask yourself what you'd like the herb to do for you and make your choice accordingly.

Here's a rundown of good herbs with recognized benefits for specific problems.

Saw palmetto. This extract from the dwarf palm tree berry relieves enlarged prostates. In Germany, saw palmetto (along with some other plant extracts) is used to treat nearly 90 percent of men suffering from enlarged prostate glands that are more formally known as benign prostatic hyperplasia, or BPH. In fact, an analysis of 18 studies found that saw palmetto was as effective in treating the condition as finasteride (Proscar), a popular prescription drug.

Saw palmetto may have a preventive effect as well. Enlarged prostates generally hit men over 50. It's thought that when men start using saw palmetto in their forties, their prostates don't swell and their libidos don't drop.

Saw palmetto works best in tablet or capsule form. Look for products standardized to contain 85 to 95 percent fatty acids and sterols, and consult with your doctor before you start taking them.

Echinacea. This natural antibiotic and immune booster is a good one to have on hand because its renowned cold-relieving properties work best when you take it at the very first sign of symptoms. That's no time to run around looking for it. It comes in many forms, but your best bet is a tincture. Avoid this herb if you are allergic to closely related plants such as ragweed, asters, and chrysanthemums.

St. John's wort. Nature's Prozac, they call it. Doctors in Europe are big on using this herb to combat mild to moderate depression. It works by stopping an enzyme that destroys feel-good chemicals in the brain like seratonin and dopamine. Be sure the St. John's wort you buy is standardized to 0.3 percent hypericin. Don't use it in combination with antidepressants unless your doctor says it's okay.

Licorice. This is a good herb to keep around because it's a great natural cough remedy. Licorice may help your cough be productive, or mucus-raising, which speeds recovery. Some studies have shown that it may even dull the central cough reflex much like codeine does. Or its sweet taste may make you swallow, suppressing an impending cough.

Lozenges can work, but make sure they offer real licorice (*Glycyrrhiza glabra*). Licorice candy doesn't work. Or try a good-tasting tea made from the cut-and-sifted root. Long-term use (daily for more than 4 to 6 weeks) or taking too much at once (more than three cups of tea per day) may be bad for your heart and kidneys, raise your blood pressure, or increase water retention. To avoid side effects, you can take a processed form called DGL, or deglycyrrhizinated licorice, also available in health food stores.

Chamomile. It's wise to have plenty of chamomile on hand since it makes a great tea when you're not using it to relieve an upset stomach. But when your stomach starts complaining, chamomile helps because it contains an oil that relaxes the smooth muscles in the stomach. Very rarely, chamomile can cause an allergic reaction. Sip your first cup very slowly and make sure your body accepts it before guzzling the rest of the mug.

Feverfew. Try this one for headaches. Feverfew contains ingredients that help constrict bloodflow and reduce inflammation. Stick to the capsule form; some people get mouth sores if they chew on the leaves.

Milk thistle. A purported liver healer and protector, milk thistle is one of those herbs whose helpful constituents aren't all water soluble, so your best bet is capsules. They must contain 80 to 85 percent silymarins.

Valerian. Does your mind race at night? Try this mild tranquilizer that's been shown to help people fall asleep without giving them the morning hangover associated with sleeping pills. The smell and taste are strong and not all that pleasant, so you might prefer capsules to a tea. Do not use valerian in any form with sleep-enhancing or mood-regulating medications, as it may intensify their effects. In rare cases, valerian can cause side effects like heart palpitations and nervousness.

Tea tree oil. Here's a good one for your herbal medicine chest. It's a volatile oil from an Australian tree that works as an excellent antiseptic. One whiff of its strong medicinal odor will convince you. Just rub it on to counteract acne, sunburn, even that nasty athlete's foot you picked up. Buy the oil in little bottles, making sure it contains less than 15 percent cineole (an irritant) and at least 30 percent terpinen-4-ol (the stuff that heals).

Herbs That Protect

Here are some candidates for your herbal shelf that are more in the spirit of your Longevity Program. That is, these are herbs that may protect you from disease and help offset the problems of aging.

Garlic. Garlic lowers cholesterol and keeps certain blood cells called platelets from clumping together and sticking to artery walls. Because of that, garlic reduces your risk of heart attacks and strokes. Clinical studies have been done on garlic powder tablets, showing that they reduce levels of serum cholesterol by about 11 percent. Your best bet, though, may be the odorless enteric-coated capsules that release the active ingredient, allicin, in the small intestine. There are lots of garlic options out there; just make sure whatever you choose is standardized to between 2,500 and 5,000 micrograms of allicin yield. Don't use garlic supplements if you're on anticoagulants or before undergoing surgery because it thins the blood and may increase bleeding. Also, don't take them if you're taking hypoglycemic drugs.

Ginkgo. Like vitamins C and E, ginkgo is an antioxidant that's been reported to aid brain function. It may help you keep that mental edge by improving bloodflow to the brain, feeding it oxygen and nutrients. That improved bloodflow, incidentally, also heads toward your penis, which is why German researchers have linked ginkgo with better erections. Check the label of any bottle of ginkgo tablets for the code 24/6, which means the product has been concentrated and contains 24 percent flavone glycosides and 6 percent terpenes. Gingko biloba doesn't mix well with antidepressants, aspirin or NSAIDs, or blood-thinning medications, so check the label or talk with a doctor before starting on it.

Grape seed extract. This one's a super anti-ager, with antioxidant activity 50 times greater than vitamin E's and 20 times greater than vitamin C's. What's more, it actually works together with E and C, helping those vitamins fight free radicals. Highly concentrated grape seed extract is easy to find in capsule form, standardized to between 80 and 85 percent OPCs, or polyphenolic derivatives.

Herbs That Get You Up and Going

Your herbal shelf can also offer you safe and healthy pick-me-ups that have been used for millennia. Here are some favorites.

Ginseng. German authorities confirm that this herb can invigorate you during down times, such as when you experience fatigue, sickness, or sluggish work performance. A lot of clinical evidence backs them up.

What you might find, though, is a confusing mishmash of products sold in

OFF THE RACK

If you have a spice rack, you have an herbal shelf. Dried kitchen spices are also healthful herbs that can or heal or prevent a range of problems. Here are some examples.

Basil. Treats bad breath and headaches

Cayenne. Eases dry coughs from colds and relieves pain; avoid taking it on an empty stomach as it could irritate the gastrointestinal tract

Dill. Treats colic and gas

Ginger. Soothes the stomach and prevents motion sickness

Oregano. Treats parasitic infections and blocks the carcinogens in cooked meat

Parsley. Aids digestion and combats bad breath

Rosemary. Eases digestion, stimulates appetite, and is rich in antioxidants

Savory. Relieves gas and diarrhea and stimulates appetite

Thyme. Treats coughs and upper respiratory infections, soothes the stomach, and prevents blood clots

every conceivable form, from liquids to chewing gum, all called ginseng. But all you have to remember are two things. First, the true ginsengs are American ginseng (*Panax quinquefolius*) and Asian ginseng (*Panax ginseng*). Second, don't buy any ginseng unless the label clearly states that the product has been standardized to contain between 4 percent and 7 percent ginsenosides, the active ingredient. Anything else is probably worthless. Both American and Asian ginseng may cause irritability if taken with caffeine or other stimulants. Don't use ginseng if you have high blood pressure.

Siberian ginseng. Though not a true ginseng, it's a less expensive relative of the *Panax* ginsengs and a popular energy-boosting herb in its own right.

Cordyceps. Take this in capsules so you won't be reminded that it's a fungus that grows on caterpillars in the Chinese highlands.

Actually, scientists are now able to grow the fungus in artificial cultures, skipping the caterpillars. Cordyceps's stamina-enhancing effects are thought to be the work of natural chemicals known as polysaccharides and nucleosides.

Decide on Other Supplements

The Day's Task

For 3 weeks now, you've been getting some fairly specific instructions to guide you down the road to health and longevity. Today we're going to leave you on your own a bit. You're going to decide which, if any, of all those other supplements on the shelves you're going to take regularly.

When you hit the supplement shelves again today (for the last time until your supplies run out, we promise) you'll be reminded that the vitamins, minerals, and herbs you've started taking aren't all that's there. There are tons of other stuff, and some of it could be right for you. Your task today is simply to think about these other supplements so you can make a decision about which ones are for you.

We'll make it even more comfortable for you: You don't even have to decide today. Just examine the other supplements. And read this chapter.

Here's a pretty good philosophy for deciding whether you want to take a particular supplement: Don't believe everything you read about a supplement, but don't automatically discount it either. Several supplements have good science to back them up. Quite a few others show promise. Others, though, are either redundant (meaning you already get plenty of the main ingredients in your diet or other supplements) or scientifically unproven. Additionally, be aware that the government does not regulate most supplements as it does over-the-counter medicines.

Taking the time to figure out which ones are right for you is a giant step in your health-and-longevity program. That's because it means you're taking charge of your own health. You're going out there and finding out what's best for you and going for it. That's what this Longevity Program is ultimately all about.

So the decision about other supplements is yours, whenever you choose to make it. It may require a little more investigation on your part, perhaps a health professional's advice. But don't panic; we're not abandoning you. We're going to walk you through some of the other supplements that you'll see on the shelves.

Proteins and Enzymes

The supplements that you can't help but notice on the shelves are the big canisters of alleged muscle builders. We'll get to protein powder drinks in Week 9; ignore them for now. But a number of amino acids (the primary building blocks of protein) are sold individually for purposes that go beyond pure muscle bulking. Here's a look at some of them and some similar compounds that your body makes.

L-arginine. This supplement is for sex. At least, that's what some animal studies indicate. In one, aging male rats that ate this amino acid for 8 weeks had significantly better erectile responses than rats in a control group. What may be happening is that L-arginine encourages the production of nitric oxide, a chemical that some urologists think is crucial to increasing penile bloodflow.

Are rat penises enough to go on? Well, a typical recommendation by L-arginine supporters in the medical community is to supplement with between 500 and 1,000 milligrams a day. But you can get that much from your diet. An ounce of Brazil nuts, peanuts, or almonds, or a half-cup of cooked lentils or kidney beans delivers around 500 milligrams. Soybeans, tofu, and sunflower seeds are good sources too. Be aware that high doses of L-arginine may cause nausea and diarrhea; for those fighting genital herpes, it may increase outbreaks.

Creatine. This supplement is all the rage these days as a training aid linked to muscle building, improved strength, more explosive power, and reduced recovery time. All this is based on the more-is-better approach. Your body produces about 1½ grams of this amino acid daily, and you get more when you eat meat or fish. But supplementing puts you way up into the 20-gram range, which is a level that creatine promoters (and some studies) contend leads to the training benefits.

Typical of the positive research on creatine is a study done at Pennsylvania State University in which those who supplemented with 25 grams of creatine improved their power output during jump squats and could do more repetitions during bench press sets. Those who got placebos did not show that improvement.

If you want to try creatine, choose the form called creatine monohydrate. It's the most effective. The product should be at least 99 percent creatine. Take 20 grams daily for 3 to 5 days to load your muscles with creatine. Then, switch to a maintenance dose of 2 to 3 grams a day. Take it with 6 to 8 ounces of grape juice or some other carbohydrate to stimulate a release of insulin, which helps get the creatine into your muscles. Be aware that for some guys, creatine doesn't go down so well, causing such unpleasant effects as nausea, dehydration, and cramps.

Coenzyme Q_{10}. Also called co-Q_{10}, this supplement strengthens your heart. It's a naturally occurring enzyme that functions as an antioxidant, acts much like a vitamin, aids in converting food to energy, and is present in especially high concentrations in the heart. Heart attack victims lose a lot of it. All of that connects co-Q_{10} to heart health, and studies have shown that supplementing with co-Q_{10} helps people with heart disease and even allows some of them to stop taking heart medications. Danish researchers, looking at eight studies of co-Q_{10} in patients who had congestive heart failure, concluded that patients who supplemented with the enzyme recovered up to 76 percent better than those who didn't.

In making your decision about coenzyme Q_{10}, you should know that your body makes the enzyme and you can get it from foods such as oily fish, whole grains, and organ meats. The co-Q_{10} supplements you see on the shelves are by no means anti-aging miracle pills, energy boosters, or slimming agents. Still, you might benefit if you've already had heart problems or if there's heart disease in your family history. Just don't think of it as a substitute for proper health care.

Glucosamine sulfate and chondroitin. Your body makes these two substances; but when taken as supplements, they show promise for the treatment of arthritis. They're often sold as a combination. If you don't already have arthritis, there's no evidence that either one can prevent it. If you do have arthritis, ask your doctor about them and any possible side effects.

Hormones

Your body's hormone production slows down over time, making you more vulnerable to the ravages of time. The idea behind supplementing with these body chemicals is to prop up their flagging levels so that (supposedly) you'll live longer and feel younger. The research is interesting but hardly conclusive on the following hormone supplements you're sure to run across.

DHEA. This hormone goes by those letters because nobody wants to say dehydroepiandrosterone. Your body produces it to convert it into other hormones, like testosterone. Since you're likely to have only about one-third as much DHEA by age 60 as you did as a strapping young man, keeping the supply steady right now by taking DHEA out of a bottle may brake the woes of aging. Indeed, several studies done on rats have linked DHEA with cancer prevention, diabetes treatment, and lowered risk of obesity. Problem is, most humans aren't rats. You would have to take dangerously high doses to get the equivalent of what the rats got, and there's no guarantee that DHEA works the same way in humans. If you take this, follow the dosage recommendations on the label. Because of serious potential side effects such as increased risk of prostate cancer, liver damage, and irregular heart rhythm—not to mention hair loss—it's smart to take this supplement only under doctor supervision.

Melatonin. This hormone comes out of the pineal gland, deep in the recesses of your brain. It regulates your body clock, leading to the belief that by taking it in supplement form you can manipulate that clock and control some parts of the aging process, not to mention insomnia. Both those benefits remain to be proven, but melatonin does have a solid track record in one area—controlling jet lag. As with so many other supplements, be aware of the possible side effects: drowsiness, headaches, nausea, depression, and, worst of all, reduced sex drive.

Nutrients

Once again, in case you missed it the first 20 times we said it: When it comes to getting nutrients, you should eat them. The vitamins, minerals, phytochemicals, and other good things in nature are best taken in their natural forms, as food.

But without exception, there are always exceptions. You've already made some of those exceptions part of your supplement routine, such as vitamins C and E, and the insurance you get from your multivitamin/mineral. You'll find a lot more proposed exceptions on the supplement shelves, including the following.

Fish oil. Ever heard of the Greenland Paradox? Neither have most people, including those in Greenland. But it seems that the Inuits in that land eat as much fat as Danes or even Americans but die from heart disease much less often. The reason for this apparent paradox is that they get their fat from fish, not from red meat. And they don't get just any old fish fat; they get omega-3 fatty acids.

Omega-3's work against heart disease by decreasing triglycerides (a type of fat found in your bloodstream), lowering high blood pressure, and keeping blood platelets from sticking together and clogging your arteries. In a study of more than 2,000 men who had just had heart attacks, one group was advised to eat fatty fish at least twice per week. After 2 years, that group had a 29 percent decrease in deaths from all causes. The other group didn't.

The down side is that some people notice a fishy odor from within after they take fish oil supplements. Possible side effects include stomach upset, easy bruising, increased bleeding, and even a rise in cholesterol levels (another paradox). It's also likely that eating a healthy diet that includes fish and flaxseed oil (another good omega-3 source) is just as good for you.

Quercetin. This is a bioflavonoid, essentially a natural chemical found in fruits and vegetables that helps give the foods their color. Quercetin is found in grapes, green tea, tomatoes, onions—and supplement capsules. Lots of people have found that it works well for them as an allergy reliever or anti-inflammatory.

Lycopene. As you may recall from Week 1, lycopene is the phytochemical reason that tomato sauce helps prevent prostate cancer. Tomatoes and processed tomato products are by far the richest food sources, but you can also get lycopene in capsule form, either on its own or combined with other carotenoids, such as beta-carotene or lutein.

The thing is, though, that most of the studies supporting the benefits of lycopene have focused only on lycopene-rich foods, not supplements. And there hasn't been any research into the long-term effects of lycopene supplementation. So if you decide in favor of lycopene capsules, stay with doses equal to about one serving of tomatoes: 10 to 15 milligrams.

Vitamins and Minerals

Your daily multi and vitamins C and E supplements should be enough for you. But you've surely noticed that those three barely make a dent in the available vitamin and mineral supplements taking up shelf space. That's partly because there are bucks to be made in selling people vitamins and minerals they don't need. But it's also because there are cases where another bottle of capsules or tablets might help. Here are some possibilities.

Calcium. Osteoporosis is not just a woman's disease, as some think. One-third of the broken hips related to osteoporosis occur in men. One good way to lessen the risk that such a thing will happen to you is to get enough calcium—at least 1,000 milligrams a day now, 1,500 if you're over 50.

With a multi and a reasonable number of low-fat or fat-free dairy products, you'll get that much calcium. But if you don't eat dairy products, you should consider a supplement.

That sounds simple enough, but when you search the supplement shelves for calcium, you'll find two different kinds. The most common (and least expensive) supplement is calcium carbonate. Take this with meals, as it's harder to absorb. The other is calcium citrate, which contains less calcium but is better absorbed than calcium carbonate. You can take this kind whenever you want.

Selenium. An antioxidant mineral that may protect you from cancer and gum disease, selenium is sold as a single-mineral supplement in a form called selenomethionine. Again, you should get enough in your diet and with your multi, but the issue here is the uncertain selenium content of the soil—and hence of the plant-based foods—in certain regions of the United States. If you live in a low-selenium area—states west of the Rocky Mountains and east of the Mississippi River—you might need more. But before you begin supplementing with more than 100 micrograms of selenium daily, discuss it with your doctor.

Targeted Combos

These supplements are the ones that jump out at you with some intriguing promises. Label reading is key here, as many of these formulas simply repackage what you're getting already. Here are some you'll probably run across.

Eyesight elixirs. You get plenty of protection already through the recommendations we've given you.

Prostate pills. The label will probably tell you that saw palmetto is the main ingredient. As you learned yesterday, that herb does indeed help treat and perhaps even prevent prostate enlargement problems that so often plague men once they hit middle age.

Heart helpers. Check the ingredient list, and you'll see some familiar names: coenzyme Q_{10}, vitamin E, vitamin B_6, folic acid, and magnesium. Except for the co-Q_{10}, you already get all you need.

Memory pills. They usually consist of ginkgo, vitamin E, and the B vitamins, all of which are good for your brain. But you can get the herb ginkgo without paying for the other vitamins, which you already get in sufficient amounts.

Manly formulas. Virility in a supplement—what a concept. But if you read the labels carefully, you'll notice that these formulas don't claim any specific benefits. You'll also see that you can get or already get the main ingredients elsewhere. Those may be herbs like saw palmetto, ginkgo, avena sativa (which is oats), and ginseng as well as vitamins and minerals. Another herb you may find in there is yohimbine, which is thought to have some sex-enhancement qualities but also too many side effects to make it a good choice.

10 Ways to Prevent High Cholesterol

1 **Getting your cholesterol count down is almost completely within your control. But it helps to know just what it is you're trying to do.** First of all, no matter how much you hear about "bad" low-density lipoprotein (LDL) cholesterol and "good" high-density lipoprotein (HDL) cholesterol, there's nothing inherently bad about cholesterol. In fact, your body makes its own cholesterol because it needs it to protect cell walls and build hormones, among other things. It's too much cholesterol that damages cells and artery walls. What's too much? A good goal is to keep your total cholesterol count under 200 milligrams per deciliter.

At the same time, though, you want to keep your HDL cholesterol count at 45 milligrams per deciliter or above because that's the kind of cholesterol that helps usher LDL out of your system. Find out your counts with any checkup that includes a blood test.

2 **Good eating is your most powerful weapon against high cholesterol.** Eat the way we've been recommending, and you'll lower your cholesterol. It's that simple. If you do nothing else but cut down on animal foods—meats, eggs, dairy products, lard—you'll have done plenty. Animal-based foods are the only foods that contain cholesterol.

Understand, though, that saturated fat, the kind that your body *converts* to cholesterol, is what sends your counts soaring. So don't be too impressed if a label screams that a product has "no cholesterol." Check for saturated-fat content, too.

3 **You don't have to shun meat completely to cut down on saturated fat.** Just lean toward the lean. Top round, bottom round, and sirloin tips are leaner beef cuts. Cut off exposed fat before you cook the meat. Throw the meat on the grill, where a lot of fat will drip off. Keep your portion down to the size of a deck of cards. Take the skin off chicken. Go for fish. And always choose low-fat or fat-free dairy products.

4 **Lots of vegetable oils are high in saturated fat, even though they contain no actual cholesterol.** Substitute oils that are mostly polyunsaturated fat (such as corn and safflower oils) or monounsaturated fat (like olive and canola oils) for those high in saturated fat (coconut oil, for example). And check labels for dangerous trans fatty acids. These fats form when manufacturers hydrogenate oils to make them solid, like in stick margarine.

5 **Try an oil you may never have thought of: walnut oil.** Or eat walnuts in moderation. Researchers have discovered that men and women in France who consume the most walnuts and walnut oil have the highest levels of HDL cholesterol. That could be because walnut oil consists overwhelmingly of the more heart-friendly polyunsaturated and monounsaturated fat. Take it easy, though. All oils have at least some saturated fat and are high in calories.

6 **Snack on apples.** Fruits and vegetables reduce cholesterol damage because they're full of artery-cleansing fiber. They're also full of phytochemicals that render LDL cholesterol less harmful. Apples and apple juice are an outstanding example because research has shown that they can reduce LDL oxidation as much as 38 percent. That's probably due to polyphenols, antioxidant plant chemicals.

7 **Another pleasant source of polyphenols is red wine.** If you like red wine, limit yourself to one to two glasses with dinner to fight high cholesterol in two ways. First, the alcohol in the wine is thought to raise HDL cholesterol. Second, the polyphenols, acting as antioxidants, keep LDL cholesterol from sticking to your artery walls.

8 **Add these foods to your eat-lots-of-them list: oat bran, rolled oats, other oat cereals (like Cheerios), beans and other legumes, and soy products.** The cholesterol-lowering secret in oats and legumes is fiber, especially soluble fiber that actually helps eliminate existing cholesterol. A number of studies have shown that a diet that includes beans reduces total cholesterol levels by 10 to 20 percent.

As for soy products, one study found that people with moderately high cholesterol levels who ate an average of 1½ ounces of soy daily reduced their LDL levels by 12.9 percent and their total cholesterol by 9.3 percent. "Soy products may also reduce or slow down a hidden prostate cancer," says Kenneth A. Goldberg, M.D., of the Male Health Center. Try these two easy ways to eat soy: (1) Crumble tofu into pasta or stir-fry dishes, and (2) make milkshakes with soy milk, lots of fresh fruit, and ice cubes.

9 **Mix a clove garlic into your meals each day.** Or take a daily a 400-milligram enteric-coated garlic capsule. Either of these can lower your cholesterol level by 12 percent or more, according to one study. Do not use supplements if you're on anticoagulants or before undergoing surgery, because garlic thins the blood and may increase bleeding. Do not use if you're taking hypoglycemic drugs.

10 **All this good eating that you're doing will get your weight down, which is good because being overweight contributes to high blood cholesterol.** Get even more benefits by adding exercise to the mix. In a large study at Georgetown University in Washington, D.C., men who jogged between 11 and 14 miles a week had higher levels of HDL than those who didn't.

10 Ways to Prevent Prostate Problems

1 **Take saw palmetto daily.** Douglas Schar, a London-based herbalist who specializes in disease-preventing herbal medicines, refers to saw palmetto as "the man's tonic" because of the protection it offers the prostate gland. Here's one theory for why it works: Prostate problems occur because as men age, their testosterone levels drop. But saw palmetto contains compounds that help testosterone stay in the body longer. Drugstores carry it in tablet, capsule, and liquid forms. However, the concentration of active ingredients can vary dramatically from product to product, so consult your doctor for a suggested brand and dose.

2 **Do not take extra zinc.** Zinc has been associated with male sexual health, but maybe it shouldn't have been. Researchers at Harvard University conducted a 3-year study of 455 men and found that taking more than the Daily Value of 15 milligrams of zinc could increase your risk of developing an enlarged prostate. "Being a man in my sixties, I would avoid any supplement containing zinc," says Dimitrios Trichopoulos, M.D., coauthor of the study.

3 **When you feel the urge to urinate, don't wait.** Logic may tell you to train your bladder to hold out as long as it can, but when your bladder is too full, urine can back up into your prostate and irritate it.

4 **Exercise at least 30 minutes a day, 5 days a week.** Researchers found that active men run a much lower risk of prostate enlargement than couch potatoes do. "Even men who walked 2 to 3 hours per week had reduced risks," said Elizabeth Platz, Sc.D., the epidemiologist at Harvard who lead the study. She suspects that exercise relaxes the overstimulated nerves in the prostate that are believed to contribute to enlargement.

5 **Take 200 micrograms of selenium.** The mineral selenium may increase levels of a particular antioxidant known to help protect prostate cells, says James Brooks, M.D., assistant professor of urology at of Stanford University School of Medicine.

6 **Get 400 IU of vitamin E each day.** Preliminary indications are that the antioxidant vitamin E also helps protect against prostate disease, says Robert Cowles, M.D., a urologist in Atlanta.

Researchers from the National Cancer Institute studied 29,000 men in Finland and found that those who took vitamin E reduced their prostate cancer risks by one-third.

Kenneth A. Goldberg, M.D., of the Male Health Center, recommends 400 IU daily. "This will provide not only for prostate but heart protection as well," he says. Because vitamin E acts like a blood thinner, consult your doctor before beginning supplementation in any amount if you are already taking aspirin or blood-thinning medication, such as warfarin (Coumadin), or if you're at high risk for stroke.

7 **Take two servings of tomatoes a week.** Cooked tomatoes are the best source of lycopene, an antioxidant that may lower your risk of prostate cancer by as much as 35 percent. Lycopene seems to stop prostate cancer cells from multiplying, says Omer Kucuk, M.D., a researcher at the Karmanos Center Institute in Detroit. Here's the best way to eat them: Have spaghetti sauce with sliced carrots or sweet yellow peppers added to it. The beta-carotene in the carrots and peppers will guide the lycopene to your prostate. Lycopene is also found in raw tomatoes, pink grapefruit and watermelon. In addition, it's available at your pharmacy or health food store in supplement form.

8 **Eat no more than 1,000 milligrams of calcium.** Researchers at Harvard studied 47,000 men and found that those who consumed 2,000 milligrams of calcium each day (about the amount in six glasses of milk) were almost twice as likely to develop prostate cancer as those who consumed 1,000 milligrams. Too much calcium can lower the body's level of a compound believed to inhibit prostate cancer cell growth, says Edward Giovannucci, M.D., one of the study authors.

9 **Eat ¼ cup of raisins each day.** In a Dutch study, men who ate 1 ounce (about ¼ cup) of raisins or other dried fruit a day had half the risk of prostate cancer of men who ate less. So pack a box in your briefcase and snack on them often.

10 **Watch your fat.** Diets high in saturated fats, common in meats and dairy products, seem to irritate the prostate and increase cancer risk, doctors say. Switching to low-fat eating may help stop the growth of microscopic prostate cancers before they have the chance to cause major problems, says Mitchell Gaynor, M.D., of the Strang Cancer Prevention Center in New York City. On the other hand, eating polyunsaturated fats—found in cold-water fish such as salmon, mackerel, halibut, and tuna—seem to protect the prostate.

10 Ways to Prevent Stroke

1 **Stop everything and check your blood pressure because nothing cuts your risk of stroke like getting that pressure down.** Untreated high blood pressure shoots your chances of suffering a stroke four to six times higher than they would be if your blood pressure were normal. Here's one reason why: The excessive pounding of blood against the vessel walls from high blood pressure can cause small tears in the vessels or stretch them like overinflated balloons. That can lead to clotting, or it can blow out the vessel walls. Or it can clog your arteries. All of those things facilitate stroke, which is simply an interruption of the blood supply to your brain because of blockage or a burst vessel.

2 **Eating lots of fruits and vegetables helps a lot, and not just because it reduces your fat intake and gets your blood pressure and cholesterol levels down.** The antioxidants in fruits and vegetables, such as phytochemicals from the carotenoid family and vitamin C, help prevent strokes. And the folate in fruits, vegetables, and beans helps reduce levels of homocysteine, a protein fragment that may be as much of a risk factor for stroke as it is for heart disease.

3 **Wash your fruits and vegetables down with black or green tea.** They're rich in the phytochemicals called bioflavonoids, which increase capillary strength. A study from the Netherlands found that men who drank more than four cups of black tea a day were 69 percent less likely to have strokes than men who drank less than three cups a day.

4 **The same high-fat diet that clogs up your arteries can impede bloodflow to your neck, raising your odds of having a stroke.** You can significantly reduce the amount of fat in your diet simply by cutting down on the oils you cook with and choosing leaner cuts of meat, low-fat salad dressings, and low-fat dairy products. When you do use oils, choose oils made from flaxseed, canola, soybeans, or walnuts. These offer a kind of polyunsaturated fat called alpha-linolenic acid that may affect blood viscosity and clotting. Studies show that men with more alpha-linolenic acid in their blood have lower risks of strokes.

5 **Exercise to prevent a stroke.** Even easy exercise like 20 minutes a day of walking, gardening, dancing, or golf cuts your risk of stroke by more than half. Strenuous exercise is even better, reducing your risk by two-thirds. Exercise inhibits the production of blood clots that cause strokes. It also

prevents diabetes because it helps you lose weight. And diabetes prevention is stroke prevention.

6 **Have a drink or two.** Moderate drinking actually reduces your risk of stroke, studies show, possibly because small amounts of alcohol raise the level of a naturally occurring clot-buster in your blood. Binge drinking, though, has the opposite effect, possibly because it spikes your blood pressure.

7 **Resist the temptation to accompany that glass of wine or beer with a cigarette.** Smoking destroys the protective layer of cells inside artery walls, causing arteries to harden. If you quit smoking, you reduce your risk of stroke by a full 50 percent.

8 **Daily doses of ½ to 1 adult aspirin have been shown to be effective in reducing the risk of heart attacks, but aspirin is only sometimes appropriate for stroke prevention.** It's not for everyone. Ask your doctor.

9 **If you're already at risk for a stroke, another topic for discussion with your doctor is whether you should take anti-stroke prescription medicine.** A study done at Wake Forest University in Winston-Salem, North Carolina, showed 27 percent reductions in stroke incidence among people who take certain reductase inhibitors such as pravastatin (Pravachol), simvastatin (Zocor), or lovastatin (Mevacor).

10 **Heed the warning signs.** Men under 65 are not immune to strokes—in fact, they're good for about 30 percent of them. Just as heart attacks can be identified by the chest pains they can cause, strokes give off warning signals. Symptoms include short-term confusion, temporary loss of vision, blurred vision in one eye, tingling or weakness in an arm or leg, and drooling from one side of the mouth. These symptoms disappear in a minute or two if the cause is a short period of reduced bloodflow to the brain called transient ischemic attack, or TIA. But TIA is still a medical emergency. And you may be having a stroke. If you can get to the hospital within 3 hours, you can be treated with clot-busting drugs, such as tissue plasminogen activator (t-PA), that improve your chance of full recovery.

WEEK 4

LEARN THE LOW-STRESS LIFESTYLE

Day 1

Improve Your Breathing

Day 2

Learn to Relax

Day 3

Get a Massage

Day 4

Work Through Your Work Problems

Day 5

Laugh—A Lot

Day 6

Become a Kid Again

Improve Your Breathing

The Day's Task

For 10 minutes today, 5 in the morning before you get out of bed and 5 at night before you go to sleep, we want you to practice what's called abdominal or diaphragmatic breathing. Here's how to do it. Lie in bed on your back, and put your hand on your belly. Breathe in slowly and deeply so that your belly pushes up your hand significantly. The inhalation should last for a slow count to four. Then, breathe out, relaxing your belly. This should also last for a count of four. Repeat this for 5 minutes, making sure every breath raises your hand. The longer and deeper the breaths, the better.

Each time you inhale a jumbo gulp of air, you give your body a gift certificate that it can spend on a number of improvements.

One of the biggest benefits you'll reap when you incorporate deep breathing into your daily life is stress relief, which is why breathing is a cornerstone of many experts' relaxation plans. As you focus on the air rushing in and out of your body, your mind turns away from the stressful thoughts bothering it. "If you can control your breathing, you can control your emotions. And if you can control your emotions, you can control your stress," says Phil Nuernberger, Ph.D., author of *The Quest for Personal Power: Transforming Stress into Strength*.

Aside from stress relief, breathing well also gives you more energy and stamina. It helps rid your body of toxins and focuses your mind. It helps you cope with pain and lowers your blood pressure.

This healing power won't cost you a penny, no matter how much air you gulp. And unless you're underwater or an unlucky miner, you'll always have plenty of it around.

You may never have thought in these terms, but we modern people are lousy breathers. We take lots of small breaths that suck in mere wisps of air

AN ALTERNATIVE BREATHING EXERCISE

Your nostrils may be identical twins, but they like to be treated as individuals. You can share a little quality time with each of them and practice a breathing method to melt away stress with the following technique.

With the index finger of your dominant hand, close one nostril and breathe in and out through the open side, says Gay Hendricks, Ph.D. Breathe slowly and deeply. Then, close off the other nostril with the same finger and breathe in and out through the open side. Alternate like this for 2 minutes, focusing solely on the air going in and out and not on whether anyone thinks you're picking your nose. Then, do it for another 2 minutes with the index finger of your nondominant hand. Finish off with another minute of back and forth with your dominant hand, then rest quietly for a minute.

at a time. This type of breathing means air gets only to the top of our lungs, instead of filling the full region, says Gay Hendricks, Ph.D., author of *Conscious Breathing*.

Only a fraction of the blood that courses through your lungs, picking up oxygen and dropping off wastes, goes through their upper area. Much more blood flows through the middle and bottom of your lungs. That is why you want to send plenty of air circulating down there.

When you fully inflate your lungs this morning and tonight, you're using your diaphragm. No sex jokes here, please—we're talking about a thin sheet of muscle in your abdomen that separates your chest from your stomach. As you breathe to the bottom of your lungs, your diaphragm will pull down into your abdomen, making your belly rise. As the air rushes in, imagine it filling the bottom third of your lungs, the middle third, then the top third. Your hand lying atop your midsection will give you a way to measure how well you're inflating yourself.

Unlike when you eat too much lasagna, your belly will stick out only momentarily. As you exhale and push out the air, contract your stomach muscles. While breathing out, picture yourself emptying the top third of your lungs, then the middle third and the bottom third.

Just like that, you've taken a step toward improving your breathing and blowing away your stress.

How to Breath Away Stress

In the closing credits of the old *Flintstones* cartoon, Fred would start pounding on the door of his home in a yelling fit after the family feline tossed him out the window. Just as our primitive ancestors had hostile, adrenalin-pumping reactions when they met angry wildlife, modern problems like work deadlines and tax auditors can flip our bodies into emergency mode.

This is the fabled fight-or-flight reaction. When faced with a sudden fear, challenge, or panic, our bodies automatically make significant adjustments, in the primal belief that they will have to react in a powerful, physical way. Our heart rates rise, our muscles tense up, our digestion halts, and our breathing becomes quick and shallow.

In primitive life, this energy often got burnt off physically in a mad dash to safety or an actual physical confrontation. But in these modern times, the challenges that trigger fight-or-flight bodily changes are usually mental and have no physical resolution. When you face them several times a day, the effect on your body is awful. The internal rushes can weaken your immune system and raise your blood pressure, damaging your heart and blood vessels and setting the stage for heart attack and stroke. These reactions may also be potentially damaging to other organs in your body. The interference with bloodflow may deprive some organs of the oxygen they need to function properly.

BREATH AND THE SOUL

If after a few sessions of deep breathing you're still not feeling the connection between the air you take in and the state of your health, crack open a few foreign-language dictionaries. In many tongues, the words for *spirit* and *breath* are the same, such as *prana* in Sanskrit and *spiritus* in Latin, according to Andrew Weil, M.D., director of the program in integrative medicine at the University of Arizona College of Medicine in Tucson.

To see the connection in English, just look at the words *respiration* and *inspire*.

That's where breathing comes in. When you incorporate today's breathing lesson into your daily life, repeatedly taking in air slowly and deeply using your diaphragm, you can control your emotions and quiet the damaging effects of fight-or-flight stress.

When your stress alarms start ringing, find a restful position (we prefer lying down with the lights off, but our boss doesn't come around too often) and focus on your breathing, says Peggy Kileff, a wellness consultant at the Institute for Preventive Medicine in Houston. Breathe in as you slowly count to four, making sure you're following the abdominal breathing method. Pause briefly, then breathe out as you slowly count to four. Do this for several minutes or until you've regained control of your stressed-out body.

As you become accustomed to this stress reliever—especially if you practice it before you get out of bed, randomly throughout the day, and before you fall asleep—you'll automatically do it when you start feeling tense.

Learn to Relax

The Day's Task

After you get home from work, go to a quiet room with a comfortable couch or bed, and lie down. Set an alarm for 30 minutes, then close your eyes and forget about time. Focus instead on your breathing. Take several slow, deep breaths in through your nose and out through your mouth. Do the progressive muscle-relaxation program detailed in this chapter. The idea is to briefly tense muscle groups around your body, then let them go loose. These are short exercises; you'll do roughly one every 10 to 15 seconds. Do the entire set of exercises three times. When you're finished, take a nap. Then, get up and enjoy the rest of your evening.

Let's be honest. Today's task is about the most unmanly assignment in the *Men's Health* Longevity Program. Most often, when we men have a high-stress day, we take matters into our own hands. We have a drink, we zone out in front of the television, we internalize, playing things out over and over in our heads, often turning silent in the process.

The problem with this is that little relaxation actually occurs. Men are not good at relaxing. That is why a formal program, no matter how un-guy-like it sounds, makes sense. This program is clinically proven to reverse the adverse physiological and mental effects of stress.

Here's why it is important to relax. Stress and muscle tension work in a vicious cycle. As soon as stress hormones hit your bloodstream, your muscles react with primal urgency, coiling like springs, ready to do battle with or propel you away from whatever is causing the stress.

If you experienced stress only once in a while, this wouldn't be a big deal. The hormones would dissipate, your muscles would relax, and you would feel fine. But modern man deals with nonstop stress everyday, explains Alison Milburn, Ph.D., a psychologist at Eastdale Psychology Group in

Iowa City, Iowa. As a result, your muscles stay tense. They get sore. They send pain signals to your brain, which triggers the release of yet more stress hormones.

Over time, stress hormones do more than cause muscle pain. They can damage your blood vessels, raise your cholesterol and blood pressure, weaken your immunity, and just plain tire you out. In short, stress can make you feel weary and older than your years.

But with today's progressive muscle-relaxation technique, you can interrupt this cycle of stress, ridding your body of tension and calming your mind. Progressive muscle relaxation is a study in paradox. It's based on the theory that, to relax, you have to tense up. And it works. If your muscles are already tight and you tense them up even more, then let them go limp, they feel much more relaxed than usual. And so will you.

The Formal Program

Progressive muscle relaxation is one of the simplest and most effective stress-reduction methods. Lie down; get comfortable. Shoo out any thoughts that don't involve relaxation. Read through the following list of motions several times so you get the hang of what you're expected to do, then begin. Here's how to do it.

1. Breathe in deeply through your nose. Raise your eyebrows and wrinkle your forehead, tensing up your whole head. Hold for 10 seconds, then relax. Exhale completely through your mouth.
2. Breathe in deeply through your nose. Squeeze your eyebrows together and scrunch up your nose. Hold for 10 seconds, then relax. Exhale completely through your mouth.
3. Breathe in deeply through your nose. Pull back your lips into a grimace, hold for 10 seconds, then relax. Exhale completely through your mouth.
4. Breathe in deeply through your nose. Hunch your shoulders toward your ears, hold for 10 seconds, then relax. Exhale completely through your mouth.
5. Breathe in very deeply through your nose. Expand your lungs so you can feel them creating tension in your chest. Hold for 10 seconds, then relax. Exhale completely through your mouth.
6. Breathe in deeply through your nose. Pull your arms in close to your body, tensing your biceps and triceps. Hold for 10 seconds, then relax. Breathe out completely through your mouth.

7. Breathe in deeply through your nose. Hold your arms out in front of you and tense your forearms tightly. Hold for 10 seconds, then relax. Exhale completely through your mouth.
8. Breathe in deeply through your nose. Make tight fists, squeezing your hands and fingers. Hold for 10 seconds, then relax. Breathe out completely through your mouth.
9. Breathe in deeply through your nose. Pull your stomach in hard and tight, creating tension in your torso. Hold your arms out in front of you and tense your forearms tightly. Hold for 10 seconds, then relax. Exhale completely through your mouth.
10. Breathe in deeply through your nose. Squeeze your buttocks together tightly. Hold for 10 seconds, then relax. Exhale completely through your mouth.
11. Breathe in deeply through your nose. Squeeze your thighs together and tense up their muscles. Hold for 10 seconds, then relax. Exhale completely through your mouth.
12. Breathe in deeply through your nose. Tense the muscles in your calves and lower legs. Hold for 10 seconds, then relax. Breathe out completely through your mouth.
13. Breathe in deeply through your nose. Scrunch up your toes and feet. Hold for 10 seconds, then relax. Exhale completely through your mouth. (If you're prone to getting cramps in your feet, skip this step.)
14. Breathe in deeply through your nose. Do an inventory of your body to find any areas that are tense. Repeat the tension-and-relaxation exercise two more times, being careful to give more attention to areas of your body that seem to be holding on to tension.

The whole thing should take only 15 minutes. When you're finished, allow yourself to doze until your alarm goes off. That cat nap should be long enough to restore your energy for the rest of the evening but not too much to leave you groggy after you awaken.

As with any other skill, it takes practice to get good at progressive relaxation. Don't expect to experience instant bliss or even a complete flushing of the day's tension. Do this a few times a week; get better at it. If you get better at it and you like it, consider doing it as often as once a day. It is surprisingly healthy.

If you indeed decide to use this progressive-relaxation method again, you may find it easier if you have a voice on a tape leading you through it. You can easily make your own.

Set up a tape recorder with a blank tape, and read through the list of numbered progressive-relaxation commands. Use a watch to measure off the right length of tension and relaxation. Keep your voice in a soothing monotone. Think James Earl Jones or Garrison Keillor. Read through the whole list several times so if you want a longer session, you won't have to stop to rewind the tape.

Talking Yourself out of It

Progressive muscle relaxation is just one of several formal anti-stress regimens. Yoga, meditation, visualization, and massage all qualify as well. All take some level of training and investment. All have been clinically proven to work.

Here's one more anti-stress system that works quite well but that you can do on your own without any studying or cost. It is called autogenics, which sounds like something a car mechanic would do but is actually a practice akin to hypnosis. Instead of tensing your muscles and letting them go slack, you simply talk yourself into relaxation.

Find a quiet room where you can lie on the floor in a comfortable position. Slowly say each of the following phrases to yourself, concentrating on their meaning and repeating them the given number of times. Pause for a few seconds after each phrase to let its meaning take hold.

- My arms and hands are warm and heavy. (Repeat 5 times)
- My legs and feet are warm and heavy. (5 times)
- My abdomen is warm and comfortable. (5 times; skip this one, however, if you have ulcers, internal bleeding conditions, or diabetes)
- My breathing is full, deep, and relaxed. (5 times)
- My heartbeat is healthy, calm, and regular. (10 times)
- My forehead is cool. (5 times)

Get a Massage

The Day's Task

Today, we put your relaxation in the strong, skilled hands of someone else. We hope you were paying attention back in The Preparation chapter in Week Zero and actually scheduled an hour-long rubdown with a massage therapist today. If you did, your task is merely to show up. If you didn't, schedule a massage, right now, for as soon as possible.

A massage is more enjoyable if you have a clean body and a full stomach, so take a shower and eat a light meal about an hour beforehand. Don't let embarrassment or self-consciousness hamper your session. Your massage therapist is a professional who has likely seen plenty of clients. But if you're feeling modest, wear a pair of boxers or gym shorts. As you lie on the massage table, clear your mind of nagging problems and concerns. Just relax; let your mind drift.

Expect to pay $45 or more for an hour-long session. It's worth every penny.

Modern Western civilization is split into two categories of people: those who will pay for a massage and those who won't. We strongly advocate that you choose to be in the first category. A good, long, slow, deep massage, done by a professional—well, it's just one of life's great luxuries. Unlike many other luxuries, it is entirely good for you.

All that grasping, kneading, and pressing of your flesh doesn't just feel good. It's actually spreading good health throughout your body. A round of massage can encourage oxygen- and nutrient-carrying blood to flow back to achy muscles. It can also increase circulation of lymph, a fluid in your body that gathers up bacteria and wastes and carries them away for disposal.

Massage is a proven stress reducer, mood enhancer, and healer. In a study at the Touch Research Institute at the University of Miami School of Medi-

RUB YOURSELF THE RIGHT WAY

If you can't find a massage therapist in your area, can't spare the money, or just don't want someone touching you, don't turn your back on massage. You can always do it yourself. Here are a couple of techniques.

- To reduce stress, softly rub your face with your hands, then press with your fingers firmly and slowly from the center of your forehead out to your temples. Press under your cheekbones from your nose to your ears, then from your mouth to the edges of your jaw.

  Next, rub the heels of your palms into your temples, with your fingertips atop your scalp. Circle your palms 10 times in one direction, then 10 times in the other. Then rub your palms in circles all around your head.

  Finally, press your hands along the back of your neck to warm it up, then use your fingers to rub deeply in a circular motion around your trapezius muscles, which are atop your shoulders and alongside your neck. Next, using your left hand, squeeze the trapezius to the right of your neck and rotate your right shoulder backward. Repeat on your left side with your right hand.
- To soothe a sore muscle or a cramp, knead the area to find the most tender spot, says Robert Edwards, director of the Somerset School of Massage in New Jersey. Once you find it, press down on the spot firmly, using both hands. Hold for a few seconds, relax, and repeat until you feel some relief.

cine, massage therapists gave 15-minute massages to workers at their job sites twice a week for 5 weeks. At the end of the 5 weeks, the workers felt less stress and less depression. Study participants even did better on math problems after massages. Other studies have found that massage therapy may lead to fewer migraine headaches and increased immune system function.

A good way to find a massage therapist is to talk to friends who've had massages or to doctors who recommend the therapy, says Marianne Bergmann, a certified massage therapist in Bethlehem, Pennsylvania. You can also use the American Massage Therapy Association's find-a-massage-therapist service by calling (888) THE-AMTA.

Once you find a therapist, ask him if he's licensed (about half of the states require licensing), where he got his training, and if he's a member of a professional association. Also, be sure to ask what types of massage he practices. Some massage styles are very soothing and gentle. Others are more aggressive and may feel uncomfortable—even a little rough—if you're not used to them. Here are some of the more common types.

Swedish massage. The practitioner will use long strokes, kneading, and friction to work the muscles closer to the surface of your skin as well as move your joints around. This is a common type of massage used in stress relief.

Neuromuscular massage. The therapist will focus on a particular muscle or group of muscles that's been giving you trouble.

Sports massage. The therapist will focus on the muscles you use and abuse in a specific sport.

Shiatsu. This style is steeped in Eastern philosophy and is similar in principal to other healing practices like acupuncture and acupressure. In shiatsu, your massage therapist prods you gently with his fingertips, looking for certain points along invisible energy pathways that are said to be flowing through your body. The goal is to remove blockages and restore complete energy flow.

What to Expect

Regardless of the type of massage you choose to have, you may still have some apprehension about exactly what will happen during your session. Here is what to expect from a typical massage.

- Before the massage, you'll probably fill out some forms and discuss any health problems you have and what you expect to gain from your session.
- If you're uncomfortable with the idea of a guy touching you, consider, again, that he's a professional. And hey, this is how the top athletes do it. If it still bothers you, go to a woman. Think she won't be able to press down hard enough? Think again. If she's a pro, her hands could well be stronger than yours.
- Your therapist won't hurt you. Often, he'll ask you use a number scale to describe any pain you're feeling. When you hit a certain number, he'll ease up.
- You'll probably fall asleep. This is natural and happens frequently, Gagnon says, so don't worry about offending the therapist if you end up snoozing. He'll probably consider it a compliment.

Work Through Your Work Problems

The Day's Task

Today's task is to take a very simple two-part test that shows you how well you keep your work life in perspective.

1. **When you arrive at your workplace today, look around and take note of how many reminders you have of your outside life: photos of your wife or girlfriend or your family and friends, a personal coffee mug that has some meaning to you, action toys that a buddy or kid gave you, knick-knacks that represent private jokes or memories—anything meaningful that you've brought in to liven up your surroundings.**
2. **When you walk into your home after work, do a similar check for items that remind you of the office. Do you have financial reports on the dining table, an open briefcase lying about, work-related reading stacked in the living room?**

The scoring is easy and pretty subjective: The more objects from the outside world you have at your workplace and the fewer work-related items at home, the more well-rounded your life. It's that simple.

||||||||||||||||||||||||||||||||||||||||||||||||||||||||||||||||||||||||||||||||||||||||||||||||

More than 11 million of America's 80 million employed men spend some of their waking hours working at home. For about half of these guys, this is either part of their job descriptions or they are self-employed. Good for them. A desk job is much easier if you get to do it in sweatpants and tennis shoes.

But the rest of us spend our days out in the workplace. And too often, we take more work home and aren't paid to do it. That's not so easy.

Then there are all the men who live with yet another overlap between their work time and playtime. They lug home work-related worries, from visions of their red-faced bosses to doubts about their capabilities. These anxieties run through their heads as they try to enjoy TV and keep them staring at the ceiling when they'd rather be asleep.

We all know overworked and overworried guys like that. Too often, we *are* guys like that.

We work longer and harder. We go in early and leave late to please the boss. Our spare time becomes just more time to do our work.

Unfortunately, the qualities that make someone a standout employee are the same qualities that can allow his job to make him miserable, says Ruth Luban, author of *Keeping the Fire: From Burnout to Balance*.

When work prevents a man from enjoying the other aspects of life, his health can pay the price. Frequent stress and overwork can lead to sleep problems, fatigue, headaches, back pain, digestive upset, or frequent infections. Excess stress also causes your body to produce hormones that can raise your blood pressure and strain your heart.

Since none of these problems are helpful for a fellow trying to lengthen his life span, your mission is to ease some of your work burdens so you can keep your life balanced.

Know Your Limits

Sometimes, when you're trying to be a productive worker, your worst enemy is you. If you pour more and more of your energy into your job, you may cut back on the after-hours activities that make life enjoyable, Luban says.

If you're heading toward burnout, you'll pass several mile markers. You'll start your job eager to show how capable you are, but as you become familiar with the work, you may sense that perhaps your goals were too lofty. Meanwhile, coworkers don't seem to be having difficulties. You try harder.

As you invest more of yourself into your job, you become more tired and irritable and less sure of yourself. You grow pessimistic about your abilities, your job, and your coworkers. If you don't take action, you'll head into despair. You may wind up feeling like a failure with nothing left to give.

To head off burnout, start by recognizing that your job is only part of your identity, Luban suggests. You don't have to be just a plumber, a lawyer, or a widget

SHOULD I EVEN BE HERE?

They're two of America's favorite sports—complaining about our jobs and griping about our bosses. As Joe Walsh of the Eagles once sang (if you can call what he did singing), "I can't complain, but sometimes I still do."

The trick, however, is to not take this too far. It's easy to become negative and self-centered, to draw a firm line between you and the evil empire under which you toil. It's that old disdainful line "I just work for them."

That's a bad attitude. If you don't believe in your company, get out of there. Not having pride in your work or your employer is bad for your mental health.

Here are some deep thoughts to keep in mind to help assess whether you are in a job that is right for you.

- A job, at its essence, is a no-emotion contract. You agree to provide strong arms or creative brain waves or impressive schmooze capabilities, and in return, the employer offers a bundle of pay and benefits. Treat it as what it is: a professional arrangement. With that frame of mind, you can assess your job situation rationally. But if you get too personal about your work, you lose your ability to see it for what it is. Remember that even at the best company, a job is not forever. You owe it to yourself to always be honest about your arrangement.
- Always do your job well, not to impress your boss or for political gain but

maker. Think of yourself also as a husband, a father, a racquetball player, a volunteer, or in other roles that you enjoy.

When you get up in the morning, don't immediately become an employee, rushing to get to the car and to work. Take a half-hour to read a book, work out, listen to some music, or enjoy some other activity that lets you be your own man.

Similarly, after you end your workday, find a transition spot between the office and home where you can hang out for a while and decompress. It could be a gym, a bookstore, or a park. Steer clear of the neighborhood pub. If your job is really stressing you, the urge to drink to relax might get the better of you.

because you believe in what you do and have the integrity to do it right. If you spend too much time working hard for the wrong reasons, you will soon learn to hate your work. Make sure you work at places that allow you to excel.

- If you are not happy in your job, it is up to you to fix it or to leave. It's a very simple equation. Either your job permits you to do the work you want to do or it doesn't. If politics, procedures, or lack of resources truly stop you from doing what you want to do professionally, either find a way to get rid of those impediments or find a job in which they aren't there. This is called being responsible for yourself.
- Everyone thinks they deserve more money, just like everyone thinks they work harder than the guy next to them. It's universal. So keep your perspective when it comes to salary issues. What pay is appropriate for your industry, your experience, your contribution? Certainly, demand what you reasonably deserve. But don't expect more than that.
- An old saying claims that your job is only as good as your boss. If you feel that you are given the freedom to do your work the way you believe it should be done, the ability to speak honestly about it, and pay that is commensurate to your contribution, well, that's about as good as it gets. You should be satisfied with that. You just can't do much better.

Work with Your Boss

Aretha Franklin has long known the key to having a good relationship with your employers: respect. If you respect your bosses and your bosses respect you, everyone goes home happier. Here are some ways to make sure that happens.

- Arrive at work in the morning as a team player who understands the company plan that passes down the ranks through your bosses and on to you, says Jeff Davidson of the Breathing Space Institute in Chapel Hill, North Carolina. Productive employees are the ones who believe in the benefits of the company's goals and strive for those same ideals. The ones who don't think in those terms can feel like outsiders and grow resentful of the team members.

- When your boss has a suggestion or criticism regarding your work, don't immediately go on the defensive. You'll usually find at least a bit of truth that you can use to better your performance, suggests Darrel W. Ray, Ed.D., an organizational psychologist in Kansas City, Kansas.
- When you're presenting an idea to your boss, emphasize how it's useful to him or the company, not to you. He's the one who needs to be sold on the idea.
- Sound off when you must. If your boss asks for your honest opinion, tell him. But remember to choose your battles wisely and voice your concerns only on the important issues. If you really have to let loose a tirade, give it to your boss in private.

Work with Your Coworkers

At work, if you want to get ahead, you have to get along. But sometimes, you'd like to take the bozo down the hall and staple his tongue to the desk so you won't have to listen to him anymore.

That approach won't work, of course, but you can't let the stress of dealing with this person make you sick either. If you feel ready to rip the guy a new out box, call a time-out so you can both go cool down. Tell him you're too angry to talk constructively anymore and you're going to go think of a better way to deal with the issue tomorrow.

Make It Through Snooze Time

One of the best parts of the day, lunch, is now just a pleasant warmth in your belly. The other daily highlight, getting off work, is still hours away. At around 3:00 P.M., you start getting sleepier than the last speaker at a hypnotist convention.

If you work for a company that doesn't mind a brief nap, you don't really have a problem. But most of us do not live in that alternate universe where work is a benevolent kingdom. So when the afternoon slump hits, try these tactics instead.

- Get up and take a 10-minute walk, preferably outside in the sun.
- Avoid the cafeteria's meat loaf special since a heavy meal can put a drag on your energy levels like a deep-sea anchor. Instead, eat something light that consists mostly of carbohydrates and protein, like a turkey sandwich. Try to keep your lunch to 600 calories or less.
- As your slump approaches, have a snack that is rich in carbs and protein. Try yogurt and low-fat fig cookies or fresh vegetables and a low-fat dip. You'll probably need to make these ahead of time and stick them in the office refrigerator.

Laugh–A Lot

The Day's Task

Your goal today is to make people laugh at work as often as you can. In so doing, you should laugh too. To accomplish this, take at least one of the following props to work.

- **The most embarrassing photo ever taken of you. Tape it to your door.**
- **The ugliest shirt-and-tie combination you can find. Wear it with pride.**
- **Several of your favorite cartoons. Copy them and post them in conspicuous places. Good sources include "The Far Side" calendar, the *New Yorker* magazine, a "Calvin and Hobbes" anthology book, and a "Dilbert" strip from the newspaper. Remember, nothing sexual or mean-spirited, or you'll get in trouble.**

When people ask you what gives, reply with a smile that you simply were in the mood for some laughs today.

During a stressful moment in the comedy *The Money Pit*, Tom Hanks throws his head back and laughs, harder and harder, until he's erupting in guffaws that a hyena would find undignified. His bathtub has just plummeted though the floor of his home and shattered on the landing below, another in a long string of household mishaps. Hanks just stands there cackling.

Perhaps he's just on the verge of going nuts, but at least he's on the right track in coping with his worries.

When stress is beating you up, hit it back with a punch line. By getting into the habit of laughing regularly, particularly in the face of frustration, you enjoy not only immediate stress relief but also physical improvements that can extend your life.

Say you're popping a bag of microwave popcorn when the snack decides to burst into flames, pouring out acrid smoke that permeates your kitchen and sets off the smoke alarm. Instead of cursing as you open the windows, take a humorous approach instead and announce that you're just telling the fire department that it's snack time, making sure the popcorn is thoroughly cooked to avoid any raw spots, or fogging the house to kill mosquitoes.

With a good laugh, your internal aggravation will sink as stress-related chemicals in your bloodstream subside. Your blood pressure and heart rate will leap, as if you were having a brief aerobic workout, then settle down lower than they were before. Also, your breathing rate will jump, putting more oxygen into your bloodstream.

And your brain, simply unable to be aggravated and amused at the same time, will settle for the latter. As for the burnt-popcorn smell, you're stuck with it until the carpet airs out.

Laughter Research

As you go through life, a good-humored attitude toward screaming children, bad waiters, and fender benders may help you live longer so you can enjoy finding the fun in life long after your crabby friends have departed.

To look at the link between longevity and humor, Richard Haude, Ph.D., and his colleagues at the University of Akron studied a group of elderly people and their deceased siblings. The average age of the living subjects was 72, and the average age of their deceased siblings was 64. The participants rated their senses of humor and their dearly departeds' on a standardized scale. The researchers concluded from the results that the living family members tended to be better-humored than the deceased ones, lending some scientific credence to the saying "He who laughs last laughs best."

It's not only that laughing is good for you; *not* laughing is bad for you. When you can't shake off chronic stress, your blood pressure can soar high and stay there, leading to hardened arteries and an increased likelihood of stroke and heart attack. In a study involving 33,000 men, researchers at Harvard University found that the more anxious the men were, the greater the chance they'd die unexpectedly of heart attacks.

University of California researchers conducting a study of 1,000 men found that the guys with severe work-related problems in their pasts were five times more likely to develop colon cancer than their calmer counterparts.

The life-giving benefit of laughter is not due merely to the aerobic workout and the burst of oxygen your body gets from gasping for breath. Studies have also shown that laughter can boost a number of cells and chemicals in your body—such as T cells, white blood cells, and interferon-gamma—that strengthen your immune system to help you fight diseases.

During stress, your body produces more free radicals, maverick oxygen molecules that ravage cells, adding wear and tear to your body. Free radicals contribute to cataracts, gray hair, dry skin, and wrinkles, points out Paul J. Rosch, M.D., president of the American Institute of Stress. If you learn how to chill out and have a chuckle, you may even keep yourself looking younger than your years.

Maybe this laughing business really *is* the best medicine, available, as always, free of charge and without a doctor's prescription. So today, when work has you stressed, aggravated, or merely bored, use the objects you take to the office—the funny photo, the ugly shirt and tie, the cartoons—to generate some laughs. Not only will you brighten your day (and, let us hope, those of the people you work with), but maybe someday in the distant future, when one of your relatives is in a study examining his ability to joke around, you'll be alive to take part too.

Keeping Your Funny Bone Active

At some point in your life, you've done something hysterically stupid. Everyone has. It's something that makes you laugh just thinking about it. Or maybe you have a book of old "Doonesbury" cartoon strips that sets you off or a CD by a favorite comedian or a tape of a classic comic song (remember "They're Coming to Take Me Away, Ha-Haaa!"?).

Having objects around that make you laugh is a good thing. But not everyone is a barrel of laughs. Many of us have lost the ability to laugh easily and often. How many jokes do you know by heart? It's a good barometer of your humor quotient.

Are you struggling to find your funny bone? When you get down to it, a sense of humor is nothing more than a reflection of your attitude on life. A *good* sense of humor is about not taking the world too seriously, or yourself or your job or your problems. It's acknowledging that life is full of contradictions, absurdities, bad managers, lousy drivers, and leaky faucets. And it's not letting any of them get in the way of enjoying yourself and leading the life you want to lead. Want to laugh more easily again? It's simple: ease up on your life attitude.

Sometimes, though, life does get oppressive enough that you need a humor kick start. When times like this arrive, try some of these recommendations for getting back your laugh.

Tear into your daily joke. Get a laugh-a-day or cartoon-a-day desk calendar for your office. Half the entries will be duds; half will actually be funny. Every now and then, they'll make you laugh out loud. At minimum, they'll adjust your attitude for a short time, and that's good enough.

Have a pillow fight. Let your opponent win. Pillow fights are the third most important usage of a bed (beaten only by sleep and sex) and, let us hope, the funniest.

Get into a tickling match. There is nothing more certain to induce serious laughter than a well-placed tickle, particularly with kids. We'll give you some help. The three most ticklish areas, according to our informal poll, are the bottom of the feet, in or near the armpits, and the sides of the belly.

Hang out with young kids. They're funny, they're creative, they're beautifully, blessedly naive. Stop trying to teach them all the time; instead, just be one of them for a while.

Make a first-laugh kit. Keep a stash of humorous toys handy at home, in the car, or wherever you may need a laugh, recommends Christian Hageseth III, M.D., a psychiatrist in Collins, Colorado. Use a pair of Groucho glasses, a red clown nose, or whatever strikes your fancy. They're hokey, but they work.

Stock a comedy library. It may not make you look as intellectual as, say, the unabridged works of Ayn Rand, but a collection of comedy videos and books can brighten your day when you're glum, Dr. Hageseth says. Let friends and family know who your favorite laugh makers are, and they'll always have options when they need to buy you a birthday or holiday gift.

Become a Kid Again

The Day's Task

This sounds more difficult and embarrassing than it is. Tonight, after dinner, take 2 hours to indulge in an activity you used to enjoy a lot as a child or teenager. Pick something legal that you gave up when you entered the responsible world of adulthood.

Climb the best trees on your block. Buy a stack of comic books from the drugstore and read them all. Shoot pool or play pinball with a buddy. Build a dinosaur out of Legos. Get yourself a model rocket, take it to an open field, and fire it off, over and over. The choice is yours.

But whichever activity you pick, do it like a kid would. Don't be self-conscious. Don't worry about getting dirty—or about getting dirty looks. Focus on nothing but the joy of doing what you're doing.

Regardless of how many of the Ten Commandments you tend to ignore, you probably still live your daily life according to a commentary from the Bible (1 Corinthians 13:11, to be exact): "When I was a child, I talked like a child, I thought like a child, I reasoned like a child. When I became a man, I put childish ways behind me."

At the risk of being blasphemers, we must report that the Bible isn't giving good counsel here. We lost something when we traded in our mud-stained T-shirts for business suits and dry-cleaning bills. Sure, we get some distinct benefits from adulthood: sex, regular spending money, and bigger, more complex toys like sport-utility vehicles and digital camcorders. But the days of climbing on jungle gyms and being filled with an upbeat sense of wonder about the world got sacrificed.

That's too bad. Acting like a kid can bring adult-size benefits. Studies show that people who are playful and optimistic live longer, healthier, and happier lives.

"It's important to distinguish between being child*like*, being spontaneous and flexible and so forth, and being truly child*ish*," says Joel Goodman, Ed.D., director of the Humor Project in Saratoga Springs, New York. "Being childish is being irresponsible and immature. But being childlike can be a very mature way of coping with and enjoying life."

And by acting like a kid, you'll be able, for at least a short time, to be king of your own little world. After all, isn't that why children have always been so dedicated to their playtime?

Kids spend hours every day being shuttled through a world they can't control, enduring cooked spinach and classroom lessons and waiting around while their parents talk about boring things. But when they play with their toys or with each other, kids suddenly have a chance to take charge and set the rules. The stuffy grown-up world fades into the background.

As an adult, you live your life taking care of other people's needs and wants. You have responsibilities to your boss, your wife, your kids, your lawn or garden. A good definition of stress, then, is lack of control over your life.

But when your tie comes off and you put your play clothes on, you become your own man. By raking up a deep pile of leaves and leaping into it, or building the world's best miniature ship in a bottle, you're the one in charge, if only for a while.

Plus, by stepping out of your usual routine with playtime, you enjoy completely new experiences that stand out from the repetitive cycle of your grown-up duties. Seek these out. Remember them. These fun times are what make life worth getting out of bed.

Between work, social obligations, and watching your own kids have their fun, you may have a hard time finding a little childlike time for yourself. Life isn't as easy as in grade school, when your recess time was as scheduled and nonnegotiable as the math hour. That's why it's important to put some playtime into your schedule, says Walt Schafer, Ph.D., author of *Stress Management for Wellness*. He suggests you set aside time for play at least once a week. You probably have a few hours to spare here and there, which you may just be blowing in front of the TV (and that's not playing, that's vegetating).

How to Be a Kid

We hope you remember. If you have kids, you have daily reminders. They make your task easier: drop the parental-unit role and be one of them. Play with them. Don't teach them, don't organize them, don't grade them—just play.

If you don't have kids and are truly stuck for something to do, call your parents or a brother or sister. They'll certainly remember what you used to like to do. It wasn't that long ago, buddy. Or consider these suggestions, all guaranteed to bring back your youth for 120 minutes.

- Take a crisp $20 bill to your local video game arcade and turn it into quarters. Don't leave until every coin is spent.
- Find a pond. Toss a piece of wood far out into the water and start chucking rocks at it. Pretend you're a major-league pitcher putting a hot one over home plate, a Navy pilot sinking an enemy submarine, or a gigantic sea monster throwing boulders at Hawaii. When you run out of rocks, creep around the edge of the pond and catch frogs. Find bizarre insects or snails. Identify the animal tracks in the mud.
- Get musical. Dust off that old guitar or drum kit and be a jukebox hero again. Raise the roof off the garage. Make the neighbors complain.
- Venture out of your neighborhood. Hop on your bike, or just walk briskly through an area that you don't normally frequent. Remember to look at the world through a kid's eyes, though. If you see a trail sneaking off into the woods, check it out. Spot a cool car parked on the street? Go look at it. Keep walking, keep looking. Stop at a convenience store and buy a soda when you get thirsty. Buy a *Mad* magazine and stick it in your back pocket, while you're at it. If you're far from home at the end of your 2 hours, call your spouse and ask for a ride. Or if you're still having a good time, ask permission to go home late.
- Do the kid sports thing. Shoot baskets. Toss around a Frisbee or a softball with a pal. Or play some mini golf.
- Draw a picture. Kids love art projects. Who cares if your human renderings still resemble stick figures? Draw a spaceship, if that's the case. Spread out lots of paper and let loose.

10 Ways to Prevent Depression

1. **Do a reality check.** As many as one in eight men may need treatment for depression in their lifetimes. You know you're heading down that lonesome road when you find yourself thinking negative thoughts like, "She hates me" or "I'm a crappy father" or "Why did I say that?" At such times you need to hit the brakes hard. Remind yourself of the things you do right and put other things in perspective. Just because your kid failed chemistry, it doesn't mean you get an F in fatherhood.

2. **Supplement with folic acid.** A deficiency in this B vitamin can bring you down, says Jonathan Alpert, M.D., assistant professor of psychiatry at Harvard Medical School. You can get more folate (the naturally occurring form of folic acid) in your system by boosting your intake of green leafy vegetables, orange juice, liver, avocados, and beans. Or try 200 micrograms of folic acid a day in pill form.

3. **Pump yourself up through exercise.** A bunch of studies have shown that weight lifting and aerobic exercise can be powerful antidepressants. Hit the road or the iron three or more times a week for 20 to 30 minutes at a time. It's hard to feel down when the stuff of life is coursing through your veins.

4. **Eat fewer foods containing refined sugar.** Studies have shown that many people who are depressed tend to consume more sugar than people who aren't. Trouble is, when you gulp down candy without any accompanying protein or fat, your body breaks it down quickly, spiking serotonin and blood sugar levels. Just as quickly, you come crashing down when you burn that stuff off. Then you're like a junkie, needing more sugar to climb back out of the hole. So slowly wean yourself off refined sugar. Take 2 weeks or so to do it. Replace it with complex carbohydrates that will keep your energy levels high—rice, corn, potatoes, stuff like that.

5. **Cut down on your daily caffeine intake.** Man, it's good to begin the day with a cup of joe. Sadly, caffeine can cause the same kind of mood swings that sugar does. If you drink more than a cup a day, try to wean yourself from the teat of the coffee pot. Slowly add decaf to your coffee quota. Every day, add a little more decaf to your cup. Then, once you're drinking mostly decaf try to get down to one cup, preferably in the morning. Give yourself a couple of weeks to make the switch. After that, you'll "perc" back up.

6 **Consider taking St. John's wort.** This herb, also called hypericum, may stop brain enzymes from destroying feel-good chemicals like serotonin, epinephrine, and dopamine, says Varro E. Tyler, Ph.D., dean emeritus of Purdue University School of Pharmacy and Pharmacal Sciences in West Lafayette, Indiana. Look for a standardized extract at an herbal store. Make sure the word *hypericin* is on the label. Do not use St. John's wort with antidepressants without medical approval.

7 **Also consider taking ginkgo biloba.** Like St. John's wort, this herb seems to work by keeping mood-enhancing chemicals in your system longer. Don't grab just any ginkgo product, though. Make sure it has the active ingredients *glycosides* and *terpenes*. Start with 120 milligrams a day and slowly increase the dose until you feel better, up to 240 milligrams a day, recommends James Braly, M.D., medical director of Immuno Laboratories in Ft. Lauderdale. Ginkgo biloba doesn't mix well with antidepressants, aspirin or nonsteroidal anti-inflammatories, or blood-thinning medications, so check the label or talk with a doctor before taking it.

8 **Eat the fruit of the sea.** If you rarely eat fish, you're missing out on those essential fats, omega-3's. Experts note that depression rates have increased a hundredfold in the last century, just as human consumption of omega-3's has declined. Today, there is a sixtyfold difference in depression rates between countries with the highest omega-3 consumption (Japan and Taiwan) and those areas with the lowest (North America, Europe, and New Zealand).

So, get fish—especially salmon, mackerel, herring, and canned white tuna—in your diet at least three times a week. Other good sources include walnuts, walnut oil, canola oil, ground flaxseed, and flaxseed oil. Fish oil capsules are also available, but they're not particularly good for people with diabetes or blood-related health problems or who use aspirin regularly.

9 **Get enough sleep.** Getting substandard amounts of sleep night after night does more than put bags under your eyes, says Michael Norden, M.D., clinical associate professor of psychiatry at the University of Washington in Seattle. It can also reduce the levels of mood-enhancing serotonin in your brain.

10 **Check your meds.** Everybody has heard of antidepressants, but how about "prodepressants"? "Our research shows that there are medications that are quite potent in creating physiological changes that can cause depression," says Scott Patten, M.D., Ph.D., assistant professor at the University of Calgary in Alberta, Canada. Here are ones to look out for: corticosteroids (used to treat inflammation), tranquilizers and sleeping pills, and medications for high blood pressure, high cholesterol, and heart failure.

If you've been inexplicably down after starting one of these drugs, check with your doctor about trying a different medication for your problem.

10 Ways to Prevent Erection Problems

1 **Use it or lose it.** An erection supplies your penis with oxygen-rich blood, making the next erection easier to achieve. So keep track of your erection frequency. You should have at least three waking erections a week, one way or another.

2 **Do what's good for your heart.** The same things that clog up your heart also clog the arteries in your penis. So follow our prevention recommendations for heart disease, cholesterol, and weight gain. Quit smoking, and you lower your probability of impotence from 56 percent to 21 percent. And cut down on stress through exercise, relaxation techniques, or breathing exercises. Stress releases adrenalin, a hormone that can stop an erection in its tracks.

3 **In particular, maintain a regimen of aerobic exercise.** When it comes to training your body to pump blood strongly and efficiently, aerobic exercise is king. By getting in at least three good sessions a week, you go a long way toward guaranteeing that your penis is getting the flow it needs to perform.

4 **Consider taking erection-friendly supplements.** We're in the age of Viagra, but there are some natural routes you might try first. One is vitamin E. If you are not already taking it as a supplement, consider 400 IU daily, says Kenneth A. Goldberg, M.D., of the Male Health Center. A study discovered that impotent men with diabetes had significantly lower levels of vitamin E in their plasma. Since vitamin E is good for your blood vessels, all men should consider taking it, not just those with diabetes. Just one warning: Because vitamin E acts like a blood thinner, consult with your doctor before taking it in any amount if you're already using aspirin or a blood-thinning medication, such as warfarin (Coumadin), or if you're at high risk for stroke.

The herb ginkgo biloba is also worth a try since it improves circulation. Start with an extract of 80 milligrams a day, taken with meals. Ginkgo doesn't mix well with antidepressants, aspirin or nonsteroidal anti-inflammatories, or blood-thinning medications, so check the label or talk with your doctor.

5 **Some evidence links zinc to potency.** That's because zinc helps your testes create testosterone, the male hormone that, among other things, helps you maintain normal muscle mass and sperm levels. The candidates most likely to benefit from a zinc supplement are those men with moderate to severe zinc deficiencies. In the quest to shed fat, many men are shunning red meat, one of the best dietary sources of zinc. Other good sources are seafood

(especially oysters), pumpkin seeds, and whole-grain cereals. Try to get 50 milligrams of zinc each day. Since it's difficult to get this amount strictly from diet, ask your doctor about supplementation.

6 **If troubles hit suddenly, determine if the problem is physiological or psychological.** The majority of erection-problem occurrences are due to stress, exhaustion, or overwork, not a breakdown or clog inside your body. To determine if the problem is linked to your lifestyle, watch to see if you are still getting nocturnal erections. Or, see if you can manually stimulate yourself to an erection. If you can answer yes to either, relax. The problem is much more easily solved because it is entirely in your control.

7 **Admit the situation to your partner.** We know it is probably the last thing you want to do. But bring up the subject anyhow. After all, it's not like she is never going to find out. Once you put it out on the table, so to speak, the problem switches from a hidden defect or taboo topic to a challenge the two of you can work on together. That in itself can be a relief for both of you and can put the whole thing in perspective. If you have more than occasional difficulty achieving an erection, well, there are an estimated 10 million to 40 million other American men in that boat with you. There are lots of solutions, but they'll work better with a team effort.

8 **Take the pressure off yourself.** Agree to a sensual session with no penetration allowed. Just lie together naked, cuddling and caressing. Add some sensual massage if you like, with oils, powders, lights, music, the whole 9 yards. You don't have to worry about getting an erection because you don't need one. What you're accomplishing here is learning to relax in a sexual environment, so even if your day was horrid you won't let your problems get into bed with you. Do this at least twice a week.

9 **See a doctor if your erection problems appear to be physically based.** A good benchmark is no erections for a full 3 weeks. Diseases and disorders like diabetes, kidney disease, chronic alcoholism, vascular disease, and atherosclerosis account for about 70 percent of impotence cases. And the medications you take for those conditions often inhibit erections. So don't consider ongoing impotence an inconvenience. Consider it a warning sign.

10 **Consider yohimbine.** Some experts believe that the bark of this African tree has sexual bite. In one double-blind study, 450 men took 43 milligrams of yohimbine hydrochloride (Yocon) a day. Within 6 weeks, 30 percent reported that their erections returned. Much research needs to happen to verify and explain the effect. For example, only synthetic versions have proven reliable in scientific studies. Some men also face side effects. Indeed, in these days of widespread Viagra, fewer doctors are interested in yohimbine. But it is natural and available without prescription.

WEEK 5

GET HAPPY

Day 1

Call Your Siblings

Day 2

Call an Old Friend (And E-Mail Five Others)

Day 3

Assess Your Marriage—And Your Sex Life

Day 4

Commune with Your Dog

Day 5

Take a 1-Day Vacation

Day 6

Reconnect with a Mentor

Call Your Siblings

The Day's Task

We hope this is an easy task, but we know that for many guys it isn't. Do it anyhow. Tonight, you are to call each and every sibling you have. Allot 20 minutes per call. Tell them you're just checking in with them. "How ya doing? How's work? How's life? Talk to the folks lately?"

Then do some talking yourself. Answer those same questions, even if they don't get asked of you. When your sibs ask why you're really calling, tell them you just felt like talking to your brother/sister. Don't ask for favors, don't try to schedule anything, don't bring up any debts or bad blood.

If your relationship with your sibling is complex or cold, you are not excused from this task. In fact, this task is especially important for you. Strategize about how to have a cordial conversation without dredging up old issues, then make the call.

By the time you're off the phone, you should feel really good.

Think for a minute about being a brother. Friends, wives, and the contents of your produce crisper can come and go. Your siblings, on the other hand, remain constant sidecar companions on this motorcycle ride called life. They've been there since birth, and they'll be there until death. How many people can you say that about?

And don't kid yourself; as uncomfortable as it may be to admit, your siblings know you better than anyone else does. They share much of your genetic code, they grew up in the same environment, they saw you go from a squalling baby to a man. They're about the most intimate support crew a fellow could have. Don't let distance, or distant slights, get in the way.

Are you still in doubt about how much they mean to you? Then chew on this: Researchers have spent a lot of time and energy tracking the dynamics of brothers and sisters because they realize the importance of this blood

THE BYLAWS OF BROTHERS

Because you're a brother, you're expected to know the bylaws that govern your relationships with your siblings. These rules mark the difference between somebody you know and somebody you're related to. Here are some examples.

- Don't take advantage. Big chores had better mean big beer afterward.
- Don't make their spouses hate you.
- Never date your brother's ex (even if it's her idea).
- Always stop your brother from calling his ex. He'll do the same for you.
- Remember your pranks. They're never funny when they show up as reruns.
- The fights you pick are yours alone—unless you're getting pounded.
- Ask for favors, but keep track. They do.
- Get up, get dressed, and go out and get them when they run out of gas at 2:00 A.M. They called you, after all.
- Know when to keep your mouth shut.
- Bust their chops, but never over the same thing twice.
- Always make your couch available if they need a place to crash.
- Never call them by their nicknames in front of the opposite sex.
- Know when what you're asking for is too much.

bond and the way it has affected every aspect of your life. Here are some of their findings.

- Studies have shown that if one sibling is an alcoholic, the others run the risk too. And it's not just an inherited trait. An older sibling may influence his younger brethren through what are called modelling processes. Basically, these processes are what you called monkey-see, monkey-do when you were kids. This influence goes both ways too. If an older brother provides a positive, healthy role model, that behavior gets absorbed by those who follow.
- Older siblings' behavior toward sex gets passed down the line. Adolescents with sexually active big brothers and sisters were found to be 2½ times as likely to be having sex as were those with sexually inexperienced older siblings. Harkening

back to our days as love-hungry teens, we refuse to take a stand here on whether that's a good thing or a bad thing. You'll have to make that judgment yourself.

- Older siblings also play a big role in teaching you how to relate to the rest of the world. While you were annoying, teasing, and making uneasy peace with each other as you grew up, you were learning an invaluable lesson: how to empathize. You figured out what you can get away with and what you can't. That's one of the most important lessons of all because it cuts to the quick of how you get along with others.
- Not surprisingly, researchers have also found that the way you get along with family stays with you throughout life. Simply put, when you have a healthy relationship with family, you get along better with others in your life, both at work and at home. If your relationship with your family is lousy, you are more likely to be socially dysfunctional and have more health problems.

The Gulf Wars

Say your relationship with your siblings is good but suffering from a bit of neglect. Let this daily task get you stoked for staying in regular contact. If, however, there are hurts and trampled feelings to mend, it's really important that you make the effort to start getting things back on track. Here are a few things to keep in mind.

Consider the situation. First, assess how important the whole grudge match going on between you is. Take a cold, hard look and be realistic. Can you even remember what you're both being surly about?

Look within, young Skywalker. It's important to take a look at your own frame of mind before tackling someone else's. Your anger may be less about their actions than about your own insecurities. Don't let yourself off the hook. If you're at fault, admit it to yourself and move on.

Put yourself in his or her running shoes. Is there anything in your brother or sister's background that might explain why he or she treated you badly? Be honest. Were you seen as the favorite son? Were you more talented, a better student, athlete, or girl magnet? Taking this into consideration is not making excuses for your siblings, but it might help you understand their behavior.

Accept. "This doesn't mean forgive and forget," says Redford B. Williams, M.D., director of the Behavioral Medicine Research Center at Duke University Medical Center. It does mean, though, acknowledging that you and your sibling both have shortcomings and that those traits are not likely to change.

If you let time, patience, and acceptance do their magic, a closer relationship with your siblings can lead to another, lesser known benefit: more workout buddies. Having a workout buddy, especially someone to whom you're close and with whom you feel a little rivalry, is a great way to help you stick to your fitness regimen. You'll even have more defined abs, regardless of whether you make it to the gym or not. It's true: During a 3-year study, people who reported the most social support from their spouses, families, and friends were the least likely to gain weight. Researchers surmise that strong family relationships reduce stress, improve self-esteem, and lead to better health practices.

Bottom line, who else knows you for who you really are—and still talks to you? Family, that's who. Keep the lines open.

Call an Old Friend (And E-Mail Five Others)

The Day's Task

You have a two-part assignment for this evening.

1. **Go through your mental phone book and pick out a friend, a good one, a real bosom buddy, the kind of guy you'd want in your platoon if crazed terrorists suddenly stormed your town. He's also probably a guy you haven't seen as much as you'd like in the past few years. Work, wives, kids, and complacency have all conspired to keep your attention elsewhere. Call him up right now and ask him to meet you at the nearest tavern for a beer. If distance prohibits meeting, each of you should go to his respective icebox, crack open a cold one, and raise the bottle to the phone. Then talk. Catch one another up on stuff. Make plans to get together—specific ones, with dates on calendars and everything.**
2. **When you're done with that, hop on the computer and whip off a quick electronic howdy to five other friends. First, concentrate on friends who are within driving distance, then branch out to buddies who may be in other states. The idea here is to use electronic mail to break the ice and get you guys talking about getting together more often.**

Why are we so concerned with getting you out with your buddies? Because it hits you right where you live: One study estimates that having pals can gain you nearly a decade in life span. People with very poor social connections live 4.5 years less than expected, while those with very good connections live 4.5 years longer.

Also consider that ignoring your friends might just bite you in the butt. Men with high levels of stress and low levels of social support had increased amounts of prostate-specific antigen (PSA) in their blood, according to another study. PSA is the stuff your doctor checks when he wants to see if you're at risk for developing prostate cancer.

Here are another few eye-openers about the value of a good friend. As you get older, your blood pressure tends to creep upward. But scientists at the University of Utah found that people with good circles of friends had lower resting blood pressures. It turned out that people over 50 had readings almost identical to people who were much younger.

Plus, researchers found that a strong social network may help you stave off cognitive decline as you age. What that means is that lonely old-timers were twice as likely to go mentally downhill as those with close friends.

As you can see, hanging out with your pals is of premium importance. Yet one survey showed that 80 percent of men say they spend more time with their mate's friends than they do with their own. "Unfortunately, men tend to rely on women for their socialization," says Royda Crose, Ph.D., associate professor at the Fisher Institute for Wellness and Gerontology at Ball State University in Muncie, Indiana. "That doesn't give them anyone to talk to of the same sex who may be going through the same things. It generally takes a crisis before men will reach out and talk to other men. Make friends, lighten up, and talk to one another, right now. You only have one life. It's better with some friends."

Making the Case to the Missus

We hate to stereotype. Well, okay, we hate to stereotype except when it's true. And one thing that seems to be almost universally true is that our wives hate our spending a lot of time with our friends. Or they just hate our friends.

If this chapter is going to work for you, you need to bring your better half onboard. There's no point in buttressing your relationships with friends if it's going to lead to calamity at home. With a little bit of diplomacy and tact, you can spend time with friends without it costing you at home.

Here's an interesting tidbit to keep in mind: She's more jealous at certain times of the month. A study published in the *Archives of Sexual Behavior* noted that women experience more intense feelings of jealousy during the first phase (days

1 to 14) of their menstrual cycles. Plan 3-day fishing trips for the last part of her cycle and see if that helps.

Also, let her know that a number of studies have suggested that men who have close friendships also have better marriages. When you're less stressed and laughing more, it's no big surprise that you're easier to be around at home.

Use a little common sense too. Don't cancel out on important things you've planned with her in order to hit the pub with your pals. You know what else goes a long way? If you bring her a little something back from your time away. Let's say you're off at a ball game. Pick up a little something for her from the stadium gift store. Tell her it reminded you of her (make sure it's not a picture of Yogi Berra). She'll be touched that you were thinking of her even while you were with pals. That's major points for next time, buddy.

The Right Stuff

There's one thing that you really don't want to be. And that's a jerk. If you find yourself with a dwindling number of chums around you, take a hard look at the way you act. The guys probably won't tell you you're being a buffoon. They'll just avoid you.

According to a survey done by DYG, a group that tracks social trends, the following attributes are some of the things that men say they admire most in other men. They're listed in order of importance. See how you measure up.

He's dependable. Perhaps the most important trait that one man looks for in another is this: If he tells you he's going to do something, he does it, come hell or high water. Among men, there really is no higher compliment than "He's a man of his word."

"This is just a bedrock of the male code," says Ronald F. Levant, Ed.D., dean of the Center for Psychological Studies at Nova Southeastern University in Ft. Lauderdale.

He's honest. This is a direct corollary of being dependable: You know that you can trust a guy to give you a straight answer. "The need to trust is such a basic emotion," says Dr. Levant.

He rolls up his sleeves and helps out. There's an addendum to this: he also doesn't brag about how hard he has worked. He comes over and helps you move that massive wall unit, but he doesn't lord it over you for weeks.

He has a good relationship with other friends and family. Yes, we admire men

MORE FRIENDLY FACTS

The case can't be stated strongly enough: Men need friends. Here are a smattering of facts to help convince you of the same.

- Friends don't let friends drive drunk. Really. As reported in the January 1, 1998, issue of *USA Today*, a survey by the National Traffic Safety Administration and the Advertising Council showed that three out of four people have stopped a friend or family member from driving drunk. Here's how they did it. Fifty-eight percent took the keys, 31 percent drove themselves, 27 percent talked the person out of driving, 10 percent asked the person to stay overnight, 5 percent had a friend drive, and 4 percent called a cab.
- A study that monitored 7,000 Californians over 17 years found that people with no social connections were two to three times more likely to die prematurely.
- A study of 292 people hospitalized for clinical heart failure found that those who were socially isolated were much more likely to have fatal heart attacks or to be readmitted for heart problems such as angina or heart failure.
- Researchers at Carnegie-Mellon University in Pittsburgh injected 276 healthy people with the cold virus and also asked them about their relationships with spouses, parents, friends, coworkers, and social groups. The people with the most types of social interactions were less likely to develop the common cold. Even if they did catch a cold, they produced less mucus.

who work hard. But we also know that there is more to life than work. Work hard, play hard is more than a moral code for us, it's genetic code. Who cares how good a guy you are if all anyone ever sees of you is your backside headed to work?

He has a sense of humor. Fortunately, this one comes easy for us. "When men get together, there's always a lot of laughter," says Paul E. McGhee, Ph.D., of the Laughter Remedy, a firm that offers programs on humor in the workplace. "We're also very good at poking fun at others." But that's a two-way street that you'd better be able to navigate. "A lot of us are good at dishing it out but not very good at taking it," Dr. McGhee adds. There's a term for that: poor sport. Don't be one.

He's authentic, not phony. We don't expect you to be perfect—far from it. Just don't pretend to be something you're not. "It's a high concern with men not to be bogus. We have to know that a guy means what he says and says what he means," says George H. Hartlaub, M.D., associate clinical professor of psychiatry at the University of Colorado Health Sciences Center in Denver.

He's a "regular guy." You hear this term all the time. But what does it mean? Here's an example. "I created a revolving shooting target out of Barbra Streisand albums and a 12-volt motor," says Todd von Hoffman, coauthor of *The von Hoffman Brother's Big Damn Book of Sheer Manliness*. "Barbra's great because all of her albums feature these huge head shots of her." It's even more fun, he adds, when he attaches exploding caps to back of the album, near her nose. "If you hit the nose, the whole thing goes sky-high," he says.

That's being a regular guy. So when the urge to do something like that strikes you, indulge it. Better yet, call up a pal and have him come over and help you with it.

Assess Your Marriage—And Your Sex Life

The Day's Task

Go get yourself shaved and showered, big fella. You have a hot date tonight. Do what you need to do to clear your schedule this evening. Call the babysitter. Think of some impromptu options for you and your wife. This should not be a preplanned event. Spontaneity is key.

If you're a bit rusty at this kind of thing, just relax and use your imagination. If it's a nice night, go buy a checkered tablecloth, a bottle of wine, some crusty bread and some cheese, and enjoy a faux-French evening under the stars. If there's a local theater group putting on a production, go see that and follow it with coffee and cheesecake. Or just take a long walk along the river, holding hands and swigging from a hip flask filled with a good 12-year-old scotch.

Above all, do not let your wife do anything to prepare for tonight except get herself ready. If there are dishes in the sink and she's horrified that the babysitter will see them, you load them into the dishwasher. If there are snacks to pick up, you go get them. Reservations to be made? Tickets to be purchased? Money to be withdrawn? You do it all. This evening is a gift to her.

We're going to propose a theory: There are two main parts of a marriage, the time you spend out of bed and the time you spend in it. Is one more important than the other, or are they equally essential to a good relationship? We believe it's the latter. That's why we want you to assess both your marriage and your sex life in this chapter. If one is not right, neither is the other.

Why are we so concerned with your love life? There are a whole slew of reasons.

HOW ARE YOU DOING?

How is your marriage going? To help get a bead on the status of your relationship, ask yourself the following questions from the book *Fighting for Your Marriage* by Scott Stanley, Ph.D., Howard Markman, Ph.D., and Susan L. Blumberg, Ph.D. If you answer yes to one or two of these, that's fine. Everyone goes through rough patches. But if you consistently answer yes to a lot of these questions, it's a very good idea to start figuring out how you can improve your marriage. Life is too short to be miserable.

1. Do routine discussions often erupt into destructive arguments?
2. Do you or your partner often withdraw or refuse to talk about important issues?
3. Do you or your partner often disregard what the other says, or do you often use put-downs?
4. Does it seem that the things you say to your partner are often heard much more negatively than you intended?
5. Do you feel that there has to be a winner and a loser when you disagree?
6. Does your relationship often take a backseat to other interests?
7. Do you often think about what it would be like to be with someone else?
8. Does the thought of still being with your partner a few years from now disturb you?

Consider first that happily married men live an average of 6 years longer than single men. And when researchers at the Veterans Administration Medical Center in Miami checked the survival rates of 143,969 men with prostate cancer, they found that those who were married lived almost 3 years longer than those who were never married or were separated or divorced. A good reason for that may be that women play a big role in men's choices to seek out medical care. Researchers at the University of California, San Diego, found that married men were 2.4 times more likely than unmarried men to seek medical care.

Also, if you decide to chuck your marriage, you'll pay for it in more ways than alimony. Researchers found that the trauma of divorce can be bad enough to negate the health benefits of remarrying (unless some really serious abuse went on in the previous marriage). Plus, other nasty things happen. The suicide rate among divorced and separated men is 2½ times higher than that of married men. And your boy won't do so hot either. A 10-year study by the National Institute of Mental Health found that, when a father leaves, it can have a traumatic, long-lasting effect on his sons.

But enough scary stuff. It's not just that you'll live longer and healthier; most important, it's that your time here on Earth will be so much more pleasurable if you enjoy the woman next to you.

So for this one day, we want you to think a lot about your relationship with your wife. Is she your friend? Can you speak freely with her? Are you harboring lingering resentments? Are you bored with marriage or perfectly happy with it? Do you love your wife as she is today? Can you be sexually free and open with her? Be honest, and be willing to act. Nothing is more worth fighting for than a great marriage.

Love the One You're With

The reason we told you to have an impromptu night out with your wife is that it smacks of something that may be missing in your relationship: romance.

Before you start cringing at the mention of that word, bear in mind that romance has gotten a bum rap. If you think it's all about cloying novels with Fabio on the covers, boring English movies where nothing ever blows up, or fat little cherubs bouncing around, think again. It's really all about sex and fun and keeping your marriage alive and strong.

So if the mere mention of the word *romance* creates an overwhelming urge to power up your buzz saw, it's time to change your attitude. And not just for her sake.

"For crying out loud, it's about being selfish," says Gregory J. P. Godek, author of *1,001 Ways to Be Romantic*. "You want to have more sex? Have more fun? Enjoy your days more? I'll tell you how to do it—be romantic." Here's a crash course in the art of romance.

Be spontaneous. "Many women, when they say they want romance, mean spontaneity," says Godek. That's why you need to surprise your wife tonight. It's the unexpected that shocks and delights. It proves to her that you've been thinking of her when she least expects it.

Work harder at uncovering the things that turn her on. One of women's biggest complaints, says Carolyn Bushong, author of *The Seven Dumbest Relationship Mistakes Smart People Make*, is that men are stone-deaf when it comes to picking

START OFF THE NIGHT RIGHT

Want to increase your chances of a warm reception when you hit the hay? Want to enjoy the evening getting there? Here are some things you can do—or not do—to secure her amorous interest in you this very night.

Do . . .	Don't . . .
Seek her out as soon as you walk through the door.	Root through the mail or roll around with the dog first.
Give her a kiss when you find her.	Ask, "Hey, when's dinner?"
Make dinner with her.	Go near the TV or sofa.
Ask her how her day went.	Get that glazed look when she actually starts to tell you.
Wash the dishes.	Forget to take out the trash.
Rub her feet while she reads.	Say her feet stink (even if they do).
Shower and shave before heading for bed.	Go near the bedroom at all without at least brushing your teeth.

up clues. When she says, "Gosh, I love purple roses," take note, literally. Write it down and slip it into your wallet so you don't forget. Surprise her with the flowers later.

Turn off the television. Try it for just a week, says Godek. See how much time it frees up in your day to spend with the woman you love. After a week, see if you want to make this a regular habit.

Be creative in the way you love her. Ultimately, you know your wife best. You have to tailor your acts of romance to best fit your relationship. You see, when it's all boiled down, the only way she knows that you love her is by the things you do. Keep at it, and you'll notice some amazing things taking place. "Do you remember how good you felt at the beginning of the relationship?" asks Godek. "That's what it can still be like."

Sex: It's What's for Dinner

Broccoli. Salmon. Carrots. These are some of the things that are incredibly good for you. Then there's sex. As far as we're concerned, sex is the most enjoyable longevity tool out there.

Researchers who studied sexual activity and mortality in a group of 918 men found that those who had the most sex had half the risk of death from heart disease compared to their less stimulated counterparts. Seeing that the average couple has sex 2,450 times during the course of their marriage, that's a lot of chances for sexual healing.

But do anything that many times, and you run the risk of your rutting becoming routine. Then it tapers off as one or both of you lose interest. Too bad, because you'll miss out on other bodily benefits, like a healthier prostate, better quality sperm, less stress, and an expanded sense of well-being. Your penis even needs lots of erections to keep it standing at attention late into life. Here are some things you can do to keep your love life limber.

Look for the new in her. Here's the thought for the day: To know her is to never stop discovering her. Deep, eh? We picked that up from a commercial, but it's a wonderful idea that the person you've chosen to be with is, in fact, this vast, unexplored territory, replete with assets, qualities, virtues, and, yes, vices that you haven't even found yet. If you think you know her completely, think again.

"People are always changing. They're always going to surprise you if you give them the chance," says Ellen Kreidman, Ph.D., author of *Light Her Fire*. So make it a quest to find out new things about your wife. Ask her what she was doing when she heard that John Lennon had been shot. Find out what her favorite candy was as a child. Even seemingly stupid questions like this can spark discussions that will lead you to places you never knew existed.

Don't criticize; encourage. As time marches on, you may be surprised to notice how many imperfections your once-perfect partner is starting to develop. (Incidentally, she's noticing the same thing about you.) Time and gravity put a bashing on us all. But don't you ever let on. "It's surprising, the nasty things people can say to one another after they've been together for years. Most people don't even realize how cruel they can be to one another," says Dr. Kreidman.

Before you say something that will put your sex life in the deep freeze for months, ask yourself how it would have sounded coming out of your mouth during your dating years. This brings up another valuable point: you *are* still dating and courting her. You're trying to convince her to spend the rest of her life with you. Remember that.

Keep in shape. We all get older. Our bodies sprout more hair, our bellies threaten to burgeon, we "forget" to take showers every day. Just to clue you in: She still wants you to be physically attractive. "It's important to women that the men in their lives take care to look nice and to stay fit and healthy. This sends a message that you care about them enough to look good for them," says Robert

Birch, Ph.D., a psychologist in Columbus, Ohio, who specializes in marriage and sex therapy.

That doesn't mean you can never wear your ratty gray sweatpants. Just keep it to a minimum. And don't let your belly hang out.

Be on the lookout for ruts. In any long-term undertaking, always remember that complacency is the killer of passion, the birth mother of boredom. Keep your eyes peeled for danger signs like always having conversations about the same things and always spending your time together in similar ways. If you see the warning signs, act.

The world is full of happy couples celebrating 50th anniversaries and beyond. They don't have any special advantages over you; they have just chosen to work together to sustain a lifetime level of interest and wonderment about each other.

You can do it too. We'd like to see the two of you on a park bench together years from now. Just don't hog all the pigeons.

Commune with Your Dog

The Day's Task

Pay close attention. We're going to ask you to do something that requires a great deal of diplomacy if you want to live through it: Carefully, delicately find a way to suggest to your spouse that she find something to do without you—again. If she asks why, tell her that this time you want to spend some quality time with the dog. An hour or two is all you'll need—as well as a dog, of course.

If you have a different pet, you're not off the hook. You still need to spend some private time with it. No pet whatsoever? Take your kids or even yourself to a pet shop to enjoy the lizards, the birds, the fish, the snakes, the puppies. Or get to a local horse farm to walk past the stalls and rub some noses.

Let's get back to those with dogs. We assume your dog likes to play outside. Go outside with your dog and the best dog toys you have. Run together. Wrestle a little. Play some fetch with a Frisbee or a branch or a tennis ball. Walk through some wilderness and let your animal be an animal. Enjoy it. Be vocal and be physical.

Last week, we attacked stress. This week, we're going the next level: retapping into the things that you enjoy most. Well, pets are astonishing in their ability to help you enjoy life.

Scientists have verified this beyond question. Several studies show that hanging out with your pet reduces blood pressure and stress levels. One study even suggests that people perform stressful tasks better with a dog present than with their spouse. Hence, our recommendation that you give your wife the credit cards and carte blanche at the mall.

You're not the only one who stands to benefit from a closer relationship with your pooch. Your dog needs quality time too. "What we sometimes do with pets is throw them occasional emotional Milk-Bones and hope that's

CHOOSE THE RIGHT DOG

If we've inspired you to rush out and get yourself a dog, what kind of experts would we be if we didn't give a few pointers (pun intended) on choosing one? So here they are.

Let him age. A puppy should be at least 7 weeks old before he leaves his mother. Any younger, and he won't finish learning the social skills he needs to be a good pet.

Search for a breeder apart. Ask kennel clubs for the names of reputable breeders. Make sure you meet the pup's parents and size up their personalities. Buy only from a breeder who guarantees the pup's health and temperament. Or go to a shelter. You'll get a great deal and save the life of an abandoned dog. Often, shelters will let you return the dog and choose another if your original pick turns out poorly.

Don't miss demeanor. The pup should be alert and should enjoy being with people and other puppies. If he cowers or runs for cover at the slightest noise, he'll likely be easily stressed.

Size up your lifestyle. Lots of people run into trouble because they get the wrong dogs for their lifestyles. Don't fixate on a Dalmatian, for example, if you don't have the time or space to let him run often. He'll chew your house apart if he is underexercised and bored. Check with the breeder or shelter to see what the breed you're interested in is like.

enough," says Marty Becker, D.V.M., a veterinarian based in Bonner's Ferry, Idaho, and coauthor of *Chicken Soup for the Pet Lover's Soul*. But they need much more from you. "And if they're given more, they thrive in that environment," Dr. Becker adds.

Take, for example, Dr. Becker's black Labrador retriever, Sirloin. "I don't recall a time when I asked Sirloin if he wanted to go out for a walk and he responded, 'You know what, I don't feel like it today,' " Dr. Becker points out.

And speaking of walks, you've just been introduced to another great reason to pal around with your canine chum. They just soak up the kind of physical activity that you need to stay healthy and live long too. Here are a couple of great ways to raise your heart rate while lowering your stress factor.

THE MILK WITHOUT THE COW

As you consider all the benefits of dog ownership, a scuttling concern might come to mind: What happens if I can't own a dog? Lots of people live in rented properties that don't allow pets. Or you simply may not want the responsibilities that come with having a full-time pet.

No problem, we say unto you. It's not necessary to put up with fur on your couch and urine on your rugs to get some of the healthful perks of owning a pooch. "Yes, you can get the stress-relieving benefits of animals without actually owning one," says Alan M. Beck, Sc.D., coauthor of *Between Pets and People: The Importance of Animal Companionship*. Here's what he suggests.

Borrow a dog. Ask friends if they will let you walk their dogs on a regular basis. Taking a stroll with a four footer, even if he's on loan, will help dispel the psychological remnants of a crummy day at work. Your pilfered pet's owner will also appreciate your giving his dog a bonus saunter through the park.

Feed the birds. Hanging a bird feeder outside your window brings Mother Nature's finest right to your doorstep. It can also give you what Dr. Beck calls the helper's high, a feeling of doing good in some small way.

Walk on the wild side. Even a day at the zoo can help you experience some creature comforts. "Studies show that people see each other more positively when they are in the presence of animals," says Dr. Beck.

Go fish. A couple of low-maintenance goldfish may be the answer if you truly want the lazy man's way out. Watch them, feed them, and zone out to the sounds of gurgling water. It's just one more connection to nature that can help relieve stress, says Dr. Beck.

Jog your dog. You need to walk him anyway. Instead of foisting the job off on your kids or wife, take the old boy out for a 30-minute jog or walk every day. You can break it up into 15-minute sessions twice a day if you and Fido are a bit out of shape.

Play simple games. In a spin on the traditional game of fetch, you can try racing your dog to the stick. Give the stick a good heave-ho, then see who gets to it first.

If he's an aging dog and you get tired of blowing his doors off, trade up to a greyhound, Flash.

Swim with him. If it's been a while since you've been swimming with your dog, man, it's time to dust off your trunks. Not only is it a hell of a lot of fun but it's also great exercise. Take along a Frisbee, and race him to it. You'll be surprised how quickly he can motor with those skinny little paws.

Canine Therapy

We mentioned before that dogs help reduce blood pressure and stress levels. There are some other benefits we'd like to tell you about, too, as you continue in your quest for a long, healthy, happy life.

- Pets fend off loneliness. It's not going to be much fun to hit 100 if you're feeling isolated all the way there. Dogs can help. In one study at the University of California, Davis, people with pets reported feeling significantly less lonely than people living alone.
- Pet ownership has been proven to have an inverse relationship to the blues, meaning that you're a lot less likely to become depressed if you have Bowser wagging his butt off every time he sees you. According to researchers, pets can fill a combination of emotional needs, sometimes even substituting for human attachments.
- Dogs can help you meet someone new. If that's your goal, then you couldn't ask for a better matchmaker than your dog. Anyone who has ever walked a happy, curious dog down a crowded park trail knows how easy it is to strike up a conversation with another pet owner or animal lover. From there, buddy, you're on your own.

Take a 1-Day Vacation

The Day's Task

Commit these symptoms to memory: congestion, high temperature, headache, muscle pains, exhaustion, vomiting, and feces that look a lot like squid parts. Pick up the phone and recite them verbatim to your boss. They're the classic symptoms of the flu. You're calling in sick today.

After you put the telephone back on the hook, sit back for a minute. Look around the house. The kids are at school. Your wife is at work. Savor this moment; breathe in the fact that you have the whole day to do whatever you want. No e-mail, no voicemail, no regular mail to sift through. Just you and the blank slate you've created for yourself.

Maybe you want to shuffle back to bed for a few extra winks. Maybe you want to sit out on the deck with a good book. Maybe you want to head out to a diner where the waitresses call you Babe, and have a leisurely brunch with the newspaper. It's up to you, bud. This day is for you.

It's a strange thing. If you really did have the flu, nobody would think twice if you wanted a day or two off. But if you want a day to replenish your batteries, your boss may view you as warily as he would Jimmy Hoffa. Well, we're here to say that you have no reason to feel bad about taking one.

"We need to balance the efforts of working, which is a necessity to provide for the things we need in life, with recovery time to care for ourselves, to replenish our supplies of energy and rejuvenate ourselves," says James Campbell Quick, Ph.D., editor of the *Journal of Occupational Health Psychology*. It's commonly called needing a mental health day.

Yet some men find it hard to enjoy themselves because they feel guilty about playing hooky. If you're one of them, you need to get over that right now. It's impossible to get the stress-reducing, life-affirming benefits of this day if you wander around feeling guilt-ridden. "One of the reasons you're

SICK EXCUSES

Maybe you've already used the flu excuse too many times in the past to call in sick when you actually aren't. Don't let that get in the way of taking a mental health day when you really need one. You just need some fresh material.

We've done the work for you. Here's a sampling of creative excuses to inspire you. Use them at your own risk.

- Constipation has made me a walking time bomb.
- The dog ate my car keys. We're going to hitchhike to the vet.
- I just found out that I was switched at birth. Legally, I shouldn't come to work knowing that my employee records may now contain false information.
- If it's all the same to you, I won't be coming in to work. The voices told me to clean all the guns today.
- The psychiatrist said it was an excellent session. He even gave me this jaw restraint so I won't bite things when I am startled.
- I can't come in to work today because I'll be stalking my previous boss, who fired me for not showing up. Okay?

taking a mental health day is that you're out of gas, emotionally and psychologically," says Dr. Quick. "You could say that, at one level, you are legitimately sick. So the day off becomes one of recovery and rejuvenation."

The European Solution

It's no wonder that you need some extra time to stress out. Consider that Americans lag way behind other developed countries in taking time off. Most of us get a measly 10 vacation days a year, or 2 weeks. If you lived in Sweden, you'd get an average of 30 vacation days, or 6 weeks, annually. In France, the average is 25 days; and in Britain, it's 22 days. Germans get an average of 18 vacation days.

Still feel bad? Then remember that it's your physical health on the line too. How effective are you going to be at work if you let stress sock you with a real illness, like heart disease?

Time away from work is one of the most powerful stress blasters in the world, says Paul J. Rosch, M.D., president of the American Institute of Stress. Most of us, he adds, don't put a high enough priority on making time away from the job a primary way of breaking up stress in our lives.

The result is that your perfectly good day off gets watered down by feelings of wasting time and angst over missing work. "It's sad that we turn what should be a soothing time into a seething time," says Steve Allen Jr., M.D., of the State University of New York in Syracuse. "On my free time, I really have to make a conscious effort to let go."

Taking Your Time

If you truly hate saying that you're sick when you aren't, you can still work the 1-day vacation into your work schedule. It's a valuable tool even if you can't bring yourself to take a spontaneous day all for yourself. Here are a few strategies to take the day you need without telling a white lie.

Plan ahead. Ask for a mental health day well in advance of when you'll need it. If you are about to tackle a difficult, time-consuming project with a short deadline, ask at the onset for a day off after the deadline. A boss who knows you are taking on a big workload is less likely to begrudge you a day to decompress. A more forward-thinking one might even take a hint and give you a comp day.

Consider telling the truth. Sure, it sounds crazy, but it just might work. When you call in sick, simply say you are fatigued and taking a day off to rejuvenate yourself. But do so only if you have a good rapport with your employer. If he screams at you to get your lazy can into work, your chances of reducing stress are shot.

Take a vacation day. This is a tough option to consider. You already know how precious vacation time is. But maybe you work for a company with a generous time-off policy. If that's the case, go ahead and take a vacation day. That way, you don't have to explain to anyone why you are taking the day off.

Be ready to work. Regardless of whether you are candid or deceptive about the true reason for your day off, the next day go back to work enthused and productive. You'll feel better about the previous day off, and your boss will too. You may even be more productive than usual during the rest of the week.

Whatever your method, do make sure you take a mental health day when you need it. Not only do you deserve it but also your body and soul require it. And if you happen to take one next March 22, look around the golf course for us. That date is, after all, International Goof-Off Day.

Reconnect with a Mentor

The Day's Task

Do you want paper or plastic? Because you have the choice here. You can either go out and buy the book *Tuesdays with Morrie* by Mitch Albom or you can head down to the video store and rent the movie by the same name.

Seriously, that's your task today. Free up a couple of hours tonight and read the book or watch the movie. It's a short book, so you should be able to finish it in an evening.

What you'll read (or see) is the true story of a man and his mentor. The titular Morrie was Albom's university professor, Morrie Schwartz, 20 years before the events being narrated. As the story unfolds, Albom hooks back up with his mentor in the fading days of the older man's life.

It will not only remind you of the affection and gratitude you felt for someone similar in your past but also convince you of the need to reconnect with that same person.

How important is a mentor, now that you're all grown up and shaving on your own? History has proven over and over again that it's exceptionally important. Sigmund Freud mentored Carl Jung. Socrates mentored Plato. Annie Sullivan mentored Helen Keller. Heck, Obi Wan mentored Luke.

And it all started with an ancient Greek legend. The first mentor was an ordinary household employee. As the story goes, the head of the household, Odysseus, was about to depart on a long journey when he asked a trusted employee to advise and counsel his young son while he was away. The worker's name? You guessed it: Mentor.

This is interesting but still doesn't answer the question of why a chapter on mentors would be in a book about living longer and healthier. The answers, of course, are pretty straightforward.

- A mentor helps you acknowledge that you are still growing, still learning, still in need of wisdom. You believe that you have yet to achieve your greatest you, that you are still on an upward trajectory. This youthful attitude alone can help add years to your life.
- A mentor helps you feel connected. You have a person—other than your wife, we hope—with whom you can speak openly and candidly. Plenty of research has shown the positive mental and physical benefits of having a person you can confide in, rather than keeping all issues and emotions to yourself.
- A mentor helps you do better in life. What's an athlete without a coach? Work life isn't that different. If you are all on your own, how can you know what's best for you? We can ask our bosses or read books, but a real-live coach who's been there and done that, well, it can make all the difference.

And speaking of sports, let us tell you a story about John McSherry. Maybe you don't immediately recall that name, but chances are, you remember how he died. National League home plate umpire John McSherry called a time-out just seven pitches into the Cincinnati Reds' 1996 season opener. He took a few steps toward the backstop and motioned for help. Then, in a horrifying moment that was broadcast again and again on the evening news, McSherry fell face first to the ground.

The 400-pound, 51-year-old umpire was pronounced dead of a massive heart attack an hour later. "He lived and died an umpire," says "Big John" McSherry's best friend and fellow umpire, Eric Gregg.

Let's rewind to the period before Big John's death. In 1971, McSherry was Gregg's instructor and mentor at umpire school. John "was like a father figure to me. He gave me a lot of advice," recalls Gregg. And of all the lessons that he learned from John McSherry, perhaps the most important one, is that life can end as quickly as a fastball crossing the plate.

Even after his death, Gregg reaps the benefits of McSherry's tutelage. In the 18 months after watching his friend die, Gregg lost 105 pounds, allowing him to cut his heart and blood pressure medication in half. He now walks 5 to 8 miles at least five times a week and swims an hour every day. Gregg no longer skips breakfast and at lunch forgoes Philly cheese steaks and burgers, replacing them with salad, a slice of bread with tuna, and a diet soda.

That's the amazing thing about mentors. When they do things right, you learn from them. And when they do things wrong, you still end up a wiser man.

How to Become a Mentor

We're hoping that today's task of reading a book or watching a movie will move you to action. Specifically:

- To get on the phone or send an e-mail to someone who mentored you in the past, and to spark up the conversation again. At minimum, just say thanks and let him know how far you've come.
- To decide if you still need mentoring in some aspect of your life. First, identify the areas where you want help. Second, identify someone from whom you'd feel comfortable receiving help, preferably someone who has weathered similar storms but who is not in the same office or situation. Third, ask that person if he or she would be willing to help you. Extend an invitation to have lunch once a week, perhaps. Don't call it a mentor-protégé relationship; just call it asking for advice. Let the relationship develop or dissolve on its own, unburdened by a formal title.
- To become a mentor yourself. We're really hoping that you'll be so impressed with the way mentors have improved your life that you'll want to do the same for someone else. If that happens, you'll be doing a very, very good thing.

In 1992 and 1993, some 959 boys and girls in 8 states took part in a historic experiment. All were between the ages of 10 and 16. Half were matched up with a Big Brother or Big Sister. The other half were assigned to a control group, where they were put on a waiting list. The matched children met with their mentors an average of three times a week.

And, brother, did those kids do well. Compared to the control group, the matched kids were 46 percent less likely to begin using drugs, 27 percent less likely to begin using alcohol, 53 percent less likely to skip school, more confident in their ability to perform schoolwork, less likely to hit someone, and more likely to get along better with their families. This was all because of people like you.

In a 1989 Louis Harris poll, 73 percent of students said their mentors helped raise their goals and expectations. Fifty-nine percent of mentored students improved their grades.

It's amazing, isn't it? Mentoring can mean the difference between success and failure for a generation of kids at risk. All it takes is for you to be yourself with your young protégé.

We haven't even mentioned how you'll benefit by becoming a mentor. And you know what? We probably don't need to. See you at the ballpark.

10 Ways to Deal With Headaches

1 **Give your head a soothing massage.** Headaches are often caused by tension or emotional states like anxiety, anger, or repressed hostility. A good way to fight back when one strikes is to massage the tensed muscles, says Fred Sheftell, M.D., director of the New England Center for Headache in Stamford, Connecticut. Feel behind your earlobes for the ridges of bone there and rub on both sides of your head for 10 minutes. Do the same with your temples, then the muscles along the back of your neck. These are major tension spots where muscles can tighten and cause headaches.

2 **When a headache hits, drink a cup of coffee.** You already knew to take a painkiller like aspirin or ibuprofen, but wash it down with a cup of coffee, says Glen Solomon, M.D., a headache expert and consultant to the Cleveland Clinic. Studies have shown that the drugs are more effective when combined with caffeine. This works well even when the headache isn't caused by tension. Several powerful over-the-counter painkillers, such as Excedrin Migraine, contain caffeine for this reason. If you are using a medicine that contains caffeine, skip the coffee so you don't double your caffeine intake.

3 **Give exercise a try to see if it works for you.** Some guys find that exercise can relieve the pain in their heads, says Joseph P. Primavera III, Ph.D., a psychologist at the Jefferson Center in Philadelphia. But others say it makes their headaches worse. If exercising actually makes your head pain worse, stop. If it does help, though, it will save you a trip to the drugstore.

Regular exercise can keep you from getting a whopper in the first place. Exercise builds up your cardiovascular system, slows your heart rate, and makes you more resistant to stress. It also bumps up the levels of serotonin, a neurotransmitter that improves your mood and helps manage headaches.

4 **As a preventive measure, sit up straight and watch your posture.** If you're hunched over a keyboard or circuit board all day, you put a lot of pressure on your neck. A headache is soon to follow. To head it off, every so often, turn your head to the left, then right. Bring it center, then move your chin down toward your chest, then back and upward.

5 **To help relax facial muscles, take a deep breath or two.** You already know that tension is the main culprit behind your throbbing noggin. You can relieve that tension and prevent the pain by using a simple relaxation technique three or four times a day, says Lawrence Robbins, M.D., director of the Robbins Headache Clinic in Northbrook, Illinois. Practice deep breathing

for a minute or so each time. Sit in a comfortable chair, rest your hands lightly on your belly, and close your eyes. Mentally count to four, inhaling for the entire time, then exhale to the count of four. Make sure you breath into your belly, not the top of your lungs. Avoid lifting your shoulders or expanding your chest; that's a sign of shallow breathing.

6 **Eat cold foods strategically.** An ice cream headache is sudden and stabbing. But you can avoid them, writes Joseph Hulihan, M.D., assistant professor of neurology at Temple University Health Sciences Center in Philadelphia. These types of headaches likely are caused by the sudden chilling of the back of your palate. So the next time you're face down in a banana split, savor the ice cream in the front part of your mouth. Let it melt a bit before you swallow.

7 **Soothe sinus headaches with a facial massage.** If a sinus cold has your brain pounding, try another type of massage, suggests Robert A. Edwards of the Somerset School of Massage Therapy. Using your fingers, massage in a circular motion starting between your eyebrows, above your nose. Slowly move the massaging motion out toward the sides of your head. Then massage right below your eyebrows, at the tops of your eye sockets. Do this several times on each eyebrow.

8 **Learn to detect the signs of an impending migraine.** A migraine often gives a useful warning signal that it's on the way, says Egilius Spierings, M.D., Ph.D., a neurologist in Wellesley Hills, Massachusetts. For example, you may experience auras, things like seeing flashing lights or squiggly lines. Or you may feel tingling in your arms and hands. When that happens, grab a paper bag. Stick your face in it and breathe for a few minutes. When you do this, you rebreathe some of the air you exhaled, building up the carbon dioxide levels in your blood. This, in turn, helps fend off migraines.

9 **Pull the shades to block out sunshine.** Since light aggravates migraine symptoms, lie down in a dark room, says Dr. Solomon. While you're lying there, put an ice pack wrapped in a towel or a cold compress on your pounding head. That will soothe swollen, pulsing blood vessels until the pain subsides.

10 **Avoid overmedicating yourself, or face a rebound headache.** Headache medications work by shrinking the blood vessels around your brain, relieving the pressure. But after the medication wears off, blood vessels swell again, which means the pain can return, causing you to pop even more pills. "People with chronic headaches who overmedicate can go from having a headache every 3 to 4 days to having headaches every day," Dr. Robbins warns. If this describes you, see your doctor to work out a program to wean you off the medications. "There are many people who have gone from, say, six Excedrin a day down to two a day and their headaches have gone away."

10 Ways to Prevent Heartburn

1 **For at least 3 hours after eating, avoid lying down.** Heartburn is caused when stomach acid leaks up through the valve dividing your stomach from your esophagus, called the esophageal sphincter. When you stay upright, gravity helps keep acid down and out of your esophagus, which isn't designed to handle it. Instead of heading to bed or crashing on the couch after supper, sit at the table with your wife and arm wrestle, actually do the dishes for a change, or get out of the house for a walk.

2 **Trim down your center.** Too much weight, especially around your midsection, may tip the scales in favor of your getting heartburn. The extra weight can weaken the esophageal sphincter, plus increase pressure in your abdomen, forcing stomach acid upward. If you trim away unneeded pounds, you may reduce your heartburn attacks. You may find that riding a bike is a good way to exercise without sloshing your belly around; if you're out of shape, start out with short distances and build up.

3 **Be sure your clothes aren't pinching into your midsection.** Tight waistbands can also increase pressure that forces acid upward, says M. Michael Wolfe, M.D., coauthor of *Heartburn: Extinguishing the Fire Inside*. If you're a size-36 man, don't just cram yourself into those 34 pants and hope for the best—buy some bigger pants or, better yet, lose weight.

4 **Avoid fatty foods.** Greasy foods make your stomach empty out slower, putting more pressure on that crucial valve, says Gary Green, M.D., associate team physician of intercollegiate athletics at UCLA. If you're at a loss for where to start, trim out fried items; they're big offenders.

5 **Become a more choosy eater.** Several specific foods can make heartburn worse, either because they weaken your esophageal sphincter, trigger too much acid production in your stomach, or contain too much acid themselves. Here's what you should avoid: alcohol, carbonated drinks, tomatoes, spicy foods, chocolate, caffeine, citrus fruits, coffee and tea (even decaf), whole-milk dairy products, garlic, onion, and mint or minty candies.

6 **Munch on some gum to head off heartburn.** Gum stimulates saliva, which pours down your throat with natural antacid properties that help quell the burn, Dr. Wolfe says. Be sure to avoid mint-flavored gum. And if you pick a sugar-free type, remember that the artificial sweetener sorbitol can cause gas and diarrhea, so you'll want to chew no more than two or three sticks containing the chemical.

7 **Quit smoking.** If you're interested enough in living a long life to read this book about it, you know plenty of reasons not to smoke. Avoiding heartburn is another one. Smoking inhibits saliva, increases stomach acid, and weakens the esophageal sphincter, contributing to heartburn. So if you smoke, stop. If you're a nonsmoker, stay that way.

8 **Eat politely.** When mom told you to sit at the table and eat like a nice young man, she was probably more concerned about her tablecloth than your future heartburn risk. But she was dispensing good health advice, say Stanley Lorber, M.D., former chairman of the gastroenterology department at Temple University, and Joyann Kroser, M.D., gastroenterologist at the University of Pennsylvania School of Medicine, both in Philadelphia. Eat small portions so your stomach won't have to create so much acid to dissolve the load it's just been given.

Eat slowly so you'll be less likely to eat too much. If you have to, eat with chopsticks or put the fork in the hand you rarely use.

Finally, chew your food thoroughly. When you put big chunks of food into your stomach, it has to secrete more acid to break it down. This acid could come up to haunt you.

9 **Boost your bed.** By elevating the head of your bed a few inches, you can help keep stomach acid from trickling back into your esophagus as you sleep, Dr. Green says. Make sure that whatever you use—be it blocks of wood, bricks, or anything else—will securely hold up your bed regardless of your activities.

10 **Drink plenty of water with your meals and between meals too.** Water rinses acid down out of your esophagus and dilutes the acid in your stomach, which can bring you temporary relief, says Norman Goldberg, M.D., a gastroenterologist at the University of California, San Diego, School of Medicine. Be sure to drink the quantity of water that experts recommend—eight 8-ounce glasses daily—so you can spread out relief throughout the day.

WEEK 6

ACTIVATE YOUR MEDICAL SUPPORT TEAM

Day 1
Assess Your Genetics

Day 2
Get a Physical

Day 3
Go to the Dentist

Day 4
Assess Your Weight

Day 5
Assess Your Strength

Day 6
Monitor Your Body

Assess Your Genetics

The Day's Task

Break out your family photo album and unwrap a fresh pack of sticky notes. For all the family members you see—we're talking aunts, uncles, grandparents, and first cousins, primarily—jot down on a separate sticky note each person's name, what significant diseases or health conditions they have, and at roughly what age they developed them. If a relative has died, write down the cause, along with the age at death.

If you need information to fill in blanks or clue you in on specifics, call your parents or other older relatives. It's odd, but they often seem to love talking about this stuff.

When you have notes on all your relatives, transfer them to a clean sheet of paper and keep it in a safe place. As you're about to find out, this information will be very useful to you.

From the moment we're born, our parents and older relatives are incessantly comparing us to the rest of the family tree. By the age of 5, you probably knew you had your grandfather's eyes, your mom's earlobes, Uncle Tommy's stubborn streak, and a host of other inherited traits. You can't blame the old folks for doing that. It gave them a small sense of immortality to see family resemblances in you. It meant that some part of them would still live on, even after they died.

But if they really wanted to do you a favor, your family should have told you that you might have inherited grandpa's high blood pressure, mom's tendency toward cancer, and Uncle Tommy's weakness for liquor. Along with the obvious traits, you've inherited a legacy that you can't see, tendencies and predispositions that exist on a genetic level and put you at greater risk for certain health problems, such as heart disease, cancer, and many other ailments.

That's why it's important to know your family's medical history. This history can give you and your doctor an idea of your future health and your family's health too. It gives you a faintly traced map of what lies ahead for you. It doesn't tell you all the potholes and sidetracks, but it does point out a few major road hazards that you can detour around, provided you have enough of a heads up about them.

Specifically, learning what conditions and diseases tend to crop up in your family can:

- Lead you to change your lifestyle and possibly avoid a hereditary ailment that would otherwise have smacked you head-on
- Arm you with valuable information for your next doctor's visit
- Show you what issues you need to watch for in your kids as they get older, and help them work with their genetic legacy

A Quick and Simple Genetic Primer

Your body is composed of billions of cells. Nearly each and every one of these cells, regardless of where they are in your body, contains an identical copy of 46 chromosomes, also known as your DNA.

Half of these chromosomes came from mom and half came from dad when you were conceived (but let's not think too vividly about that). Each chromosome, which looks like a long thread, contains about 80,000 genes. These genes determine a great deal of what you look like, who you are, and how well you'll age. That includes what sort of ailments will come your way too.

To some degree, virtually all diseases have a genetic link, says Reed E. Pyeritz, M.D., Ph.D., professor of human genetics at Allegheny University of the Health Sciences in Pittsburgh. Alzheimer's disease, heart disease, stroke, and most types of cancer are some of the most common and the most dangerous inherited illnesses, but they're by no means the only ones.

How do invisible little genes contribute to, say, cancer? Let's look at a hypothetical friend, whom we'll call Bob. One of the genes in Bob's cells is supposed to produce replacement cells as part of normal body maintenance. But the gene and a few thousand others like it turn out to be faulty. They makes cells faster and faster. Cells start to pile up and can eventually grow into a tumor.

But even if Bob has inherited some haywire genes, it doesn't mean he's destined to die of cancer. "Genes cock the gun, but the environment pulls the trigger," says Jan Breslow, M.D., professor of genetics at Rockefeller University in New York

City. That means Bob can take steps to protect himself if he knows what to watch for. You can, too, if you start keeping track of your family's medical history.

Putting History to Work

Once you've put your family health information on paper, be sure to use it to your best advantage. Here's how.

- Take it to your doctor. When you go in for your next physical, be sure to take your family history with you. Your doctor will be able to use it to determine which medical tests and screenings you need to undergo, which lifestyle changes you need to begin, or even which preventive drugs you should start taking.
- Don't pull your triggers. If colon cancer runs in your family, be sure to eat a low-fat, high-fiber diet. That means less ice cream and more beans, fruits, and wheat-bran cereals.

  If you have a lot of diabetics in your family tree, you have an extra responsibility to keep your weight down and avoid high-sugar, high-fat foods.

  If cancer runs in your family, it's really time to ditch the cigarettes. Actually, that should be a priority even if the disease doesn't pick on your family. There's no need to make yourself the first victim.

  If heart disease among the kinfolk worries you, start yourself on the path to healthy living. Don't smoke. Eat more fruits and vegetables and fewer fatty foods. Exercise at least 30 minutes a day, and practice stress-relieving techniques. These strategies will do you more good than will worrying about your genes, suggests Ichiro Kawachi, M.D., Ph.D., associate professor of health and social behavior at the Harvard School of Public Health.
- Pass it on. The genetic material you inherited didn't stop with you. Your kids have some of it too. Use what you know to guide them into healthy eating and exercise habits. Teach them to watch for signs that may indicate they've inherited a health problem.
- Finally, for the love of God, *don't* throw yourself headlong into bad habits just because you think a hereditary disease is going to get you anyway. If you're going to make a self-fulfilling prophecy, predict that your healthy practices will let you age well, despite whatever obstacles your forefathers put in your path.

Get a Physical

The Day's Task

Way back in the beginning of this book, we asked you to set up an appointment for today with your family doctor for a thorough health checkup. If you did this, then we are . . . stunned. If you didn't, today is the day to do it. Get on the phone and ask for an appointment, even if you feel great, even if you have a deathly fear of long needles, even if—horror of horrors—your insurance doesn't cover it. It is that important.

The tests you'll receive will vary, depending in part on your age and the last time you were examined. Use this time with the physician to discuss any symptoms you've been having, however minor. Ask for pointers on ways you can improve the way you're taking care of yourself. Ask about all those alternative remedies your wife or girlfriend has been taking. Get your money's worth out of the visit.

Physicals are never going to be as jolly and fun as those heartwarming doctor's office scenarios that Norman Rockwell was always painting. But checkups take up just an hour or two of your time each year, and they can save you from a world of hurt later.

You can think of it like Plato did when he declared that "the life which is unexamined is not worth living." But we'd rather use a car metaphor: Most guys don't wait to maintain their cars until the engines lock up or the brakes start screeching, says Kenneth A. Goldberg, M.D., of the Male Health Center. Instead, we take them for regular inspections and oil changes. It's smarter and cheaper in the long run. Same goes for your body. It's better to, say, bring down high cholesterol than perform a double bypass.

So your mission for today is to let the doctor check your signs, make sure everything is still working smoothly, and help ensure that your body will be running for years to come. The following maintenance schedule gives you an overview of the tests you should anticipate as you age. Your doctor may recommend different tests at earlier times if your symptoms, your personal health history, or your family tendencies call for them, Dr. Goldberg says.

Physical Examination

We hate to scare you, but physicals these days often require two visits to the clinic. Visit one can be termed the fluid-extraction day: you'll give blood samples and pee in a cup. You may have an electrocardiogram to map your heart pattern (we'll explain more about this on page 192). The idea here is to run the basic, universal lab tests so that when you meet with your doctor, he'll already have the results.

Once you get to the doctor, he or she will examine your vital signs and your medical history and discuss your health habits and any medical problems that run in your family. (The family information you compiled yesterday will be very useful now.) You can expect the doctor or a nurse to start by checking your weight, pulse, and blood pressure.

Your physician will likely also make sure your eyes and ears are working well, listen to your chest for heart or lung troubles, inspect your skin for signs of cancer, and prod your abdomen to check the condition of some of your internal organs. The doctor is also likely to feel the areas where your lymph nodes are clustered to check for swelling; check you for a hernia; examine your testicles and penis for growths; test your reflexes and muscle strength; feel your chest for lumps; listen to the pulse in your neck; and feel your thyroid, also in your neck.

Be sure that you tell your doctor all your health complaints and symptoms. The physician is probably the only person who truly cares, other than maybe your mother, and this is the best time to tell him.

You'll need a physical exam every 3 years in your twenties and thirties, every year or two in your forties, and every year from then on.

Blood and Urine Tests

From just a few squirts of your fluids, your doctor can check you for high cholesterol, diabetes, and problems in your liver, prostate, and kidneys. You can also find out if your blood is brimming with the right number of platelets and red and white blood cells. Your doctor can check for HIV if you want too.

A test of your levels of homocysteine, an amino acid that appears to contribute to heart disease by helping cholesterol build up in your arteries, may become common in the near future, Dr. Goldberg says.

Get these done every 3 years in your twenties and thirties, every year or two in your forties, and every year from then on. You should have your blood tested for the prostate-specific antigen (PSA), which points to prostate problems, every year from your fifties onward, suggests Dr. Goldberg.

Electrocardiogram

When your heart beats, it puts out a faint electrical signal that your doctor can observe with equipment hooked to electrodes taped to your body. You'll learn if your heart is beating properly and even if you've previously had an undiagnosed heart attack. You may be asked to walk on a treadmill while hooked up to the machine to test your heart while it's under the stress of exercise.

You should have one of these done every 4 years in your forties and every 3 years from your fifties onward. If you're at high risk for heart problems, get one in your twenties and one in your thirties as well.

Rectal Exam

Gulp. Set aside the embarrassment and discomfort of this test for a moment and remember that a regular rectal exam can save you from major discomfort and serious illness over time.

With one very perceptive (and gloved) finger, the doctor can check you for hemorrhoids, rectal cancer, and prostate problems. Your doc can also remove a bit of stool to test for hidden blood that can point to colon cancer or polyps.

If you get this done as part of your visit, do it first so you won't dread it the whole time you should be concentrating on working with the doctor. As it begins, relax your entire body and ponder the following thought: "By doing this, I'm helping to ensure that I'll be around to spend my retirement savings." Repeat a few times and it'll be over. You need this exam annually after you turn 40.

Blood Pressure Exam

High blood pressure, known in lab-coat terminology as hypertension, is a silent disease with no symptoms. But leave it unattended, and you're just asking for all sorts of serious complications like hardened arteries, eye damage, stroke, heart attack, and kidney failure.

Here's a quick blood pressure decoder. The top number is a measurement of the pressure when your heart contracts and sends blood out into the arteries. It should be 140 or less. The bottom number measures the pressure as your heart refills with blood. It should be 90 or greater.

Avoid coffee before this test, as it can boost your numbers by as much as five points. Have your blood pressure checked at least every 2 years throughout your life.

Tuberculosis Test

This bacterial disease was a real killer back in the days when they called it consumption, but for a while mankind had nearly vanquished the bug. Unfortunately, it's back with a vengeance, and now it's more powerful since many strains have become resistant to drugs.

You can take a simple test in which the doctor pricks your skin to see if you've been exposed to tuberculosis (TB). If you've been infected, you can start taking medications to get rid of it *before* you get sick.

Get a TB test every 5 years, starting in your twenties.

Sigmoidoscopy

You can learn a lot about the inside of a house by looking through the back door, and that's the principle at work behind this test. The doctor will insert a flexible scope into your rectum and lower colon to observe your inner landscape on a TV monitor and look for polyps, growths that can lead to cancer. If it makes it easier, distract yourself with the thought we suggested for the rectal exam.

Get this every 3 to 5 years in your fifties and beyond.

If polyps are discovered during the sigmoidoscopy or if you have symptoms or a family history of colon cancer, your doctor likely will schedule a colonoscopy. This is done under anesthetic and involves an exam of the entire colon.

Chest X-Ray

If you smoke, stop. Until you quit, get a chest X-ray every year after you turn 45. If you don't smoke, great, you're off the hook on this one.

Shots

Regularly introducing your body to a hypodermic-wielding nurse can help you avoid several maladies. Get a flu shot each October and a tetanus booster every 10 years. Also, ask your doctor if you have a particular need for a pneumonia vaccine, which is typically recommended for people ages 65 and older.

Go to the Dentist

The Day's Task

Today's task is particularly easy, and we hope you've had a lot of practice. Pick up the phone, call your dentist's office, and make an appointment for your regular cleaning and checkup. Ask for the next available appointment, even if it's early in the morning. Then go. Your exam should include a check of your entire mouth, including your gums, your tongue, and the top of your throat, especially if you use tobacco.

Be sure to make your time in the chair an interactive experience. Ask the dentist and hygienist for any advice they can offer on better ways you can brush, floss, or use other techniques to keep your mouth healthy. Ask that they watch you as you practice the techniques right there in the office. Finally, ask about any irregularities that you've spotted in your mouth.

Don't feel silly asking for help. After all, you're paying for their time. And the information they give you can add years to your teeth and quite possibly your life.

Before you leave the office, make another appointment to come back in 6 months.

Not too far back in our history, keeping your teeth wasn't such a serious issue. Until the last few generations, losing a few choppers—or even all of them—was just another fact of life. Not so coincidentally, up until the early 1900s, men were lucky to see the age of 50. Make no mistake, their dental health and, just as important, their attitude toward dental health played a role.

It's a simple, logical progression. The healthier your mouth is, the more teeth you keep. The more teeth you keep, the more balanced a diet you can eat. The better you eat, the healthier you stay and the longer you live.

Dentistry has evolved in a few ways since you were a child. Today, the goal of dentistry is to help patients keep all their natural teeth for their entire lives. To help achieve that, dentists place more emphasis on gum health than a few decades ago. In fact, some dentists say that for adults, flossing, which benefits gums more than teeth, is just as important as brushing. That's a shift. The reasons are compelling, as you'll see below.

The goals of dentistry have shifted for many patients as well. In these modern times in which so many of us are in more interactive, entrepreneurial jobs, personal hygiene and appearance are of far greater importance to our careers than in the more industrial days of our fathers. Whether we like it or not, our teeth make a major statement about who we are and how we care for ourselves. It's no wonder that most dentist offices now have posters and promotions for teeth-whitening services hanging on every wall and door.

One other shift that has occurred is responsibility. It is up to the patient, not the dentist, to take control of his dental health. As with any type of health regimen, it is the daily actions you take that matter, not the once-in-a-blue-moon dentist visits. This is why we say you can and should talk to your dentist and his staff during your infrequent visits. Granted, it's hard to carry on a conversation at the dentist's office, what with you lying prone in the chair while latex-covered fingers and metal tools poke around your mouth. But when you can speak, you should ask questions—lots of them.

"Too many people don't really feel they have a lot of ownership of their teeth. They take themselves to the dentist's office and absolve themselves of any responsibility," says Matthew Messina, D.D.S., consumer advisor for the American Dental Association. "But I try to create an environment in my office where it's okay to be more involved and to ask questions."

A proactive dental patient is most likely to keep his teeth in his head for the rest of his life. A passive guy leads to passive dental care, and that's the fast track to dental disease, which, trust us, you don't want.

When Bacteria Bite Back

Because all sorts of things go into your mouth, it's easy for roving bacteria to get a foothold in those crevices between your teeth and under your gumline. Once they do that, they'll grow. Before you know it, the bacteria form a sticky film called plaque that can harden into a substance called tartar. Left long enough, plaque and tartar can irritate your gums in a condition called gingivitis.

Gingivitis isn't fun. Your gums might bleed when you floss, and they might ache from the infection. But it gets worse. Left to fester, this minor gum disease can work itself into a major periodontal problem, dissolving the bones beneath your teeth, causing them to loosen and fall out or turn rotten and require pulling.

The situation can get even worse than that. When you have gum disease, bacteria can easily enter your bloodstream, contributing to blood clots and narrow blood vessels and increasing your risk for a heart attack. Research has clearly confirmed this.

But if you can avoid all of that by asking your dentist to, uh, drill you on the finer points of oral health, can you think of any reason why you shouldn't? Neither can we.

Brushing and Flossing 101

Since you see your dentist only twice a year, we thought we'd include some tips for the other 363 days you'll be caring for your teeth solo.

Brushing. Brush your teeth twice a day with a soft-bristled toothbrush that you use gently. Using a stiff brush and a strong forearm may be good for, say, cleaning burnt sauce off your barbecue grill, but it's not good for your teeth. Too much power while brushing can wear away your gums, making your teeth more sensitive and opening an entrance for invading bacteria. That's what you're trying to avoid in the first place. One effective trick is to hold your toothbrush like a pencil. That pretty much guarantees the right amount of pressure.

A quick once-over with your toothbrush isn't going to do the job. Each time you brush your teeth, go at it for 2 to 3 minutes. Squirt on some fluoride toothpaste, which helps prevent tooth decay, and follow the American Dental Association's brushing directions.

1. Place your toothbrush at a 45-degree angle against your teeth, with the brushing surface pointed toward your gums.
2. Gently move the brush back and forth in short strokes.
3. Brush the outer tooth surfaces, the inner sides, and the chewing surfaces.
4. Use the tip of the brush to clean the inner sides of your front teeth, using an up-and-down stroke.
5. Brush your tongue to dislodge bacteria.

Flossing. Flossing hits the areas between your teeth, where the toothbrush can't reach. If you want to avoid gum disease, you're going to have to floss at least daily, along with brushing. It doesn't matter which kind of floss you choose—

waxed, unwaxed, plain, or flavored. Experiment to see which kind you like. If you do all your mouth work at one time, floss first, brush second.

Here's how to use floss.

1. Take about 24 inches of floss and wrap most of it around one of your middle fingers. Wrap the rest around the middle finger of your other hand.
2. Pinch the floss between your thumbs and forefingers. With a gentle rubbing motion, guide the floss between your teeth. Don't snap it forcefully into your gums; that causes unnecessary bleeding, and it hurts.
3. Curve the floss into a C shape against one tooth and slide it into the space between gum and tooth.
4. Press the floss tightly against the tooth and rub it up and down, essentially cleaning crud off it like scraping dead bugs from your windshield with the squeegee at the gas station.
5. Repeat on the rest of your teeth, including the very back ones.

Here are some other hints to keep your mouth in mint condition.

- For a super blast of germ-nuking power, use a shot of hydrogen peroxide. After brushing to break up the plaque, swish a bit of peroxide over your teeth. Then, spit it out and rinse your mouth with plenty of water. The peroxide doesn't taste too bad and has the same foaming effect as when you pour it on a cut. Just make sure not to swallow any of it.
- Eat plenty of foods rich in vitamin C, like fresh broccoli, peppers, pineapple, oranges, and grapefruit, suggests Irwin Mandel, D.D.S., director of clinical research for dentistry at Columbia University School of Dental and Oral Surgery in New York City. Scientific evidence suggests that the vitamin can strengthen weak gum tissue and make the gum lining more resistant to bacteria, which makes swelling, bleeding, and tooth loss less likely.
- Consider using an electric toothbrush or mouth-cleaning device. The American Dental Association gives its formal approval to gizmos that work well, so look for an endorsement on the package. However, understand that electronic mouth-cleaning tools won't do a better job than a good old-fashioned brushing. Their value lies solely in the convenience. If they make teeth cleaning easier for you, that's the benefit, which is plenty good enough.

Assess Your Weight

The Day's Task

Get a pencil, a tape measure, a sheet of paper, a bathroom scale, and a calculator. You're going to figure your body mass index, a number that can help you determine if you're overweight or underweight.

First, measure how tall you are. Stand against a wall in your bare feet and hold a thick, hardback book on your head. Stand as straight as you can, and be sure the edges of both book covers are touching the wall. Hold the book in place against the wall and make a small pencil mark under the lowest cover. Measure the distance between the pencil mark and floor with a tape measure, and write down the number in inches.

Then, weigh yourself and write down the number.

Using the calculator, find the square of your height in inches (multiply the number by itself). Divide your weight by this number. Next, multiply by 704.5. That gives you your body mass index, or BMI.

It's not as complicated as it sounds. Here's an example: A man who's 5 foot 11, or 71 inches, would take the square of that number, 5,041, and divide 175 (his weight) by that number. Then, he'd just multiply the result of that by 704.5 and get a BMI of 24.5. Simple, right?

Because we're all made up differently, it's hard to declare what weight to consider fat, scrawny, or just right. But the BMI gives you a pretty good idea. According to the National Institutes of Health (NIH), if your BMI is between 18.5 and 24.9, your weight likely isn't a health issue.

In a large study looking at more than a million American adults, researchers from the American Cancer Society found the lowest rates of death from all causes in men with BMIs between 23.5 and 24.9. The risks weren't significantly higher for guys with indexes between 22 and 26.4. But when

WEIGH YOUR OTHER OPTIONS

If your calculator is broken and you can't figure your body mass index on paper, or if you just want more ways to assess your weight and related risks, give these a try.

- Estimate your body-fat percentage. Sit in a chair with your feet flat on the floor and your knees bent. Gently pinch the skin on top of your right thigh with your thumb and index finger. Measure the thickness of the pinched skin with a ruler. If it's ¼ inch or less, you have about 14 percent body fat, which is ideal.

  If you gather up an inch, you're probably closer to 18 percent body fat, which is getting high. With anything more than an inch, you're at a higher risk of diabetes and heart disease than a trimmer guy.
- If the circumference of your waist, measured at belly-button level with your stomach relaxed, is more than 40 inches, you have too much fat in your abdomen. When fat accumulates in your midsection (leading to an apple shape, as opposed to the pear shape that occurs more commonly in women), you can be at a greater risk for diabetes, heart disease, stroke, and high blood pressure.
- Check your shirt collar. Put on a dress shirt and run your finger around the inside of the collar. You most likely had at least a half-inch of clearance between your neck and collar when you bought the shirt. If it's tight now, you've probably gained weight.
- Compare your neck to your waist. Measure your waist, then your neck. Subtract your neck size from your waist size. Do this again every month. If the number goes down, you're losing fat. If it goes up, you're gaining fat.
- Here's the least scientific tactic of all, but it's very, very effective. Get naked, and stand in front of a full-length mirror. Take a hard look. Are you happy with what you see? Any ribs showing? Any muscle definition? Any tapering from shoulders to waist? Then, look straight down at your penis. Without bending over, can you see the entire expanse of flesh from your chest down to Mr. Happy? Or is a belly roll blocking your vision? Enough said.

guys who'd never smoked or had a history of disease hit BMIs of 30, their risk of death really leaped.

"The evidence is solid that the risk for various cardiovascular and other diseases starts to rise at a BMI of 25," says F. Xavier Pi-Sunyer, M.D., chairman of the NIH panel on obesity.

Working the Numbers

The NIH has developed some guidelines about your BMI.

- If your BMI is 18.5 or less—for instance, if you're a 6-foot guy who weighs 136 pounds—your *lack* of poundage is putting your health at risk. Talk to your doctor about healthy ways to add weight, preferably in the form of muscle.
- If your BMI is between 18.5 and 24.9, you probably don't need to make any major changes to your weight. Just focus on keeping a healthy lifestyle. In 2 years, check your index again to be sure you're still doing well.
- If your BMI is 25 to 29.9, you're classified as overweight and may want to talk to your doctor about your health risks. But don't go calling Richard Simmons just yet. Losing weight will be more important to your health if you have heart disease, high blood pressure, osteoarthritis, sleep apnea, diabetes, or high cholesterol or triglycerides. You also have extra reason to lose weight if your waist measures more than 40 inches around, you smoke, or you have a family history of weight-related ailments.
- If none of these other issues describe you, then you may be fine just watching your weight to ensure that it doesn't go up any more and adopting healthy eating and exercise patterns.
- If you do need to drop some, the NIH suggests that a reasonable goal is to lose 10 percent of your body weight over the course of about 6 months. For a 6-foot guy who weighs 210 pounds, that would be a loss of less than a pound a week, or cutting out the equivalent of a medium order of French fries per day.
- If your BMI is 30 or greater, your weight puts you at high risk for diabetes, high blood pressure, and heart disease. And if your waistline is also more than 40 inches, your risk goes even higher. Talk to your doctor about your weight and any health problems you have, and work out a plan for shedding some pounds.

Assess Your Strength

The Day's Task

Find an open spot on the floor and assume the pushup position: Your hands should be on the floor directly under your shoulders, fingers pointing forward. Your legs should be together and fully extended. With a simple, slow pushup test, you're going to assess the strength of your chest, shoulders, biceps, and triceps.

Keeping your body in a straight line from your feet to your head, *slowly* lower yourself until your chest and nose nearly touch the floor. Take 3 full seconds to lower yourself. Hold for 2 seconds, then push yourself up quickly.

Do as many as you can at that pace. It's key that you don't do these any faster; otherwise, your momentum will do some of the work and you won't be getting an honest assessment of your strength. If you can do 21 or more pushups at this rate, your strength is excellent; 16 to 20 is still good; 11 to 15 is average; and 1 to 10 shows that you have room to improve your upper-body strength.

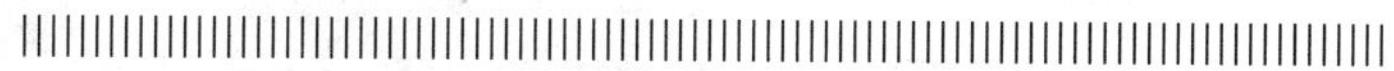

Do you know how strong you really are? Your automatic answer is probably yes, but stop and think about it. How do you really know? If you only base your strength on the exercises and activities you do, you're not getting an accurate picture of your true strength. *Of course* you're going to perform well at the things you enjoy doing—you do them all the time. Your body has been specially trained to excel at them. But to get a truly accurate picture of your strength, think about the things you don't do.

If you have a barrel chest but half-pint thighs, you may be hell on the bench press, but we bet that a few squats or calf raises would leave you trembling like a leaf. Perhaps you avoid those exercises, but in doing so, you get a completely inaccurate idea of your strength, says Michael Mejia, a personal trainer in Plainview, New York. You don't learn about where you need to improve your strength. When you have to put the full measure of your body's capabilities to a *real* test—say, pushing a stalled car to the service station or shoveling 3 feet of snow from your driveway—your system may not be able to deliver the goods.

Along with helping you stay fit now, regularly monitoring your abilities as you can with the slow pushup test will help you correct shortcomings and stay strong when you're in your later years. Nowadays, you may measure your life in terms of how steep a slope you can ski down or how many times you can curl your barbells. But not too far in the future, your quality of life will be measured in achievements that will be much different but every bit as important to you.

Will you be able to tumble around the yard with your grandkids? Will you be able to carry four bags of groceries up a flight of stairs without hassle? Will you be able to hang out on the floor and then get up without groaning? This will depend, in part, on how well you keep tabs on your body as it changes.

Test Yourself

Exercise, including strength training, can slow natural muscle loss and bone deterioration as you age. In Week 10 of this program, we'll discuss in depth how you can get stronger. Here, you'll learn how to tell which body parts and systems show room for improvement so you'll know where to focus your attention while getting more fit. Retest yourself monthly and change your workouts to address your weak areas.

Upper-back and shoulder muscles (1). Lie on the floor under a barbell on a squat rack. Grab the bar with an overhand grip and pull yourself up while holding your back straight. Time how long you can hold your chest against the bar. If you have high blood pressure, skip this exercise.

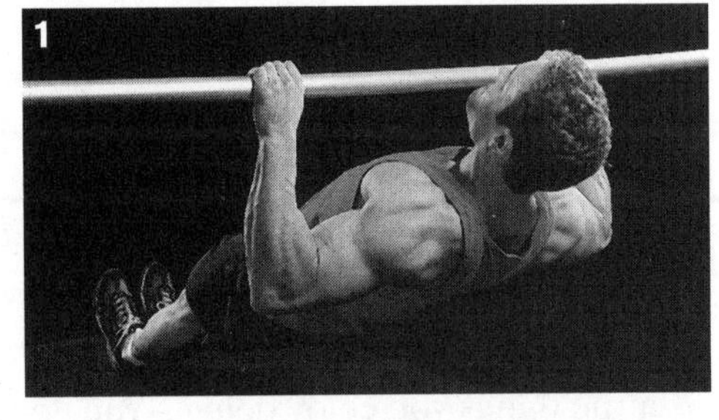
1

If you can hold it for at least 31 seconds, you're doing great; 21 to 30 seconds is good; 11 to 20 seconds is average; and 10 seconds or less isn't so hot.

Abdominal strength (2). Lie on the floor with your hands under the small of your back, then raise your feet straight up in the air, keeping your legs straight. Holding your legs together, slowly lower them as you press the middle of your back against the floor. When you feel your back starting to rise away from your hands, note the position of your legs. If you envision yourself on a clock face,

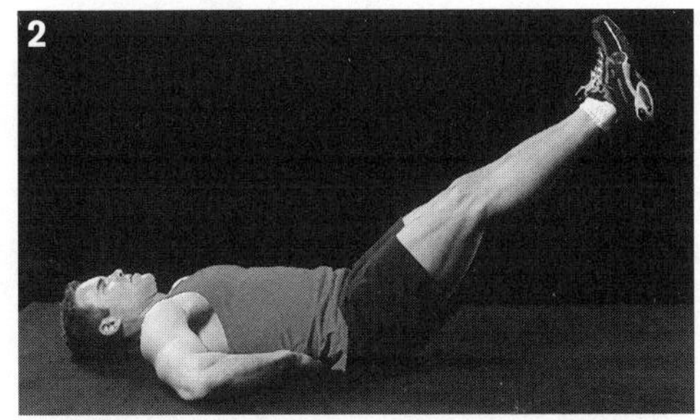
2

holding your legs straight up in the air is 12:00, flat on the floor is 3:00, and an angle halfway in between is 1:30.

If your back comes up off the floor at 3:00, that's great; 2:00 is good, and 12:00 to 1:00 is poor.

Aerobic fitness for beginners. If you're not accustomed to working out, try this test. Find a solid step about 8 to 10 inches high. Step up and down on it rapidly for 3 minutes. Then, calculate your heart rate by putting two fingers on the inside of your wrist to find your pulse, counting the number of beats for 15 seconds, and multiplying by four.

If you're between ages 30 and 40, a count of 143 or lower is excellent, 144 to 151 is average, and 152 or higher is poor. For men ages 41 to 50, 135 or lower is excellent, 136 to 143 is average, and 144 or higher is poor. For men over 50, 125 or lower is excellent, 126 to 135 is average, and 136 or higher is poor.

Aerobic fitness for active people. This test from the Cooper Institute for Aerobics Research in Dallas is designed for healthy, active people.

Head out to your local track for a 1.5-mile run. If it's a 440-yard track, that will be six laps on the inside lane. Run as fast as you can, but don't push yourself to complete exhaustion.

If you're in your twenties, a superior time is faster than 8:13, good is 8:14 to 12:51, and poor is slower than 12:51. If you're in your thirties, superior is faster than 8:44, good is 8:45 to 13:36, and poor is slower than 13:36. If you're in your forties, superior is faster than 9:30, good is 9:31 to 14:29, and poor is slower than 14:29. If you're in your fifties, superior is faster than 10:40, good is 10:41 to 15:26, and poor is slower than 15:26. If you're in your sixties, superior is faster than 11:20, good is 11:21 to 16:43, and poor is slower than 16:43.

For a refresher on improving your aerobic fitness, check out Week 2 of this program.

Lower-body strength (see photo 3 on page 204). Stand with your feet shoulder-width apart. Cross your arms over your chest and align your head with your upper body. Keeping your feet flat on the floor, bend your knees and *slowly* squat toward the floor. Keep your torso straight and don't let your knees pass your toes. Take 30 seconds to squat to the point where your thighs are as close to parallel to the floor as you can comfortably get them. Take another 30 seconds to raise yourself back to the starting position. If you don't feel like you can last the full minute, go faster, but try to do the entire motion.

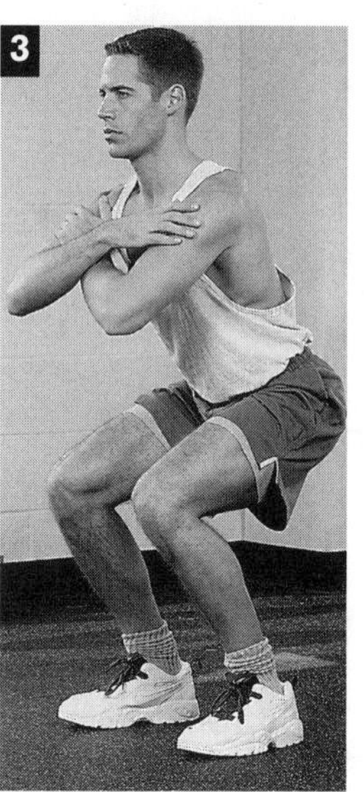

The more slowly you can squat and rise back up, the stronger the muscles in your lower body. On average, if you're in your twenties, you should be able to go the full 60 seconds; in your thirties, 52 to 55 seconds; in your forties, 44 to 50 seconds; in your fifties, 38 to 45 seconds; and in your sixties, less than 40 seconds.

Assess Your Stretch

If you listen to conversations in the weight rooms and locker rooms of America, you'll rarely, if ever, hear guys talk about their flexibility. But this attribute is a crucial measurement of your fitness. You'll tend to lose flexibility earlier than you experience other age-related changes. In fact, if you don't work to keep your muscles loose, you can start feeling creaky even in your thirties.

As your longevity propels you into your later years, stretching can give you more freedom of movement to do fun things. It would be most disappointing to hit 85, when women outnumber men by a ratio of 2 to 1, and not be able to sweep all those ladies off their feet with your dance moves.

Look at your flexibility now. This test helps you measure your nimbleness.

Flexibility (4). Sit on the floor with your left leg stretched out in front of you and your right foot tucked against the inside of your left thigh, near your knee. With your back straight, bend over at the hips and reach for the toes of your left foot.

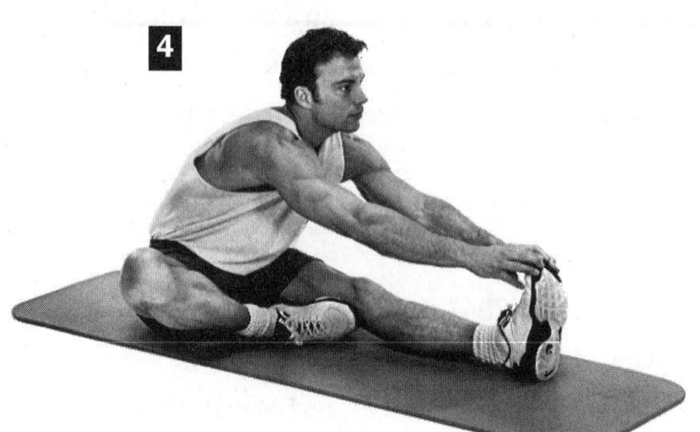

If you're between the ages of 20 and 40, getting your wrist to your toes is good; fingertips to toes is average; fingertips to ankle is fair; and fingertips to sock line is poor.

If you're between 41 and 60, fingertips to toes is good; fingertips to ankle is average; fingertips to sock line is fair; and fingertips above sock line is poor.

Monitor Your Body

The Day's Task

After you get out of the shower today, use a mirror or a helpful spouse to examine every inch of skin on your body. Take special note of every mole and blemish that dots your personal landscape. You'll accomplish two goals: (1) finding any signs of skin cancer and (2) observing the pattern of marks on your skin, in case anything changes later.

While you can do most of the skin-surveying yourself, the spouse or mirror will help you examine hard-to-see areas like the small of your back, the back of your neck, and, well, your backside in general. Just make sure a pair of eyes takes a look at all 17 square feet of your skin, from head to toe.

If we watched out for our bodies as well as we do for our homes, we might stay healthier. Most of us would call in a roofer if we noticed the ceiling leaking after a storm. Most of us know to clean up a dropped bowl of chili before any stains set in the carpet. But when it comes to our own health maintenance, we tend to ignore our bodies' warning signs. Sometimes, we just don't spot the subtler signals because we don't know what it is we're looking for.

It pays to learn. Did you know that if you spot a type of skin cancer called a melanoma and have it removed early enough, you have a 90 percent chance of being around 5 years later? But if it spreads to nearby lymph nodes, your odds of another five birthday parties drop to 50-50.

You *can* catch this and other types of problems early with just a bit of preventive maintenance. What follows is a battery of easy self-tests you can conduct in the privacy of your own home. They take only a few moments, but they can add years to your life if you perform them regularly.

Your mission starts today, as you take a look at the largest organ on your body. No, not that one. We're talking about:

Skin. As you inspect your hide, watch for any mole that triggers the ABCD warning: It's Asymmetrical, meaning the two sides don't match; its Border is irregular, with ragged edges; it has a varying Color instead of a uniform shade; or it has a Diameter of more than 6 millimeters, which is as big around as a pencil eraser. All these characteristics are possible indicators of melanoma.

Other signs may point to forms of skin cancers that are less deadly but more common. Watch for spots that look flat, scaly, and red or areas that are raised, shiny, and waxy and tend to bleed. You may also find blue, brown, or black places in them. Another alert is a growing lump with a rough surface or a flat reddish patch.

If you come up with any suspicious places today, head to the doctor. If your skin appears to be problem-free, great. Make plans to inspect it on the first day of every month or some other memorable date, such as mortgage-payment day.

While you're at it, check the following areas at least every month too.

Testicles. While you're enjoying a hot shower and your scrotal skin is loose, take a few extra seconds to check yourself for testicle cancer. This is the most common of all cancers in men from ages 15 to 35, but it can hit any man, from child to senior citizen. It's also a very curable form of cancer, particularly if you find it early.

Your testicles should feel like shelled hard-boiled eggs as you gently roll them between your fingers and thumb. Their surface should feel smooth and firm. Take note of any hard lumps; changes in size, shape, or consistency; pain or heaviness in your scrotum, or dull aches in your groin or abdomen. You may feel a small, firm area near the back of each testicle, but that's normal. It's called the epididymis, and it's where sperm mature and are stored.

Penis. Check here for any odd spot or blemish; it could look like a rash, bump, or wart. Check from base to tip, front and back. If you notice anything suspicious, visit your doctor promptly.

Your ailment could be trivial, like an inflamed hair follicle, or more serious, like a sexually transmitted disease. It could also be penile cancer, which is rare, affecting only one man out of 100,000 in America, but a fearsome malady for any guy to contemplate.

Lymph nodes. Use your fingertips to press around your neck, groin, and armpits to feel for anything amiss. If the nodes are normal, you'll have trouble finding them. But if your fingers come across one that's swollen and tender, you'll notice it.

These bean-size nodes, parts of a gland system that spread throughout your body, act as filters to grab bacteria, infection, and other unsuitable debris from your body. A swollen gland likely means just that your body is fighting an infection somewhere. But swollen lymph nodes can signal a type of cancer called lymphoma. If you spot any, it's best to let a doctor know so you can learn what's causing the inflammation.

Breasts. Whether you think of them as powerful pecs or a chiseled chest, the facts remain that guys have breasts and we can get cancer there. The way you'll monitor them is similar to the way women do. Each month, press the area around your nipples with your fingertips to feel for lumps. All the tissue should be of the same consistency and should feel the same from month to month. Pressing shouldn't cause pain, and squeezing the nipple shouldn't produce a discharge.

Other warning signs to watch out for are nipples that are red, scaling, or inverted and dimpled skin on the breast. If you find anything that's not right, make a doctor's appointment.

Cardiovascular system. Once a month, before you get out of bed, take your pulse. Use your first two fingers to find your pulse under the edge of your jaw or in your wrist. Count the beats for 15 seconds and multiply by four. Write down the number.

If you notice a big change in your pulse, faster or slower or irregular, mention it to your doctor on your next visit. It could signal the beginning of cardiovascular disease.

Urinary/digestive systems. These are areas you should monitor for problems every day. Fortunately, it's almost impossible not to while you're in the rest room. Rectal bleeding or blood in the stool can be a sign of a minor problem, such as a hemorrhoid, but it could also indicate colon or rectal cancer.

Similarly, blood in the urine can be a sign of a simple ailment like a bladder infection, but it could also point to bladder cancer. You may see just enough blood to tinge the urine yellowish-red, and there may not be any accompanying pain.

If you see any blood where it's not supposed to be or notice unexplainable changes in your bowel or urinary habits, take your observations to the doctor.

Tongue. If you smoke, chew tobacco, gnaw on rocks, drink toxic chemicals, or just want to be careful, inspect your mouth once a month by running your tongue over your palate, along your cheeks and gums, and even inside your lips. You're looking for bumps or sores. If you find something that shouldn't be there, ask your doctor or dentist about it. Cancer of the mouth happens, as do viral outbreaks.

10 Ways to Prevent Heart Disease

1 **We have to start with the most obvious: Not smoking is the most important thing you can do to prevent heart disease.** Smoking is the number one risk factor for heart disease. If you smoke, you practically double your risk of heart attack.

The fact that smoking is dangerous isn't exactly a stop-the-presses health revelation. But that's the thing about heart disease and heart attacks: Most of the preventive measures are well-known. Trouble is, they're not that often put into practice. So if you pay attention to this list, you'll be way ahead of most Americans, even if heart disease runs in your family.

"Know, monitor, and change controllable risk factors," says William Castelli, M.D., medical director of the Framingham Cardiovascular Institute in Massachusetts. "If all Americans did this, heart disease would be eradicated, just as polio was." Instead, cardiovascular diseases (that is, diseases of the heart and circulatory system) kill approximately 2,600 Americans a day, about 1 every 33 seconds.

2 **Avoid a fat-loaded, protein-rich, fiber-poor diet that ignores fruits and vegetables.** This is the quickest route to all the things that cause heart disease: overweight; high blood pressure; high levels of bad, low-density lipoprotein cholesterol and the fat called triglycerides; low levels of good, high-density lipoprotein cholesterol; and high levels of the amino acid homocysteine.

So go the other way. Eat lots of fruits and vegetables, eat more fiber-rich whole grains and beans, go easy on the animal protein, and go very easy on the fat. "Eating a heart-friendly diet is one of the most effective ways to prevent artery-clogging heart disease," says Julie Avery, R.D., a registered dietitian in preventive cardiology at the Cleveland Clinic.

3 **Lower your total blood cholesterol levels.** Your risk of a heart attack goes down 2 to 3 percent with each 1 percent drop in total cholesterol. Cutting down on animal foods, such as meat, high-fat dairy products, and lard, is the best way to get your cholesterol count down, since they're the only source of dietary cholesterol and the top source of saturated fat, which your body converts to cholesterol.

4 **Be friendlier.** A lot of typical male emotions aren't much to be proud of, among them social isolation (à la Clint Eastwood), hostility (à la Sylvester Stallone), cynicism (à la Humphrey Bogart), and depression (à la Woody

Allen). They're also almost as devastating to the heart as lunching on lard. For example, one 5-year study found that people who were socially isolated (including your classic brooding loners) were three times more likely to die from heart disease than those who were more social.

So get sociable and tame that ongoing anger. One recommendation is to have a dialogue with yourself about it. Ask yourself if your anger is justified. If it is, think about an effective response to what's causing the anger, and act on it. If the emotion is not justified, tell yourself that it isn't doing any good. Just by reasoning with yourself this way, you can often manage your anger. Other heart-helping emotional strategies are to drop grudges and help others.

5 **Do 30 minutes of moderately intense aerobic exercise—like jogging, biking, or playing basketball—three times a week.** It keeps your weight down. It tones your heart muscle. It widens your blood vessels, reducing blood pressure. It helps remove lesions from your arterial walls. It helps drain the anger we just talked about. And it reduces your risk of heart attack by 35 percent.

6 **Stay slim.** We've mentioned the dangers of being overweight a number of times already. Here are the numbers to go with it: By maintaining your ideal weight, your risk for heart attack drops 35 to 55 percent.

7 **A moderate amount of alcohol daily—one or two drinks a day—can reduce your risk of heart disease by as much as 40 percent.** Your best choices are dark beer or red wine because they also contain plant chemicals called polyphenols that act as heart-healthy antioxidants.

8 **If your blood pressure is too high, you can cut your risk of heart disease by 2 to 3 percent with each percentage point that you lower it.** Among the ways of lowering your blood pressure are losing excess weight, exercising regularly, managing stress, reducing your salt intake, eating garlic, and eating more fish.

9 **Downing a baby aspirin or half of an adult aspirin tablet daily can cut your chances of a heart attack by 33 percent.** That's because aspirin keeps blood components called platelets from clumping and contributing to clots.

10 **Vitamin E may lower your risk considerably.** In a study of more than 2,000 patients with heart disease, those who took 400 to 800 IU of vitamin E daily reduced their risks of heart attack by 75 percent. That may be because vitamin E is an antioxidant that protects against cholesterol accumulation as well as the dangerous oxidation of that cholesterol. Vitamin C, by the way, does much the same thing. Because vitamin E acts like a blood thinner, consult with your doctor before beginning supplementation if you're already taking a daily aspirin or a blood-thinning medication.

10 Ways to Prevent Cancer

1 **Each day, eat at least five servings of fruits and vegetables.** An extraordinary amount of research has confirmed that free radicals, unstable oxygen molecules in your body, can cause significant damage to cells. This cellular damage may set up your body for cancer, which is essentially a rapid mutation of the cells of a particular body part.

The way to neutralize these free radicals is with antioxidants, which provide the free radicals with the extra electron they need to become stable again. And as we've already noted, perhaps the best source of antioxidants is fruits and vegetables, says Paul Engstrom, M.D., a medical oncologist at Fox Chase Cancer Center in Philadelphia.

All fresh produce offers antioxidants, and a smart course is to eat a diversity of colors and types. But clearly, some fruits and vegetables are cancer-fighting stars. Eating three slices of pizza with tomato sauce a week can slash your risk of prostate cancer by 35 percent. In one study, those who ate the most onions had the lowest rates of stomach cancer. Preliminary test tube evidence suggests that a compound in grapes may slow tumor growth. Broccoli contains compounds that appear to reduce the risk of colorectal cancer. And in yet another study, people who ate the most apples were the least likely to get lung cancer.

2 **Dominate each plate of food with vegetables and grains.** A good rule of thumb is that meat should never take up more than one-fourth of your plate. But far better is to have several meals a week with no meat at all. You should learn to begin looking at meat as if it were chocolate or ice cream, something you have on occasion for a treat, perhaps just one serving each week, says William J. Catalona, M.D., chief of urologic surgery at Washington University School of Medicine in St. Louis.

Beef and other red meats are full of saturated fat, which has been linked to development of cancer. In one study, the men who ate the most red meat were 2.6 times more likely to develop advanced prostate cancer than men who avoided meat. Limiting meat in your diet will help you limit fat. The National Cancer Institute recommends you stick to a diet of less than 30 percent calories from fat.

3 **Eat one serving of soybeans a day, in any of their various forms.** Eating soy foods appears to be associated with a reduced risk of cancer,

says Lianne Latkany, R.D., nutrition research manager at Memorial Sloan-Kettering Cancer Center in New York City.

In one study, people who ate soy at least once a week had half the risk of developing growths in the colon that are precursors to colon cancer than people who didn't eat soy. A soy-rich diet may also help reduce the harmful effects of testosterone, the hormone that is thought to fuel the growth of prostate cancer cells. Researchers speculate that the key to soy's healing power is a class of compounds called phytoesterogens.

Shoot for about 1 cup of soy milk or ½ cup of tofu each day. Snack on roasted soy nuts or toss some in your salad.

4 **Get into a regular vitamin regimen.** Popping pills won't get you out of eating fruits and vegetables, but it can provide extra insurance that you are getting all the nutrients your body needs. Take a standard multivitamin/mineral supplement with 100 percent of the Daily Value for most nutrients, says Julie Parsonnet, Ph.D., associate professor of medicine at Stanford University. Just be sure the multivitamin doesn't have iron. One study showed a link between high levels of iron and cancer; moreover, men just don't need the mineral, though women do.

Of course, multivitamins only make sure you are getting the minimums you need to be healthy. For prostate-problem prevention, consider serious antioxidant boosts such as 1,000 IU a day of vitamin E and 200 micrograms a day of selenium, both potent antioxidants. Because vitamin E acts like a blood thinner, consult with your doctor before beginning supplementation in any amount if you are already taking aspirin or a blood-thinning medication, such as warfarin (Coumadin), or if you are at high risk of stroke.

5 **Develop a taste for green tea, the subtle, aromatic tea often associated with Japanese cuisine.** People who drink about four cups of green tea a day seem to get less cancer. That's why green tea continues to be studied for its cancer-fighting benefit. Its anti-cancer power may be due to nutrients called catechins or a compound called EGCG, a powerful antioxidant. Granted, the suggested four cups of tea is a lot to drink. If this is unrealistic for you, try green tea supplements instead. One pill has the same amount of catechins as 2 to 4 cups of tea.

6 **Consider taking one aspirin a day.** Considerable research has shown that an aspirin a day for a few decades may lower your risk of colon cancer. But aspirin is not benign. It is an acid and can hurt your digestive tract if taken in excess. It's important to ask your doctor if aspirin therapy is the

right choice for you, says Bandaru Reddy, Ph.D., of the American Health Foundation.

7 **Exercise for at least 30 to 40 minutes each day.** This standard advice is reiterated by Leslie Bernstein, Ph.D., professor of preventive medicine at the University of Southern California School of Medicine in Los Angeles. One study of nearly 48,000 men found that the ones who ran 4.5 miles a week at a 10-minute-per-mile pace had half the risk of colon cancer of those who exercised the least. Regular, moderate exercise has been shown to reduce the risk of prostate cancer as well.

8 **Stop smoking.** Smoke contains more than 43 carcinogenic, or cancer-causing, substances. Moreover, each inhalation generates millions of free radicals, making smokers particularly susceptible to oxidative tissue damage and aging.

The risk of developing many cancers, including those of the lungs, mouth, kidneys, and pancreas, begins to drop as soon as you quit smoking. Fortunately, there are more tools than ever before to help you kick the habit. Check out some of the chewing gums, skin patches, and smoking-cessation programs.

9 **Protect your skin when in the sun.** Direct sunlight causes significant free radical damage to your skin, making the sun the primary cause of skin cancer. So when venturing out under the bright blue sky, wear long-sleeved shirts and put on a hat, especially if there is little hair on your head. Experts also recommend wearing sunscreen with a sun protection factor (SPF) of 30 if you're fair-skinned and 15 if you're dark-skinned. Be sure it offers protection from both UVA and UVB rays and contains either zinc oxide, titanium dioxide, or Parsol.

Don't just save the sunscreen for days on the beach either. You should wear it every day on areas that get exposure, like your face and hands. Also, use a sunscreen lip balm with an SPF of at least 15; and, in general, try to stay out of the sun between the hours of 10:00 A.M. and 2:00 P.M., when the sun's intensity is strongest.

10 **Schedule a physical every few years, and specifically ask for cancer-related screenings.** "Screening for colon cancer is simple, easy, and effective, and it is sensational in preventing the disease," says Alfred Neugut, M.D., Ph.D., associate professor of public health at the Columbia University College of Physicians and Surgeons in New York City. You can also get screenings for risk factors for stomach cancer, skin cancer, and prostate cancer.

WEEK 7

KICK-START YOUR BRAIN

Day 1
Learn Something

Day 2
Get Creative

Day 3
Listen to Music

Day 4
Jump-Start Your Senses

Day 5
Get a Good Night's Sleep

Day 6
Book Your Next Vacation

Learn Something

The Day's Task

Sometime this evening, go to a bookstore. Head over to the fiction section to see if they have a classics department. Find a book by a world-famous author—Dickens, Tolstoy, Hemingway, Melville, García Márquez—whose work you have never read. Pick something that the world has already declared brilliant.

You have until the end of the *Men's Health* Longevity Program to read it. That's 6 weeks. No excuses. Don't tell us it's not possible. Just do it. Fifteen minutes a night is probably as much as you'll need. You will thank us for helping you rediscover the joy of great, thoughtful writing.

He was rich and powerful, the founder of his own town, the father of the modern American lead pencil. For other men, that would have been enough. But not for the fictional Emil Faber. Despite all his success, the one thing that gnawed at the business titan was that he had never graduated from college. So in 1904, he founded Faber College. Years later, this venerable institution of higher learning would be immortalized in the cinema verité classic *National Lampoon's Animal House*.

In the film's opening sequence, the camera slowly zooms in on the statue of Faber that graces the campus. Inscribed there are the words that have inspired generations of students and filmgoers: "Knowledge is good."

Yes, it is. Pointy-headed intellectuals may snicker at Faber's homespun wisdom, but those three simple words convey a profound truth: Knowing stuff is better than not knowing stuff. Especially for guys. Learning and exercising our innate sense of curiosity are essential to our health and happiness.

Researchers from Menlo Park, California, who conducted a 5-year study of 1,118 men between the ages of 60 and 86, proved this. They found that those who were still alive at the end of the study had significantly higher levels of curiosity than those who had died.

PLAY HEAD GAMES

Brain-teasing board games, books, and word puzzles were probably a part of your rainy-day repertoire as a kid, and it's still a good idea to haul them off the shelf and dust them off occasionally. The following activities are great for sweeping the cobwebs out of your cranium and keeping your memory sharp.

Exercise your ability to remember words. Crossword puzzles and Scrabble are old favorites that will give your memory a workout. Newer ones to try include Scattergories and Taboo.

Test your ability to remember names. Read novels that feature many characters. *One Hundred Years of Solitude* by Gabriel García Márquez is especially tricky because many of the characters have the same name. If you want something less weighty, try *The Lord of the Rings* by J. R. R. Tolkien, which showcases enough dwarves, elves, and hobbits to feed a battalion of dragons.

Improve your ability to remember where you parked. Orienteering, an adult form of the hiking you did in Scouts, is a great way to get in the habit of paying attention to your surroundings. To find your way to an orienteering event, look in the yellow pages or write to the U.S. Orienteering Federation at P.O. Box 1444, Forest Park, GA 30298.

Not only is curiosity a driving force that keeps your gray matter stoked but, maintained over time, it also can help you find suitable ways to cope with the myriad challenges that life throws your way, says Gary E. Swan, Ph.D., director of the Center for Health Sciences at SRI International in Menlo Park. "Older adults should attend as many continuing-education classes as possible because they provide the environmental support for you to solve problems creatively, to try new things, and to listen to new ideas," he says.

Let's get into the nuts and bolts of your noggin for a second to explain why the idea of lifelong learning is much more than a community college advertising slogan. There are rootlike parts of nerve cells in your brain called dendrites that carry information into the cells for processing. When you're young and learning at breakneck speed, these dendrites keep adapting to all the input they receive, creating webs of nerves that help your brain work more efficiently.

These webs will hold up throughout your life, but only if you keep fertilizing them by thinking about challenging things, says Bob Jacobs, Ph.D., associate professor of psychology at Colorado College in Colorado Springs. The idea is to learn something that plays to your weaknesses, he explains. In other words, do something you don't normally do. Never been musically inclined? Take up the saxophone. If your job is physically demanding, take up brainier stuff like reading and writing. If you're desk-bound all day, learning a new sport might be the ticket.

You don't question the fact that your muscles need to be used, stretched, and worked hard to stay healthy. You need to view your brain the same way. Consider that the powerhouse in your head can store information equivalent to 20 million books the size of this one. A bookshelf holding all those tomes would be 631 miles long. Not bad for a head that holds about 3 pounds of spongy mush.

Think in terms of a high-performance automobile. If you drive a 5.0-liter, V8 engine at 20 miles an hour all the time, what do you think is going to happen to it? It's going to seize up and get clunky. You need to take that baby out on a quiet highway every now and then, open it up, and blow the dust out of the cylinders. Your muscle car of a head is the same way.

"There are people over 100 years old who are functioning very well, mentally," says Vernon Mark, M.D., coauthor of *Reversing Memory Loss*. "One of the reasons for this is that they don't retire from life. They keep challenging themselves in new ways. That's important because the brain abhors boredom. You need to keep it stimulated."

And don't even begin to give us the old line about an old dog not being able to learn new tricks. Leo Tolstoy, the famed Russian novelist, had his first bicycle lesson when he was 67. Queen Victoria starting learning the Hindustani language when she was 68. Grandma Moses didn't even begin to start painting until she was in her seventies. And the Buddhist scholar Bhanddanta Vicittabi Vumsa recited 16,000 pages of Buddhist canonical texts when he was 63. These feats make any excuses you might have seem pretty pale, eh?

Sharpen Your Wits

No matter what you choose to learn, whether it be flying a plane or casting a fly, you'll have an easier time of it if you keep your mind nimble. Here's a good overall brain workout.

THINK LIKE LEONARDO (NOT THE FEATHERWEIGHT ACTOR—THE OTHER ONE)

In his 67 years, Leonardo da Vinci managed to pioneer the sciences of botany, anatomy, and geology. He drew up plans for a parachute, a helicopter, and other flying machines and invented the telescoping ladder that's still used by firefighters today. Somehow he also found time to paint the *Mona Lisa* and the *Last Supper*. Here's how you can learn to learn like Leo, according to Michael J. Gelb, author of *How to Think like Leonardo da Vinci: Seven Steps to Genius Every Day*.

Ask questions. Throughout their lives, great minds ask confounding questions with a childlike intensity. For instance, "How do birds fly?" The answers can lead to discoveries.

Carry a notebook at all times so you won't forget your brilliant ideas. Da Vinci's notes, by the way, were written backwards. Some think it was because he was protecting his ideas from being stolen. Or maybe it was just his way of stretching his brain.

Challenge your long-standing opinions. You may have formed many of your views during or immediately after important childhood events. Ask yourself whether those conclusions still make sense.

Use your eyes and ears. Focusing on the parts of an object or scene, not just the whole, can help expand your perception. Instead of simply looking at a mountain, notice the rock formations and trees.

Try to write with your nondominant hand. Taxing the opposite side of your brain can help you think in a different way. (And people reading your notes will think you attended medical school.)

Test your brain at the market. The next time you go grocery shopping, leave your shopping list in the car, says Michael Chafetz, Ph.D., author of *Smart for Life*. Before you go into the store, take a minute to memorize six to eight items that you need. Once you're in the store, get a cart and pick a starting point. Go get your first item, then return to the starting point. Get the rest of the items one at a time, returning to the starting point each time. That's all there is to it. This simple exercise strengthens your memory and improves your ability to create a mental map.

When you do this regularly, you'll find that you can remember more and more things—not only groceries but also tasks you need to do at work or home.

Turn off the television. There's a good reason it's called the boob tube, and it has nothing to do with breasts. Researchers at Kansas State University, Manhattan, found that people who watched just 15 minutes of television had diminished brain wave activity, an indication that their minds were turning off. How else could you sit through a rerun of *Eight Is Enough*?

"For the most part, the images on that screen just flow through you without enhancing your life," says Dr. Chafetz. He recommends making at least one night a week a no-television night. That might be a good time to take a night class.

Pick up a good book. Nobody's saying that being brainy is about learning pi to the 27th decimal place. Sometimes, it's simply a matter of picking up the latest bestseller. Reading is a time-honored brain booster that helps improve language skills while keeping your memory strong, says Dr. Chafetz. Spend at least 15 minutes a day with a book of your choice.

Practice your math skills. It wasn't that long ago that you did math problems either in your head or with a slide rule. Then came cheap calculators, and now you're lucky if you can count your toes. When you're at the cash register, make a game of figuring out the change you're due before the clerk punches the sale button. Balance your checkbook in your head. Check it with a calculator afterward until you're sure of yourself. "If you use a calculator every time you have to add three numbers together, your mental abilities are going to suffer," says Thomas Crook, Ph.D., director of Memory Assessment Clinics in Scottsdale, Arizona.

Try tongue twisters. You thought you left those tongue twisters back in elementary school, didn't you? Well, drag them back out. They not only improve speech but also help you improve your concentration abilities. At least once a day, practice a tongue twister like "Fresh fried fish don't flip like fresh fish flip." Say it quickly five times in a row.

Build an imaginary house. You can quickly improve your powers of thinking with a technique called mental imagery that you can practice in bed, in the shower, or on the pot, says Dennis Gersten, M.D., author of *Are You Getting Enlightened or Losing Your Mind?*, who has studied ways in which American prisoners of war kept their minds active. One of the simplest forms of mental imagery involves focusing on an image or situation, then using your imagination to embellish it with as much detail as you possibly can. "The prisoners of war in Vietnam who survived the best were the ones who created problems in their minds and

HOW GOOD IS YOUR MEMORY?

How much of the stuff that you learn will you retain? Test yourself with this quick and easy peek into your memory capacity. Read over this list for 1 minute, then try to recall as many of the 10 words as you can.

Pickle	**Artist**	**Button**	**Table**	**Balloon**
Mailbox	**Lipstick**	**Shovel**	**Engine**	**Nickel**

The average number remembered for each age group is eight or nine for people up to age 30, seven or eight for those 30 to 39, six or seven for those 40 to 59, five or six for those 60 to 69, and four or five for those 70 and older.

If you did better than the average for your age group, great. We'll look for you at the blackjack table in Vegas, next to Rainman. If you didn't do better than average, don't panic. There's great variability in how people perform on memory tests. If you totally bombed, see your doctor to rule out any organic problems.

worked on solving them," says Dr. Gersten. "One man built a two-story house in his head. He imagined the process in such great detail that he would actually discuss the color of the tile in the bathroom with his cellmate. When he was released, he built that house in a Midwestern state, exactly the way that he had pictured it in his mind."

Here's a version that doesn't involve spending time in the Hanoi Hilton. Picture a cube in your mind, imagining that each side is a different color. In your head, turn the cube from side to side, memorizing the colors as they appear. Then, rotate the cube again and predict the colors before they appear. "There's a lot of mental effort involved in picturing a cube and consciously trying to rotate it," says Dr. Gersten. "You're really forcing your mind to work in a very active way." Do this for 5 minutes twice a day, and you'll substantially improve both your memory and your ability to think more clearly. Plus, you'll have no problem solving the Rubik's Cube if it ever makes a comeback.

Get Creative

The Day's Task

Allow us to do you a favor. We're about to give you a few million bucks.

You're welcome.

Now that you're a rich man, what do you want to do with your days? Will you write a memoir for your kids? Hike into the woods with an easel and palette? Pick up the saxophone you put down in high school and cut loose? Will you create the ultimate woodworking shop?

Ponder this question all day. This evening, your job is to get started. Seriously. If it's the Great American Novel that you're after, write the first page. If it's the feel of clay squishing between your fingers that you crave, go out and buy some pottery supplies. If it's flower arranging that speaks to you, say hello to Myrtle at the floral shop for us.

But no matter what your new pastime, do not go to sleep tonight without investing at least 30 minutes in it, even if you just browse the lumber section at the hardware superstore or the drum section at the local music shop.

Perhaps you've never really thought of yourself as a creative person. We're here to tell you you're wrong.

"One of the great myths in our country is that creativity is something special, that only some people have it," says Dean Keith Simonton, Ph.D., professor of psychology at the University of California, Davis. "Studies show that the main difference between people with talent and those without is that those who have it have spent time developing that talent."

Before we go further, we need define to *creativity*, a word that we use all the time but have difficulty explaining. Probably the best definition of creativity is the ability to make connections between seemingly unconnected things or ideas. Creativity is Vincent van Gogh using intense swirls of color

CREATIVITY KILLERS

Some days, you feel so artistic you'd make a beret look good. Other days, you feel like you couldn't make it through a paint-by-numbers. "Creativity is a fragile commodity that can be suppressed or impaired much easier than it can be turned on," says Teresa Amabile, Ph.D., professor of psychology at Brandeis University in Waltham, Massachusetts.

The secret to getting the blood of Botticelli surging back through your veins is to avoid the following creativity killers.

People who say your ideas will never work. Constructive criticism is one thing—if you ask for it. But the knee-jerk reaction of a dour-faced smart ass is wholly unnecessary. Tell your brother-in-law to beat it.

Drugs and alcohol. There is no good scientific evidence that creativity can be chemically enhanced. In the long run, overuse of these substances has the potential to damage your creativity abilities far more than it could enhance them. Have you heard Keith Richards come out with anything worthwhile lately?

to depict a starry night or Apple Computer engineers putting little trash can icons on their computer screens for people to use for deleting files.

Creativity is a way of thinking. It is as much a part of everyday life for chemists, corporate managers, basketball coaches, and salesmen as it is for artists.

Age is no excuse. Studies show that many people get more creative as they get older. Sophocles wrote *Oedipus Rex* at 70—or at least, that's what our mothers tell us. The great German poet Johann Goethe finished his epic *Faust* when he was 82.

Unfortunately, many of us have stuffed our creative sides down into the abyss that swallowed our Cheryl Tiegs posters. Maybe we did it because some dimwitted instructors laughed at our drawings of space battles, or maybe we just got busy with other things. "There are a lot of people out there who have a lot of creativity that they're not utilizing at all," says Dr. Simonton. That's too bad because research finds that people who express their creativity in whatever ways they choose find greater satisfaction and meaning in life than those who never explore their creative sides. Remember, we're talking about not only extending life here but making it a better ride along the way.

Material motivation. Most creative motivation comes from within, but extrinsic motivators like money, fame, awards, and acceptance can drain your creative juice.

Keeping score. The pressure of having to score points, meet certain standards, or live up to others' expectations can seriously stifle your creative abilities, says Dr. Amabile. Your creations are for you and you alone. Remember the words of actress Tallulah Bankhead: "Nobody can be exactly like me. Sometimes even I have trouble doing it."

Creating in a crowd. How creative could you be if you knew your crabby third-grade teacher or stickler of a boss were peering over your shoulder every minute? Dr. Amabile's research has shown that such environments have a dampening effect on creativity. Find your own out-of-the-way place to do your thing.

Too little time. We're trying to coax the Muse out of hiding here. She can't be rushed. Don't set ruthless time limits on your projects. Work at a comfortable pace. If it takes a while, so be it. Deadlines are for the office.

Sharpening Your Creative Edge

If you're feeling a little creatively constipated, you'll be relieved to hear that there are ways to throw a little bran into the system and get things flowing again.

Turn off the self-filtering system. Your brain has two modes of thinking, critical mode and creative mode. You spend the vast majority of your time in critical mode: analyzing, making decisions, getting things done, working within established rules and structures. When you drive a car, for instance, you're always assessing oncoming traffic, figuring out when to change lanes, watching your speed. There's no creativity. (Imagine the repercussions of deciding that, for the fun of it, you're going to drive the whole way to work in reverse.)

Creative mode is much different; it is your brain operating without analysis or critique. It is taking an idea, and then building on it, twisting it, growing it, expanding it. This is an awfully fun and exciting mode to be in, but too often even when you need to be creative, you remain in critical mode. Throw out a potential solution at a workplace meeting, and everyone pounces. ". . . It's too expensive. . . . The boss would hate it. . . . There's no staff to handle that."

If you want to think creatively, you have to let your ideas run unimpeded. Like popcorn popping, ideas come slowly at first, then burst out in a short, intense flurry, then taper off. Wait until the ideas taper off before you start assessing viability. Then, look for the good in the ideas that you can preserve, rather than completely tossing out ideas because they don't stand up to scrutiny on their own. This approach to thinking applies as well in the workplace as in the workshop.

Practice the following exercise. Choose a problem or project that interests you, consciously tell yourself to enter creative mode, and then fill up sheets of paper for 15 to 20 minutes, without self-censure. If you start saying things like, "That won't work" or "That one is stupid," give yourself a whack. As creativity experts will tell you, the best idea often comes shortly after the most absurd idea.

Consider the waffle cone. Ask yourself, "What could the world really use right now?" Posing this question may just lead your innate sense of inventiveness to new creations, says Ellen J. Langer, Ph.D., professor of psychology at Harvard University. Quickly write down a whole host of ideas. Don't prejudge them, just get them down on paper. From there, you can branch off into different directions.

Sometimes, a great idea is simply an old idea turned on its head. For example, ice cream was once served on top of a flat waffle. Some confectionery genius got the idea to fold that waffle into a funnel and, bingo, the waffle cone was born.

Take another look at failures. Whether it's a home-improvement project gone awry or a philosophy attempt that turned out more kindergarten than Kierkegaard, mistakes and unexpected results can yield hidden gold. The 3M company thought a new glue they invented was a bomb because it wasn't sticky enough. But they turned it into Post-it Notes and are now counting their billions.

Improve on the best. Stimulate your own creativity by studying the work of the geniuses in your chosen field. Read your favorite writers closely, paying attention to the way they structure language. Visit a museum and get the guides to explain how the works were created. You can build from that, picking up where others left off.

Explore the world. Most of us draw inspiration and creative energy from the greatest creation of all, the universe around us. The sight of a sunset, the sound of a train whistle, the feel of the forest floor, the manic bustle of Manhattan—these things are the stuff of life. Get out there and get dirty.

Above all, explore yourself. A creative man must be willing to delve into places where others fear to tread. Novelist Erica Jong said it best: "Everyone has talent. What is rare is the courage to follow the talent to the dark place where it leads."

Listen to Music

The Day's Task

Block off an hour at home for yourself. Turn on the answering machine and turn off the ringer. Send your significant other, your kids, and your pets to the store. This is private time, fella.

Stand in front of your CD, cassette, vinyl, or, god forbid, eight-track collection. Which album always sucks you into the music as soon as you put it on? Which album makes you mellow while at the same time heightening your senses? Choose that one.

Sit or lie down. Dim the lights, if you care to. Do nothing else for the length of the album except concentrate on what's happening in the music. Do not read the mail. Do not eat a sandwich. Just listen. Pay attention to both the foreground and background of each piece. Pick out an instrument every now and then and follow it through the melody. If you find yourself thinking about something else, redirect your attention to the music.

While you're sitting there getting all tuneful, some pretty cool things are happening in your body. Your anxiety level is dropping. Your blood pressure and heart rate are heading downward. Your tolerance for pain is increasing. Your creative juices and ability to concentrate are rejuvenated. Even your immune system is getting a great shot in the arm. "It's like vitamins in the airwaves. You can enhance your immunity by choosing music that evokes your relaxation response," says Steven Halpern, Ph.D., president of Inner Peace Music in San Anselmo, California.

It doesn't take much imagination to see how a few minutes with madrigals each day can help your body and mind hang in there for the long term. No one is exactly sure why we respond so well to music, but it looks like our brains are hardwired to thrive on it. In fact, the right song can act like an overall tonic for the things that ail you.

10 GREAT ALBUMS TO HELP YOU CHILL OUT

1. *Talking Timbuktu*, by Ali Farke Toure and Ry Cooder: American blues meets African rhythms: slow, sensuous guitar-based music
2. *Handful of Beauty*, by John McLaughlin and Shakti: One of jazz's greatest guitarists takes on the music of India: complex yet hypnotic
3. *Kind of Blue*, by Miles Davis: Arguably the most beautiful jazz album ever made
4. *The White Album*, by the Beatles: Nothing need be said
5. *Greatest Hits*, by Billie Holiday: Astonishingly emotional, soulful vocals
6. *Pachelbel Canon and Other Baroque Hits*: Lilting, moving orchestral music
7. *Hejira*, by Joni Mitchell: Songs of wanderlust and yearning: one of her more daring albums
8. *Passion: Music for The Last Temptation of Christ*, by Peter Gabriel: The soundtrack to the movie: Middle Eastern themes, anguished, beautiful music of the Sahara
9. *Hawaiian Slack Key Guitar Masters*, by various artists: Some of the most interesting acoustic guitar music you'll ever hear
10. *John Coltrane and Johnny Hartman*: Sultry, romantic jazz vocals surrounded by achingly beautiful sax playing

"We know music is so incredibly complex; it has tempo, rhythm, melody, harmony. And so it stimulates the brain in many ways at once," says Alicia Ann Clair, Ph.D., a board-certified music therapist at the University of Kansas in Lawrence.

Don't fret too much over what constitutes the "right" song. "Many years of research have shown me that there is no set prescription, no particular piece of music that will make everyone feel better or more relaxed," says Suzanne Hanser, Ed.D., chairperson of the music-therapy department at Berklee College of Music in Boston. "What counts is familiarity, musical taste, and the kinds of memories, feelings, and associations a piece of music brings to mind."

Music not only helps you get to the later years in life, it's a super tool to have when some pitfalls happen along the way. Music, you see, is developing a great reputation as a healer as well as a sustainer. Research shows that our brains respond to music as if it were medicine.

Here are a few cases in point. Researchers at Colorado State University found that people who had had strokes and people with Parkinson's disease walked more steadily and with better balance if they practiced while hearing a metronome or a piece of music with a strong, steady beat.

Another study of 20 depressed people ages 61 to 86 found that moods rose and depression fell when they listened to familiar music and practiced stress-reduction techniques. If you've found yourself singing the blues, put music to work for you. Choose some upbeat, energetic tracks. You may even find a few to which you can belt out the lyrics. It's tough to be down in the dumps when you're wailing with James Brown.

Insomnia is another beast that music soothes. Classical and New Age music helped 24 of 25 people with sleeping problems nod off more quickly, snooze for longer periods of time, and get back to sleep more easily if they woke up in the middle of the night. If you have sleep struggles, simply slip in a CD of softer music about a half-hour before bedtime. Continue listening in bed.

Even pain can be diminished with the help of music. Take a puck in the chest? Have your wisdom teeth out? Slip on the cat? Anything from postoperative pain to chronic aches can be eased with flowing melodies and distracting rhythms, say music therapists and researchers. One study found that people who listened to their favorite music while awake during a surgical procedure needed smaller amounts of sedative and pain medications. "Music won't eliminate the need for pain relievers, but it may help them be more effective," says Dr. Clair. To reap the rewards, find some gentle, soothing selections and concentrate on them for at least 15 minutes as you sit or lie comfortably. Give the music your full attention.

Health without Handel

So what happens if you're just not a music-loving sort of person? Fret not; you can still use sound to get many of the same benefits. If symphonies aren't your suit, buy a babbling brook instead. Or try an ocean or forest.

Nature's sounds can be exceptionally relaxing, says Dr. Halpern. "Use whatever natural sound makes you feel comfortable." You can buy tapes with the above-mentioned sounds, or you can even find clock radio-like machines that electronically generate Mother Nature's voice. From crickets in the night to

SET UP YOUR SYSTEM FOR MAXIMUM SOUND

Whether you have state-of-the-art surround speakers or punky garage sale specials, you need to position them properly or your sonic experience will be muffled. Keep these hints in mind.

- The speakers should be at least 6 feet apart, ideally at each end of the longest wall in the room.
- The tweeter (that is, the small speaker that produces higher-pitched sound) should be positioned around ear level. Remember that you're usually sitting when you hunker down with some tunes, so take that into consideration. A set of speaker stands will do the trick.
- Sound emits from the backs of the speakers too, so keep them in front of similar structures. For example, don't put one in front of a fish tank and the other in front of a venetian blind.
- Keep the area around the speakers clear. Music sounds rotten filtered through your hibiscus plant.
- There's a "sweet spot" about 6 to 10 feet in front of the speakers, centered between them. If you can, slide your couch or lounge chair over there.

chirping birds, it's all there. Or you can just get the blazes out of the office and away from town for awhile and immerse yourself in the real thing.

You don't have to be a music lover to appreciate the therapeutics of a simple beat. When you're under pressure, take a pen or pencil and go to town on your desk, your computer, a soup can, or whatever gives you a good beat. The drumming gets a flow going, says Dr. Halpern, and it allows you to get your frustrations out on an inanimate object instead of, say, your boss.

Jump-Start Your Senses

The Day's Task

Today's task is more like a science experiment than anything else. It will seem a bit odd but will take only 30 minutes or so, and it should be rather revealing.

Gather together the following items: your old baseball glove, a can of Play-Doh, a stick of cinnamon, an after-dinner mint, your wife or girlfriend's perfumed lingerie, and a container of baby powder.

Don't feel bound to use those exact things. If you don't have one or two of two, substitute something else with an aromatic smell. Take the items into your bedroom or study, draw the blinds, and sit down in a comfortable chair.

One by one, take each item and hold it under your sniffer. Close your eyes and deeply breathe in each scent. Let your mind wander through the memories that each smell brings with it. Notice how you feel with each one. Are some stimulating? Are some wistful? Are others relaxing? Make a mental note, and let yourself be pleasantly surprised.

That, friend, is the tremendous power of your senses in action.

There's a school of philosophical thought called empiricism that you should know about. Basically, it says that you and everything you know are products of your senses. Imagine yourself completely sense-free: no vision, no hearing, no smell, taste, or touch. You'd be an inert blob, incapable of knowing anything and probably named Bluto.

When you think about it, empiricism makes a lot of sense. Your whole belief structure, your knowledge of the world around, and your ability to function in that world depends entirely on the input funneled through your five senses.

It is odd that people spend so little time cultivating their senses. Sure, we sometimes give our senses a treat—a great meal, a concert, a wilderness walk. But how many of us can claim to have truly refined senses of taste or hearing or sight?

Some hobbies are all about this, things like wine tasting, cooking, avid music listening, even massage. If you have a passion for something of the senses, we salute you. You are, by definition, a sensuous person, a phrase that registers well with women and speaks to your love of life. But if you are one of the many who do nothing at all for any of their senses, you might wish to change your ways.

With practice, you can see better, smell better, taste better. We'll provide advice on optimizing these three senses (the massage you got on Week 4, Day 3 and the music you listened to yesterday covered touch and hearing). But first, a few comments. Your brain can concentrate hard on only one sense at a time. Sure, all five are always functioning. But only one fills up your front-of-consciousness thinking. You either watch an orchestra closely or listen to its music closely, but not both. So as you practice your senses, be aware of sensual distractions. Perhaps the best way to hear a song better or taste a wine more carefully, for example, is to merely close your eyes. Visual stimulation often dominates other forms of sense stimulation.

To practice this division of your senses, take a walk in an unfamiliar neighborhood and throw your whole sensory system into learning about it. Are there any landmarks nearby? What colors are around you? What are the sounds, the smells? Touch the fire hydrant next to you. Note the texture of the sidewalk beneath you. Notice all this, and you will be amazed at how well you remember your way around the next time you pass through.

The Power of Sight

It makes perfect sense that when the big fella upstairs wanted to set all of creation rolling, the first thing he did was turn on the light. Few forces in our world carry the importance of light and the sight that depends on it. You read with it, drive by it, jog in it, and face the urinal with it. Here's how to use it better.

Try some eye and vision exercises. Here are a few.

- Focus on 10 different objects in 10 seconds by scanning around the room. Then, try to name the objects in the order in which you saw them. This will improve your eyes' ability to work together and to shift more rapidly.
- Tape a page of newsprint to a wall at work, about 8 feet from where you sit. Stop what you're doing every 5 to 10 minutes and look at the newspaper. Bring the

headline into focus, then look back at your work. Do this five times, then get back to work.

- To sharpen your ability to track a moving object, play catch using a ball or beanbag marked with letters and numbers. As it comes toward you, call out the last letter or number that you see before you catch it. Keep the speed down and the spin limited at first so you have a fighting chance of seeing something.
- Practice peripheral vision. Lock your eyes straight ahead, but try to see as much as you can to the sides. Don't cheat; keep your eyeballs motionless.

Research has shown that the colors that surround you can have a decided impact on your moods. Put that knowledge to use by controlling the use of color wherever you can. Use lighter blues, greens, and mauves and eggshell white in places where you want to be mellow, says Cam Busch, R.N., a certified art therapist in Chattanooga, Tennessee. Use brighter colors in rooms where you need to be juiced up, like your office. Red and orange are both stimulating colors.

Go natural. It's no accident that Ansel Adams is a big seller in the office-art department. Pictures of nature tend to have restorative effects on your state of mind. Hang a big wall calendar with a different nature scene for each month, or tack up a favorite nature poster, suggests Deborah Good, Ph.D., chairperson of the art-therapy program at Southwestern College in Santa Fe, New Mexico.

Liven things up. Paper isn't the only way to strew nature around you. Chunk some potted plants and flowers in your office too. Seeing real live flora around you is important. That's why so many hospitals are adding "healing gardens" to their facilities, both indoors and out.

Get out of the dark. For some people, a lack of seasonal light is a lousy thing. It's called seasonal affective disorder, and it can make you feel depressed, lethargic, and fatigued in the gloomy winter months. If you're one of the 6 percent of people who are affected by this, use your sight to pull you back out. Get a couple of extra incandescent lamps for each room in which you spend a lot of time. The extra lumens can reenergize you. And get out for a daily 45-minute walk during the day, ideally in the morning, when your biological clock is more receptive to sunlight.

Eat for your eyes. Fruits and vegetables containing vitamins C and E and beta-carotenes can slow cataract growth and promote eye health. For C, try strawberries or cantaloupes. For E, chow down on almonds, peanut butter, and shrimp. Beta-carotene aplenty is found in white, yellow, and orange fruits and vegetables.

Keep up the maintenance. When was the last time you had an appointment with an eye doctor? Even if you have good vision and no history of problems, you should still go at least once every 3 years. If you wear contacts or glasses, you'll likely see an eye doctor about once a year.

The Power of Smell

As you can tell by the experiment we had you try earlier, smell is a big deal. And it's something you need to take care of if you want it to hold up. "Your sense of smell declines by about 10 percent between age 40 and age 60, and by as much as 50 percent more by age 65," explains Alan R. Hirsch, M.D., neurological director of the Smell and Taste Research and Treatment Foundation in Chicago. Besides being at higher risk of dying in gas explosions or contracting food poisoning, guys with blunted sniffers can face erection problems.

In fact, one study found that 18 percent of people who lost their ability to smell developed sexual dysfunction. "Your ability to smell your partner seems to be very important to arousal," says Dr. Hirsch. Here are a few ways to keep your snout supple.

Take sniff therapy. "Studies have found that if you expose people several

GET A WHIFF OF THIS

You know that your sense of sight is directly related to your sexual turn-ons—hence the success of the Victoria's Secret catalog. But did you know that your nose also plays a role in your sexual arousal? Certain smells have been found to increase bloodflow to your penis, according to Alan R. Hirsch, M.D. Those odors are not, however, the perfumed, womanly scents that you might expect.

In one study, Dr. Hirsch found that a combination of pumpkin pie and lavender elicited a 40 percent increase in penile bloodflow. Second place went to a cross between black licorice and doughnuts (there was no mention of how many cops took part in the study).

If you want to try an experiment at home, use the above smells or try to recall the scent of a particularly fond experience that you shared with your partner. Re-create it with whatever materials necessary—scented candles, incense, perfume, motor oil.

times a day to a scent they can't detect, they'll develop the ability to detect it within 3 months," says Dr. Hirsch. This sensitization is a good practice to get into even if you don't have problems detecting smells. Just like your muscles, your olfactory membranes need workouts to stay sharp. Remind yourself to savor the bouquets of things like herbal tea, that new-car smell, and the nape of a woman's neck. And always, when outdoors, reserve a few moments to smell the air, preferably with your eyes closed, and discern its flavors. Oak? Grass? Horse manure?

Avoid allergens. Chronic sinus infections and allergies account for one-quarter of the cases of smell loss. If you suffer from allergies but don't know what's causing them, get tested by an allergist.

The Power of Taste

You don't have much interest in eating sawdust, do you? Then you need to care for your tastebuds every bit as carefully as you do your other senses. Your sense of smell controls a large part of your ability to taste, so if you don't care for the former, the latter slides downhill too. Food will start getting blander and blander. As a result, you'll start craving sweeter and saltier foods, which are easier to taste.

That's part of the reason that most men put on weight as they age, says Dr. Hirsch. Once your sense of smell weakens, you generally shovel down richer food and more of it before you feel satisfied. Here's how to fight back.

Masticate for pleasure. Chew your food twice as long. "The more you chew, the more aroma reaches your nose," says Dr. Hirsch. "That can help heighten your sense of taste and trick you into feeling fuller, faster."

Cleanse your palate often. Take a drink of water or a bite of plain cracker between bites of food. That way, your tongue becomes a clean slate before it experiences each new flavor.

Enjoy hot food. The more you heat food, the more you agitate flavor molecules within it. So for maximum taste, eat meals quickly after they emerge from the oven or stove.

Use your entire mouth. Different parts of your tongue register different flavors. If you want to experience the full flavor of a wine or food, be sure that the food spreads out over your entire tongue. The first time you try this, you might discover that you have been ignoring parts of your tongue as you've eaten and drunk over the years.

Nix the smokes. Smoking damages the tissues that are responsible for taste. "It

EAT YOUR MOTHER-IN-LAW'S COOKING WITHOUT FEAR

If boiled liver is your mother-in-law's culinary specialty and she invites you for Sunday brunch, reschedule. Go at 7:00 P.M. instead. Your tastebuds tire out later in the day, so you may not notice what you're swallowing. "If you have to eat something unpalatable, do it as late in the day as possible," says Alan R. Hirsch, M.D., of the Smell and Taste Research and Treatment Foundation.

If it's midnight and you still can't choke it down, you may be one of a rare group known as supertasters. Researchers are finding that this category of people tend to turn up their noses at a lot of foods because the tastes are too intense. A higher number of tastebuds than average may be the culprit. Here's how to tell if supertaste is one of your superpowers.

1. Use cotton swabs to paint the front surface of your tongue with blue food coloring.
2. Find a piece of notebook paper with binder holes in it. Visually divide your tongue in two. Center a binder hole on one side or the other, placing it as close to the front of your tongue as possible without touching the tip.
3. Ask a willing participant to use a flashlight and magnifying glass to look for little pink circles on your tongue that didn't pick up the blue dye (hopefully, you freshened your breath before you dyed your tongue). Count the circles. If there are more than 30, you're a supertaster. If there are fewer of these telltale dots, stop whining and eat your liver.

is well-documented that smokers have lower sensitivity to both taste and smell," says David V. Smith, Ph.D., vice chairman of the department of anatomy and neurobiology at the University of Maryland School of Medicine in Baltimore. Once you stop smoking, a lot of the sensual acuity that you lost will come back.

Get a Good Night's Sleep

The Day's Task

Go to the supermarket or a pharmacy that carries herbal remedies and pick up a package of valerian tea. This evening, fix yourself a cup, come back to this book, and enjoy the tea while you read.

You don't hear a lot of men bragging about how much sleep they got last night. In fact, you probably don't hear any men bragging about that. You only hear guys bragging about how they went without sleep for 3 days in a row in college or how they've been burning the midnight oil all week.

But the importance of sleep has been recognized throughout the ages. Shakespeare called sleep the "chief nourisher in life's feast." Keats referred to it as the "soft embalmer of the still midnight." And, according to Ralph Waldo Emerson, "health is the first muse, and sleep is the condition to produce it."

So when you brag about how little sleep you've been getting, you might as well brag about how much you've been smoking lately. "Sleep quality affects your immunity, cardiovascular health, growth rate, and a lot of other things conducive to a long life," says Bob Ballard, M.D., director of the National Jewish/University of Colorado Sleep Disorders Center at the National Jewish Medical and Research Center in Denver. "Illness and sleep patterns go hand in hand. When you don't get enough sleep, you are more prone to illness because there is a circadian rhythm in keeping immunity strong. Your body needs to rest through sleep in order to stay healthy."

The ABCs of Zzzs

There are three things you need for a good sleep: the ability to fall asleep with minimum effort, the ability to sleep soundly through the night, and the ability to wake easily and feeling refreshed. Let's take a look at how you can do all of these.

A TALE OF WRETCHED INSOMNIA

W. C. Fields was a man of many odd habits, including sleep habits. Having insomnia, he sometimes found sleep by sprawling out on pool tables or, because he enjoyed haircuts, seated in a barber's chair while wrapped in warm towels. On his worst nights, he could reach the Land of Nod only by lying under a beach umbrella while a garden hose sprayed the canvas above him with water, imitating the sound of rain.

Fall asleep. Your valerian tea will help. It's a natural sedative. And unlike prescription sleeping pills, it has virtually no addictive qualities. Feel free to down a mug each night. If you want to branch out, try a cup of chamomile tea on alternate nights. It has many of the same properties as valerian. In rare cases, these teas cause side effects or allergic reactions. Read the package they come in for appropriate warnings. Do not use valerian in any form with sleep-enhancing or mood-regulating medications, as it may intensify their effects.

After you've finished this nightcap, take a hot shower or bath. The warm temperature heats you up and, as you cool, your body knows it's bedtime.

Another technique is to go to bed at exactly the time you're feeling sleepy. If it's close to bedtime and a wave of tiredness comes over you, don't ignore it while you finish up whatever you're doing. Your body operates on a 60- to 90-minute sleep cycle. If you don't catch the beginning of that cycle, you'll be up for another hour and a half.

Turn the thermostat down to 65°F. That's the temperature your body naturally craves when sleeping. If you find it too cold, use extra blankets instead of hiking the heat.

Finally, when you're lying in bed, shift your mind into low gear. Take a deep breath and release it slowly. As you do this, relax your fingers, your shoulders, and your jaw. You can't be tense when these areas are relaxed.

Stay asleep. Make sure your pillow provides the right amount of support. If it doesn't, you'll move all night long, trying to get more comfortable. To test your pillow, fold it in half and put a shoe on top. If it springs back, it's okay. If it doesn't, it's incapable of giving you proper support.

Also, keep your home well-humidified. Especially during winter months, dry air can make breathing difficult for snorers and other mouth breathers. If it's too dry, you wake up to get water and rub your nose and mouth.

Avoid any stimulants like coffee and smokes right before bed. Stimulants floating around in your system make it tough to sleep soundly. You'll also want to move your exercise time to before supper. If you exercise within 3 hours of bedtime, it can interfere with your sleep quality. But if you hit the road before the evening meal, your metabolism will gradually slow down all evening until it hits downright sleepiness at just about bedtime.

Wake up refreshed. What rouses you from slumber is increased bloodflow to your brain that is triggered by stress hormones. But this mechanism is competing against another drive, the one pleading for more rest. "It's a teeter-totter effect," says Timothy Roehers, Ph.D., of the sleep disorders and research center at Henry Ford Hospital in Detroit. The outcome of that battle can determine the course of your whole day.

You need an incentive to overcome the sleep drive. Plan a great breakfast, promise your wife a morning romp in the bed, or set the coffee pot on automatic timer so your java is waiting for you when the alarm goes off. If you have something to look forward to, you'll wake up with more zip.

Also try moving your bed so it faces a window. Sunlight is your body's main signal that it's time to get up. That's why it's so easy to wake up early when you're camping. The sun blazing down on your tent lets your brain know that it's time to rise and shine. To let even more light in the room, raise your shade halfway before you go to bed.

Make sure that you're not trying to force yourself out of bed too soon. Being just an hour or two short on high-quality slumber can make you exhausted. "Many Americans force their bodies to run day after day on 5 to 6 hours of sleep, when they really need 7 to 8," says Mary A. Carskadon, Ph.D., professor of psychiatry and human behavior at Brown University in Providence, Rhode Island. Even 1 hour of sleep deprivation makes a big difference. The day after the start of daylight savings time, when people have lost an hour of sleep, traffic accidents increase by 7 percent. The day after the return to standard time, accidents decrease by 7 percent.

But don't start sleeping in on the weekends to try to catch up on lost sleep. You throw your biological clock out of whack and end up screwing up your sleep during the work week. If you get up at 7:00 in the morning Monday through Friday, do the same on the other two days of the week. "Just as your body prefers

SIGNS THAT YOU HAVEN'T BEEN SLEEPING ENOUGH

Some people have been sleep-deprived for so long that it's become a way of life. They truly can't tell if they need more winks. Here are some indications that you need more pillow time.

- You're so exhausted that you fall asleep the instant your head hits the pillow.
- You sleep late on the weekends.
- You fight sleepiness during the day. "Some people think it's normal to frequently be sleepy off and on during the day. It's not," says Dave Dinges, Ph.D., chief of the division of sleep at the University of Pennsylvania School of Medicine in Philadelphia.
- You fall asleep during meetings, while reading, or when watching television.
- You find yourself nodding off right after supper.

to eat at certain times, it also prefers to sleep and be awake at certain times," says Donna Arand, Ph.D., clinical director of the Sleep Disorders Center at the Kettering Medical Center in Ohio.

Finally, if you have to get up in the wee hours to go to the bathroom, do it in the dark. Flicking a light on, even for a brief moment, disrupts your body's production of the sleep hormone melatonin and makes you wake feeling crabby and poorly rested. If you keep missing the bull's-eye, buy a dim night-light to help you out. And invest in a good tile cleaner.

Book Your Next Vacation

The Day's Task

Take this book over to your computer. Log on to the Internet and head to a search engine. Do a search for the word *vacation*. If your results are like ours, you'll get about three million hits.

Obviously, you're not going to go through all those sites—this is just to get your wanderlust stirring. Do, though, spend one full hour clicking on the sites that catch your eye. Don't rush. Let your imagination drift off to places you've never been and people you've never seen.

Then, log off and grab a pad of paper. For 15 minutes, ponder the following, taking notes as you go: When can I take my next vacation? What is the absolute best vacation I can imagine? What about that vacation is most alluring? What vacation can I actually take that fulfills those needs?

Be aggressive. Often, we rein ourselves in when it comes to vacation planning. Go one level beyond your comfort zone when it comes to cost, time, and distance. Most important, be sure that the vacation you plan can easily fulfill your fantasies, whether they revolve around food, adventure, relaxation, sunshine, sport, or privacy.

Now, go tell your favorite traveling companions that it's vacation time.

We know what's going through your mind. You're swamped at work, the dog needs to be looked after, your car is in the shop, whatever. You can't possibly afford the time off right now.

You're not the only one thinking that way. One survey found that one-quarter of all American employees do not use all their allotted vacation time because they are too busy. Another survey found that 47 percent of executives who take vacations take work with them, and 22 percent even admit passing out business cards during their last vacations.

Add to that the miserable fact that America trails virtually all developed

PACKING FOR ADVENTURE

Adventure travel has become a hot phrase. It basically refers to vacations in which you go into the wild and do something mildly dangerous, exotic, or physical, like mountain climbing or rafting or overnight cycling.

If you are planning this type of vacation, understand that what you pack should be dramatically different from your ordinary vacation gear. Most adventure travelers pack too much and then become miserable when they have to lug it around. Here are a few things that you should pack for your wilderness trip. View anything else with a wary eye and ditch it if you can.

Essential toiletries. Pack a couple of rolls of toilet paper, toothpaste and a toothbrush, an antidiarrhea medication, aspirin, antibiotic ointment, and moleskin for blisters.

Fast-drying clothes. You want clothing that dries quickly and wicks moisture away from your body. Wool and some synthetic materials work well. Tencel is one of the synthetics that tends to be lightweight and fast-drying. Try to stay away from cotton. It's going to get wet, and it never dries.

A head lamp. You need this for camping or if you'll be traveling in a country with unstable electricity. It leaves both of your hands free to do what you need to do at night.

A small shortwave radio. Some aren't much bigger than a deck of cards. A radio can literally be a lifesaver when you need to find out precisely what is going on in the region where you're traveling. If there's a violent demonstration by revolting students, you can avoid that area.

nations in the average number of vacation days granted by employers. All this makes you a prime candidate for stress and burnout. Even worse, skipping your vacation can quite literally kill you. A study of 12,338 men showed that the more times they blew off their annual vacations, the more likely they were to die.

"I think it's inhuman that people have to work for a company and all they get is 2 to 3 weeks a year. Worse yet, most companies don't even want them to take those weeks all at once," says Roger Dawson, a professional lecturer, business consultant, and international negotiating expert in La Habra Heights, California.

Pack the Bags, Leave the Stress

Okay, we've convinced you that you need some real time off. But there's a trap that you really need to avoid: taking your office and home worries with you as well as adding new ones during your trip.

"Vacations can be the world's most powerful stress blaster for some people and a most powerful source of stress for others," says Paul J. Rosch, M.D., president of the American Institute of Stress.

Some vacation stress is inherent. Merely getting packed and out the door can be utter hell. Then, there are going to be airline delays, flat tires, surly cab drivers, haggling vendors. Treat them as part of the adventure. Above all, put the office out of your mind. Here are a few techniques that can help you enjoy your time away as well as make a seamless reentry to work.

Don't worry about wasted time. It's easy to think of a vacation as misspent time. But you earned it by the sweat of your brow. Remind yourself of that.

Run interference. If your boss wants a way to contact you, give him the phone number of a close friend or family member and leave your emergency number with that person. That way, your designee can weed out what's really important from what's only modestly so and call you if it's a real catastrophe.

Take a phantom day. On your voice mail message, say that you'll be gone a day longer than you actually will be. This will forestall a firestorm of phone calls when you get back and give you time to re-acclimate.

Recruit a spy. Call a coworker the day before you return. He'll update you on the current emergencies and boss tirades. You'll be prepared when you walk in the next morning.

Go back on a Tuesday. It's less hectic than a Monday in most offices, says Mitch Marks, Ph.D., a San Francisco organizational psychologist. A short workweek will keep that vacation feeling alive a little longer.

No More Excuses

All right, we've given you the incentive and the trip tips. It's up to you to follow through. Don't minimize the importance of a vacation, and don't try to whittle it down to a long weekend. You need a week off, minimum. You need pure, extended rest. And the thing is, you'll come back revitalized and more efficient at your job than you were before you left. Your battered brain will have recovered, your spirits will be higher, and your energy levels will be back to normal.

See you at the beach.

10 Tips to Prevent Memory Loss

1 **Pour your drink down the sink.** Since alcohol can easily get between your mind and the information you want to remember, you should cut back on drinking if you're having trouble with your memory. While we still don't know the exact effects of just a few drinks a day on your recall, drinking until you're tipsy definitely puts you at risk for memory loss, says Barry Gordon, M.D., Ph.D., author of *Memory: Remembering and Forgetting in Everyday Life*.

2 **Catch up on your sleep.** When you get plenty of sleep, you let your brain work most efficiently at processing and storing information, Dr. Gordon says.

But when you're tired, you have more trouble keeping your attention focused, and your memory can pay the price, says Janet Fogler, coauthor of *Improving Your Memory*.

No standard formula can tell you how much sleep you need, since the amount varies for each person. However, if you're drowsy during the day or require an alarm clock to wake up, you should get to bed earlier. Keep going to bed a half-hour earlier each week until you wake up before your alarm rings.

3 **Collect your thoughts before bedtime.** As you're lying in bed awaiting a full night's sleep, let information that you really want to remember run through your head. Researchers at the Israel Weizmann Institute of Science in Israel have found that sleep helps the brain consolidate information, and the body's circadian rhythms during sleep help the brain retain new facts.

4 **Stick with your best thinking method.** Some people learn facts best when they hear them. Some people learn them best when they see them. Others store thoughts by acting on them or writing them down, says Kenneth Manges, Ph.D., a Cincinnati psychologist. Ask yourself which style suits you best, and use it every time. Maybe you need to hear someone repeat her phone number an extra time, maybe you need to write it down, or maybe you need to say it to yourself several times.

5 **Give your memory a workout.** You can keep your memory strong by memorizing lists whenever possible instead of writing them down, says Alan S. Brown, Ph.D., a psychology professor at Southern Methodist University in Dallas. While helpful, written lists can be a crutch that reduces your ability to remember information. The next time you make a grocery list, leave several items off and try to keep track of them in your head.

6 **Give your body a workout too.** Sedentary people can sharpen their minds by getting aerobic exercise, Dr. Gordon says. In fact, exercise can improve some mental abilities by 20 to 30 percent. So don't forget to get out and swim, run, bike, and move your body however you like—in fact, if you do enough of it, you may not be able to forget.

7 **Get help from ginkgo.** The herb ginkgo biloba may give your memory the boost it needs by promoting better bloodflow to your brain, allowing it to get more oxygen and nutrients. Ginkgo has shown some promise in helping relieve symptoms in people with memory-robbing Alzheimer's disease, and it may help those with mere absentmindedness too. "It's good for those of us who forget where we put our car keys," says Victor S. Sierpina, M.D., assistant professor of family medicine at the University of Texas Medical Branch in Galveston.

Take 120 to 240 milligrams of ginkgo biloba extract daily in two or three doses; expect to take it for at least 8 weeks before seeing an improvement. Look for a ginkgo product with "24/6" on the label, meaning it contains 24 percent flavone glycosides and 6 percent terpenes, which are both active ingredients. Gingko biloba doesn't mix well with antidepressants, aspirin or nonsteroidal anti-inflammatories, or blood-thinning medications, so check the label or talk with a doctor before taking it.

8 **Pay attention in conversations.** The common courtesy of looking people in the eye can help your memory. When your gaze wanders from a person during a conversation, so does your attention. Thus, you're more likely to remember what people say if you keep eye contact as you talk to them, says Tora Brawley, Ph.D., a neuropsychologist at the Duke University Medical Center.

9 **Learn to handle information overload.** If you have trouble remembering information because torrents of it are pouring on you from all directions, try this exercise a few times this week. Read a book with the volume on a nearby television turned up. Put the book down and watch TV for several minutes. Then, read the book some more. After 10 minutes of switching your attention, turn off the TV, put down the book, and see how much you remember from each source, says Fran Pirozzolo, Ph.D., a Houston neuropsychologist. Gradually, your ability to keep out distractions should improve.

10 **Organize your surroundings, and your mind may follow.** Choose designated spots for everyday items like your mail, your car keys, your glasses, and your newspapers, Fogler suggests, and you'll remember where they are without having to search for them. In addition, toss out old magazines, newspapers, and other unneeded items to cut down on household clutter and distractions.

WEEK 8

OVERHAUL YOUR LOOK

Day 1

Inventory Your Closet

Day 2

Buy Some New Clothes

Day 3

Start Caring for Your Skin

Day 4

Fix Your Face

Day 5

Get a Haircut

Day 6

Get an Attitude

Inventory Your Closet

The Day's Task

This Saturday or Sunday morning, when you have no other plans or distractions, take everything out of your closet and throw it on the bed or floor. Item by item, one by one, try on your duds. Model them in front of someone with enormous patience and brutal honesty—your wife or girlfriend, your sister or daughter, anyone whose sartorial taste you trust. Clothes that look good go back in the closet. Those that don't, place in a trash bag. Be ruthless. If your only reason to keep something begins with a phrase like, "But this is the shirt/belt/jockstrap I wore when I met you/got my parole/dislocated my knee sliding into home," it's not clothing, it's memorabilia; and it has no place in your closet.

When you've finished, your closet should contain only stuff that looks good on you. Take the trash bag to a Salvation Army or Goodwill store and make a charitable deduction. As for the memorabilia, do what they do at those theme bars: frame it. Then, hang it in the den.

This week, we are focusing the Longevity Program on matters of style. Not fashion, mind you, but style. Fashion is the ever-changing runway craziness. Try to use fashion to convince people you are young, and you will surely fail. That's inevitable. But style . . . style is timeless and enduring.

Style, of course, entails many things. Certainly, it includes a sharp sense of dress. That is why this first day's task is about assessing your clothes. Style also means smart grooming. But more than anything else, style is about demeanor. A man of style carries himself with dignity, with strength, with purpose, with confidence. These are not overtly visual attributes like a suit of clothes, yet you see them instantly in a stylish man. It is how he carries his head, shakes hands, or uses eye contact; it is how he smiles or laughs; it is how he fits into any situation so naturally, so quickly. Ultimately, style is about

HOW TO WEAR A SCARF—MANFULLY

If you live in Ft. Lauderdale or San Diego, you may never need a scarf. But those in colder climes should bear in mind that the scarf should always complement your overcoat. That doesn't mean you have to find a perfect color match to your coat. Check and plaid scarves work well with almost any neutral, solid topcoat. But don't wear a patterned scarf with a patterned coat.

Wear your scarf in a simple, straightforward style. Just cross it over the front of your neck and let both ends hang down the front, inside your coat. Do this, and you will always look good.

being yourself. It is about knowing exactly who you are and then crafting a look that projects that, without compromise or bending to the winds of fashion or peer pressure.

What does this have to do with longevity? More than you may think. Self-confidence, pride, independence—these are outstanding mental attributes. Moreover, if you look good, you will feel good, others will feel good about you, and so you will be motivated to continue looking and feeling good. It is a never-ending cycle with never-ending rewards. Stated simply, style is a life-enhancing, life-celebrating habit.

Back to the Clothes

Step one in this style transformation, of course, is fixing your wardrobe. We know you're too busy to keep current on the latest fashions, and that's fine. In fact, it's probably preferable. As a rule, men's clothing styles change slowly, so keeping up isn't that hard. What's more, certain types of traditional men's wear never become passé. So if you lean toward a traditional look, you'll always be in style, even as you grow older.

You have to be prepared to discard those contents of your wardrobe that belong to a younger, less wise era in your life, no matter how much sentimental value you've attached to them. Yes, that includes the rhinestone-studded shirt you wore during your urban-cowboy phase.

Following is an item-by-item, season-by-season plan for remaking your closet into a monument of timeless style. Once you have cleaned your closet, take out a pad of paper and write down any of the listed apparel that you are missing.

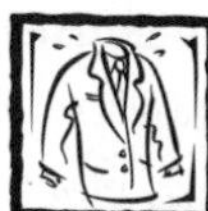

Fall/Winter Wardrobe

The contents of your closet must be dictated, of course, by your lifestyle. If you're an investment banker, you'll own more suits than a machinist. If you're a priest or in the military, your fashion options are greatly simplified. Keeping this in mind, we offer some guidelines on what clothes to have in your closet for the fall and winter months.

Shirts (long-sleeve): Cotton turtleneck; flannel shirt (plaid or print); corduroy shirt (solid or print); button-down cotton oxford (solid or striped); pinpoint oxford (white or blue; button-down or spread collar); solid or white dress shirt, cut fuller (variety of weaves and collars); denim work shirt (button-down or straight collar); three-button knit polo shirt or heavy-gauze rugby shirt

Sweaters (ribbed, cable knit, fancy pattern, or solid): Wool V-neck, crew neck, cardigan, turtleneck

Pants: Jeans (blue or black), khakis (plain front or pleated), gray flannel (pleated, cuffed), plaid or houndstooth, black wool blend or gabardine (pleated, cuffed), corduroys (fine, medium, or wide wale)

Sport jackets: Tweed (Harris or houndstooth), blue blazer, camel hair or cashmere (luxury item)

Suits: Pinstripe worsted and blue, brown, tan, or gray worsted

Shoes: Black dress (wing tip or cap toe), brown semidress suede oxford, walking, slip-on (black, brown or cordovan; penny loafer or tasseled), hiking or work boots, athletic shoes (depending on your sports: tennis, running, basketball, and so on, or cross-training)

Coats: Waist-length ski jacket or parka, long wool, raincoat or trench coat with removable lining

Accessories: Hats (knit stocking cap or Irish walking hat), scarves, gloves, earmuffs, sleeveless down vest, belts

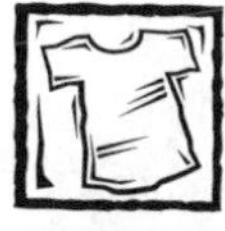

Spring/Summer Wardrobe

The weather is warmer and your wardrobe is cooler in the spring and summer. Here are some basic items you may want to have in your closet.

Shirts (short-sleeve): Polo shirt, button-down or straight collar cotton dress shirt (striped or print), linen, fun and wild print (Hawaiian-style)

Sweaters: Cotton crew neck, mock turtleneck (high-quality cotton, silk-cotton blend, or silk knit), boat neck, sleeveless vest, cotton sweatshirt

Pants: Linen, khakis (plain front or pleated), tropical wool dress trousers, shorts (mid-thigh or to knee)

Sport jackets: Blue blazer and cotton, linen, or silk (variety of patterns)

Suits: Earth-tone gabardine and light shade of poplin (cotton-polyester blend, also called wash-and-wear)

Shoes: Oxford lace-up (buck or suede), athletic shoes (depending on your sports: tennis, running, basketball, and so on, or cross-training), casual slip-on, boat or deck shoes, sandals, cloth or canvas shoes (lace-up or slip-on)

Coats: Denim jacket, light windbreaker, washed silk or microfiber, zip-front, golf-style jacket

Accessories: Swimsuits (boxer trunks), belts (rope-style)

As you can see, your spring/summer wardrobe has a more casual feel to it. But there is a fine line between being casual and being a slob. You can still look natty, not ratty, if you follow these rules.

Know your cotton. You spend much of the warm-weather months wearing cotton, so learn what's primo and what isn't. Labels that say "100 percent combed cotton" or "mercerized cotton" and have tags boasting of double-yarn construction or a special cotton variety such as pima are all good bets. "Mercerized" means that once a cotton thread is spun, the extra fluff is removed. This gives a shirt a smooth, polished feel and sharper color. This stuff looks good under a summer sport coat.

Decide what to dry clean. Some of the garments you should regularly take to

BIG-FOOT FACT

If that pair of shoes you bought 6 years ago seems tighter now, it may be that they are. Your feet can continue to expand in length and width throughout your life. Carrying all that weight above them can stretch ligaments and tendons enough that your feet may grow one full size by the time you turn 50.

To give your feet a break, measure them every trip to the shoe store. And spend more time in shoes with laces. They keep your feet from expanding better than slip-ons do.

the cleaners are khaki shorts, linen shirts, and chinos. Dry cleaning is inexpensive, and you'll get your clothes back crisp and as wrinkle-free as a supermodel's face.

Be wary of linen. A short-sleeve linen shirt provides a classic look at a Fourth of July picnic. But linen pants or a linen suit for business wear is riskier. The reason is *mucho* wrinkles. Silk and rayon are summer fabrics with similar risk factors, so determine the wrinkle quotient for a particular garment by wearing it in a no-pressure weekend setting. If it holds up, work it into your weekday rotation.

Don't bare too much. If you've worked out diligently and are proud of your body, summer clothes offer the best opportunity to strut your stuff. Enjoy the admiring glances, but don't turn them into rolled eyes by going too tight, too bare, too often. If your body is still more fluff than buff, you need to learn what is flattering and what isn't. Avoid horizontal stripes and anything form-fitting, and you ought to be okay.

Office Decorum

There's a revolution in office wear. Thanks to those bad boys of the Internet industry, where every day is Hawaiian shirt day, never before have so many workers tossed off their ties and loosened their clothing inhibitions. Today, casual-dress offices are pretty common—and we're talking about every day, not just on Fridays. It's no surprise that there are plenty of casual-clothes casualties out there. Many workers grapple with what's appropriate under the new rules. Here are some tips to help you avoid a fashion faux pas.

- Take your wardrobe cues from this chapter. Observe how your company's movers and shakers dress. Then, dress a bit more conservatively than that because rank has its privileges. If you change jobs, don't assume that what you wore at your last job still passes muster. Standards vary from region to region, from company to company. Remember that it's safer to look a little too dressy than to be underdressed. You can always dress down by removing your jacket, loosening your tie, or rolling up your sleeves. But you can't go the other way.
- Use caution in wearing a T-shirt. At some companies, they are out of the question. Even if your employer permits them, limit yourself to a solid-colored shirt, maybe with a single chest pocket. Don't wear a tee promoting a concert, a beer, a girlie bar, or anything else.
- Consider wearing a blazer or sport coat. It spiffs up even the most casual garb, including jeans. And if it's too dressy, you can always take it off.

- Safe shirts for casual wear include polo shirts, solid colors or muted prints, banded-collar shirts, denim shirts, nearly pressed oxford button-downs, and stylish rugby shirts. Chambray, denim, and flannel give a softer look than standard starched cotton.
- Safe pants for casual wear are dress slacks and khakis. Jeans might be okay—review tip one again—if they're crisp and clean and dressed up with an oxford shirt and blazer.

Workout Wear

Finally, while you're taking stock of your wardrobe, you may as well survey your gym gear. If you belong to a health club, you already know they've become as glitzy as gambling casinos and turned into places where men and women are often as intent on ogling one another as in getting or staying fit.

Even if your interest is in dumbbell curls rather than girls with curls, it behooves you to look sharp at the gym. Exercising is a good way to socialize, even to network and conduct business. So do you really want to look like the gym equivalent of a guy wearing black shoes with white socks? If not, keep the following guidelines in mind when you're packaging your gym bag.

Scrap the skintights. If your shorts are so tight that you're the butt of jokes, it's time to go to bigger sizes.

Be fabric-conscious. If your gym clothes are made of polyester or acrylic fabric, ditch them. They don't look good and, worse, they don't wick away sweat. Replace them with garments made of microfiber, such as Lycra, which look great and breathe easier.

Lose the logos. Don't wear anything to the gym with prominent slogans or logos. Solid, crisp colors are always in style. If you insist on wearing a printed fabric, make sure it's a small, subtle print.

Go vertical. If you've added girth to your gut, again, ditch the horizontal stripes. They make you look even wider than you are.

Think about your location. What may be hip in a California health club could elicit giggles and guffaws in New Jersey. Generally, the farther east you go, the safer you'll be dressing in a conservative and simple shorts-and-t-shirt combo.

Buy Some New Clothes

The Day's Task

Yesterday, you came up with a list of clothing that you need to round out your closet's offerings. There's no need to buy it all in one day, of course; that would be expensive, mind-numbing, and utterly miserable. So prioritize your shopping. Figure out what you need soon, what can wait. Schedule much of your shopping for the end of January and early in August. That's when you'll find the best deals, just after the holiday rush and just before the fall fashions hit the shelves.

But be sure to leave something to buy today, for it's time to learn how to shop. Here are the first lessons. Take your list, and stick to it. Don't browse or impulse buy; you'll end up with stuff you don't need and spend more than you intended. Dress for your shopping trip based on what you're looking for. If you need a sport coat and dress shoes, for example, wear a button-down shirt and thin socks, not a bulky sweater and thick sport socks.

Stereotypes aside, clothes shopping need not be torture for men. You just have to know what you want and how to get the highest quality, quickly. You have your list, so the battle is in good part won. The next step is to know quality when you see it. To do that, you need a sense of fabrics, patterns, and color schemes. That's where this chapter comes in.

Why do you need to know this stuff? It's simple: To look good, you have to know what matches and what clashes. That's pretty obvious where colors or patterns are concerned. But a discerning eye is also needed for fabrics. Regardless of color, some fabrics—because of their texture or how they're made—just do not go with other fabrics. And even clothes made with the same type of fabric can vary widely in texture and quality. Knowing how to spot what is quality and what isn't makes all the difference between buying

SUITABLE ADVICE

Next time you buy a suit, remember the following.

- As your midsection expands, so does your waist size. If you don't buy bigger pants, you'll end up with pants that hang low in the front, giving you an aging, sagging-crotch appearance. Have the pants tailored to fit your dimensions.
- If your shoulders start sloping, you'll find that your jacket rides up in back. So when you have your jackets fitted, don't suddenly develop military-perfect posture. Just stand the way you normally do.
- Don't wear your new suit with an old tie from the back of your closet unless the widest part of the tie is the same width as the lapel of the jacket. Or, to avoid guessing games, treat yourself to a new tie when you buy the suit.

a wardrobe that will look good on you for years to come and buying one that makes you look like a rumpled, threadbare old man.

Finding Fine Fabrics

The clothing you buy will have either a hard finish or a soft finish. Hard finishes are flat, smooth, and closely woven. They feel thin and durable. Examples include 100 percent wool or blends of wool or cotton and synthetic fabrics.

Soft finishes are thicker and bulkier. They look and feel warmer. They trap heat and are better for winter and casual wear. Flannel is one example of a soft finish.

Hard-finish fabrics hold creases better, while softer fabrics don't hold creases unless they're fixed with synthetics.

Trust your touch more than your eyes when deciding whether to buy a particular garment. Since most guys no longer wear undershirts, texture is especially important when buying a shirt, which will brush your skin. Look for a comfortable cotton shirt, a soft fabric that breathes.

Here's the scoop on the major fabrics and their qualities:

Cotton. Cotton goes by more names than a check forger: chambray, chino, corduroy, denim, poplin, seersucker, terry cloth, and velvet. Cotton is king for good reason. It not only looks good, but its porous quality absorbs body moisture, keeping your skin dry. It washes easily, especially in cold water, without damage to its fibers.

Wool. No need to feel sheepish if you don't know this, but wool fiber is, first and foremost, flexible. It will bend up to 20,000 times before it breaks. That's more than 6 times the resiliency of cotton and more than 10 times sturdier than silk. That's why nearly 9 out of 10 suits and three-quarters of all sport jackets are either 100 percent wool or wool blends.

Wool comes in two types of yarn: woolen and worsted. Woolen yarn is used in the winter fabrics: flannels, tweeds, and meltons. Worsted yarn is finer and more tightly twisted than woolen. An example is gabardine. Worsted wool is terrific for moderately warm climates and helps give you a refined look.

Synthetics. Now a half-century old, polyester was one of the early man-made, or synthetic, fabrics (nylon was the first). It's made by heating two petroleum-based chemicals and forcing the resulting molten liquid through tiny holes to form fibers.

Synthetics' best qualities are that they are wrinkle-resistant and can take endless beatings in a washer and dryer. One of their drawbacks is that they don't breathe, so they don't wick moisture away from your body. Still, their overall quality has improved greatly. Brand names include Dacron, Lycra, CoolMax, Supplex, Tactel, and ThermaStat.

Picking a Pattern

As a general rule, finer, tinier, and more subtle clothing patterns are considered dressier. Louder, bigger, and bolder patterns are more suitable for casual wear. You have three basic choices, with slight variations.

Solids. If you're in doubt as to what type of pattern to go with, solids are always a safe, albeit conservative, choice. The safest of the safe are blue, gray, and beige.

Stripes. Vertical stripes make heavy guys look slimmer and short men appear taller. There are many types of striped shirts: narrow versus wide stripes, evenly spaced versus intermittent, high contrast versus low contrast. The bolder the stripe, the more informal the look. Only you can determine whether you look right in a particular pattern.

Plaids/checks. As with stripes, there are several varieties of plaids and checks. Glen plaid, also called glen check, is a boxlike design formed by lines crossing at right angles. Tartan plaid consists of a series of checks superimposed over each other to form a larger check. Houndstooth is a broken check that resembles a four-

SHOP TALK

Here are some guidelines to follow when you shop for clothes.

Belts. They should be 2 inches larger than your waist.

Jackets. A sport coat should be long enough to cover your butt. If you're taller than 6 feet, buy a long.

Shirts. The thinner the stripe is, the dressier the shirt.

Pants. Avoid those with loose strings or shiny fabrics. Be sure there's ample fabric so that you'll be able to let them out if you develop an ample waistline.

pointed star or a dog's teeth. Tattersall check is a pattern of regularly spaced lines in two different colors that cross each other like a game of tic-tac-toe.

Other patterns that don't fall into any of the above categories include paisley, herringbone, and polka dots. Regardless of the pattern, the tricky business for you, the clothes buyer, is to mix and match patterns in a way that doesn't cause a wave of migraine headaches among people you meet.

You can mix and match in any of four ways. (For the purposes of this exercise, we'll assume you're coordinating a jacket or suit with a shirt and tie.) The first way is to buy three solid colors. Try to make one of the colors vivid enough to jump out from the others. The second method is to mix two solid colors with one pattern. Next is to combine two patterns and one solid. Be sure the sizes of the two patterns aren't the same. The fourth and most difficult way to mix and match is with three patterns. Use two of one pattern and one of another, for example, two checks of different sizes and one stripe, or two stripes of different sizes and one small plaid or check.

Color Bind

Wear clothing in colors that flatter you, and you'll look healthier, more powerful, and vital. Choose the wrong colors, and you'll appear older and sickly.

Men with muted or softer complexions look better in hazy colors that have a touch of gray or are faded. Those of us with darker complexions and hair look better in bright, crisp, rich colors. If you're in doubt as to where you fall, buy clothes in colors to match your eye color—a foolproof technique.

Start Caring for Your Skin

The Day's Task

Open your medicine cabinet. Check the cluttered little cupboard jammed below the bathroom sink. Scan any shelves on the bathroom walls that hold various and assorted sundries. If you don't find the following items there, go out and buy them. Start using them immediately. Make it a lifelong habit.

- **An all-over moisturizing lotion**
- **A body scrub**
- **Deodorant**
- **A really good bar of soap**
- **A cooldown product**

Wait! Don't stop reading because you think only frivolous fops and pretty-boy models give a dermis about their skin. Truth is, ever-increasing numbers of men are spending money on cleansers, moisturizers, anti-aging supplements, and other products aimed at keeping their skin young. This is not a bad thing, and here's why.

Healthy, youthful-looking skin looks good. Looking good projects an image of vitality. Women, children, potential bosses, and fellow airplane passengers like that. Healthy skin also feels good. You don't need to itch, scratch, or rub. You are comfortable.

Taking care of your 14 to 18 square feet of skin just makes sense. And it doesn't cost too many cents. Moreover, it makes the statement that you give a damn about how you look and how you feel. It is a self-indulgent pleasure that confident men aren't embarrassed about enjoying.

The proof of this is that more men are devoting time and money to skin care. One study estimated that sales of toiletries such as deodorants, scented soaps, shower gels, and facial and body scrubs geared to men exceeded $44

SKIN-CARE FARE

Even though the average person uses at least seven different skin care products a day, most men give them no more thought than they would pimples on their butts. Understandably, our knowledge of skin care products is about as comprehensive as that of Albanian literature. Read on for help.

Astringents. These products remove oils and soap residue from your skin. They are generally drying; witch hazel is one example. If you have dry, sensitive, or irritated skin, you may feel itching and burning after using an astringent.

Moisturizers. These lotions prevent water loss by coating an oily substance over your skin to keep water in or by drawing water from the inner skin layer to the outer skin layer.

Lanolin. This wool grease is sometimes used as a moisturizing ingredient in skin care products. Products labeled "hypoallergenic" often contain lanolin.

Sunscreens. You know what they are, but how do they work? They contain chemicals that either absorb, reflect, or scatter light.

million in 1998. The Clinique cosmetics company even has a "For Men Only" area on its Web site where guys can get a skin-type analysis and other skin care information.

So let there be no arguments. Ignore skin care only if you dare. For the straight scoop on face goop, check out Day 4 of this week. For tips on enhancing the rest of your bod, read on.

Your Skin-Care Arsenal

You may think that just because you wear long pants and a long-sleeved shirt to work, you needn't concern yourself with the skin beneath your clothes. After all, who's going to see it, right?

The thing is, however, if you're lucky enough to get naked for some indoor calisthenics now and then, your lady friend will see—and feel—your hide. If it's rough or flaky, *you'll* want to hide. And except in the gym or when you're playing a sport, how your skin smells is important too. Here's more info on the stuff you need to look and smell your best.

- An all-over moisturizing lotion keeps your skin looking younger. Typically, you use it after a shower. Squeeze a teaspoon or so into your hand, and rub it into your arms, legs, shoulders, back, wherever. If you have oily skin, choose a moisturizer that has a larger percentage of water than of emollient. If you're a dry guy, select a lotion that has a higher percentage of moisturizer than water.
- A body scrub is a cleanser that contains abrasive particles, such as—don't laugh—apricot pieces. It is usually heavier than a facial scrub; it has bigger, more abrasive particles than face scrubs. In either case, the abrasives help remove old or dead skin cells. Rub it on wet skin and rinse.
- Deodorant kills bacteria and leaves a nice smell. You may prefer an antiperspirant. It prevents sweating.
- If you have dry skin, use a mild soap or soapless cleanser. Use as little soap as possible, shower or bathe in cool water, and apply a moisturizer immediately after toweling down. Guys with oily skin can use a nondeodorant soap. An antibacterial soap may also be a good choice because it kills bacteria and may prevent breakouts in the process.
- If you sweat like an NBA player or have trouble bringing down your body temperature after exercise, several cooldown products may help. Jovan BodyTonic Refreshing Aftersport Body Cooler is a gel that uses marine extracts to cool your overheated engine. Tommy Hilfiger sells Body Cooling Gel with menthol.

Skin Repairs

As your body's biggest organ (no jokes, please), your skin is a broad target for numerous ailments and diseases. Here are some of the most common, along with ways to head them off in advance or treat them when they occur.

Dry skin. Unless you're auditioning for the part of the Elephant Man, you don't want itchy, scaly skin. You can try to avoid the condition by showering or taking a bath in warm, not hot, water. If the water is too hot, it melts lipids that protect your skin. Afterward, put a capful of mineral oil on a wet washcloth and apply to areas that tend to be dry, such as your arms, legs, and torso. Avoid your face, underarms, and groin.

Then, add a good, unscented moisturizing cream like Eucerin to your arms and legs. Using a moisturizer twice a day, especially right after showering, should help a lot if you already have dry skin. And if you live in a dry climate or it's winter and the heating system in your home or office dries up the air, use a humidifier to keep yourself moist.

Age spots. Sometimes called liver spots because of their color, these blemishes occur most often on the backs of the hands, the forearms, the shoulders, and the face in people over 55. They are due not to aging but rather to years of accumulated sun damage to the skin.

As with skin cancer, you can minimize the number of these noncancerous spots by wearing sunscreen, a hat, and sunglasses. The sooner in life you start, the better off you'll be later on. Also consider tinting your car windows, if your state's laws allow this. Otherwise, even with the windows rolled up, you won't be shielded from ultraviolet radiation.

Boils. Ugly and painful, boils are infections that originate deep in the layers of a hair follicle or pore in your skin, then rise to the surface. If you have one, apply an antibiotic ointment containing bacitracin zinc. You also should apply warm compresses. Soak a washcloth in warm water and place it on the boil for 15 minutes three times a day. That may bring the boil to a head, and it will drain naturally. Keep the area clean by washing with an antibacterial soap. As tempting as it might be, don't try popping it. You'll run the risk of reinfection.

To avoid boils in the future, use an antibacterial soap on a regular basis and

THE SENSITIVE GUY

Certain drugs and even some colognes can make your skin more sensitive to the sun's ultraviolet rays. Avoid the following products if you work or play outdoors a lot. If you must use them, slather on plenty of sunscreen.

- Aftershaves with musk scents
- Diuretics such as chlorothiazide (Diuril), chlorthalidone (Hygroton), and hydrochlorothiazide (Oretic)
- Antibiotics such as sulfonamides (Bactrim) and tetracycline (Sumycin)
- Painkillers containing ibuprofen or naproxen
- Antihistamines such as diphenhydramine (Benadryl), clemastine (Tavist-1), pseudoephedrine (Actifed), and chlorpheniramine (Chlor-Trimeton)

THE SKINNY ON SKIN

Skin accounts for 16 percent of your total weight. A square inch of it has about 600 sweat glands, 100 oil-secreting glands, 60 or so hairs, 20 blood vessels, and a whole lot of nerve endings.

powder areas of your body that may rub uncomfortably against clothing or equipment (like a bike). Otherwise, friction can injure the skin at that spot and create a prime breeding ground for boils.

Insect bites and stings. A variety of pests ranging from mosquitos and chiggers to bees, wasps, and spiders can leave your skin itchy, red, and swollen. Don't scratch the irritated area. It could become infected. Do buy an over-the-counter lotion such as After Bite and a pain reliever such as aspirin or acetaminophen to soothe the sting. If you can stand to do nothing, the discomfort should go away in a few days.

Rashes. Redness caused by the dilation of blood vessels in your skin may be due to your working with a substance that is irritating. But if you also have a fever, a headache, joint pain, or trouble breathing, go to a doctor at once. You may be having a severe allergic reaction to something. For an isolated rash, however, wash the offending substance from your skin. Then, you can cover the rash with a 1 percent hydrocortisone cream to calm the itch. Other remedies include soaking in an oatmeal bath product in water as cold as you can stand and applying cornstarch powder to the affected area.

Blisters. When a shoe or a shovel handle rubs repeatedly against your skin, blisters may raise their ugly, painful heads. If you've popped the blister, keep the "roof" intact—don't rip it off. For an open blister, clean the area and apply a layer of antibiotic cream. Then, cover it with a bandage. Reapply the cream every time you take off the bandage or put on a new one. Whenever possible, expose the blister to air to help it heal faster. If you have a blister on your foot, for example, slip into flip-flops when you get home from work. A 20-minute soak in lukewarm water will also speed the healing process.

Fix Your Face

The Day's Task

This morning, give yourself the perfect shave. To make sure you have all the things you need on hand, read these instructions thoroughly before you start. If you don't have all the necessary equipment, buy it today.

1. **Put the following items by your bathroom sink: your razor, equipped with a brand new blade; a tube of shaving gel or lotion (but not shaving cream in a can); a clean washcloth; and a good-quality skin or aftershave balm for men (make sure it does not have alcohol; instead, seek healthy skin ingredients like alpha hydroxy acids or aloe vera).**
2. **Take a hot shower. When you're done, towel down quickly and get in front of the mirror.**
3. **Lather up your face evenly and fully. Leave the lather on for a minute or two while you brush your hair, put on deodorant, and trim your nails.**
4. **Get back to the mirror. Using a light and smooth stroke, start the shave with your cheeks so that more sensitive areas such as your neck and Adam's apple have more time to soak up moisture from the lather. Unless you need your chin to shine like a bowling ball, shave only in the direction that your hairs grow. Going against the grain may get you a closer shave, but it also gives you a far greater risk of razor bumps, scrapes, cuts, and ingrown hairs. Rinse your blade frequently.**
5. **When you are done (a careful shave takes about 2 minutes), run some warm water onto the washcloth and wipe down your face.**
6. **Rub a dime-size dab of aftershave lotion evenly into your cheeks and neck as well as around your mouth.**

What do you see when you look in the mirror in the morning? A face you've known all your life, sure. And yet, it's not really the same face you had 10 or even 5 years ago. Living on a planet that has gravity and orbits a sun takes its toll. In some cases, it's a toll you don't mind paying. A little gray hair lends a certain gravitas, even as well-placed creases and wrinkles lend your face character and authority.

At the same time, you can't help but notice the ways time has slapped you in the face. Wrinkles around your eyes can make them look sallow and sunken. Skin that once accented a sharp jawline now appears to dangle. Physical imperfections and blemishes of all kinds seem to stand out. But spending hundreds of hours and dollars on concealing facial imperfections feels, well, feminine. What's a man to do?

There are good reasons why we commenced our discussion of facial appearance with the topic of shaving. First, it's the one grooming task you have to deal with most every day. Second, nothing affects your facial appearance more than the state of your whiskers. A bad shave—or no shave—makes you look haggard; a freshly shaved face gives you a youthful glow. Third, a shaven face allows other facial features, such as a strong chin or a nice smile, to stand out.

The theory of shaving that underscores the instructions on the previous page is that the more moist your facial skin, the easier and better the shave. In fact, some believe that the best shave is to be had during your shower, with hot water streaming down your head and steam filling your tiled cubicle as you do the razored nasty. Try it one morning. Near the end of your shower, without any cream or gel or anything applied to your face, shave as you would at the sink. You'll be surprised at how smooth it can be.

Moisture is at the heart of many of the other steps you can take to improve your facial appearance. Here are some quick tips for minimizing or eliminating some of the negatives of your face and accentuating the positives. We promise that none of them involves makeup.

SHAVING FACTS

Here is more than you'll ever need to know about shaving.

- Most guys begin shaving between the ages of 15 and 16.
- A man's beard grows an average of 15⁄1,000 inch a day, or 5½ inches a year.
- Over the course of his life, a typical man will lop off 27½ feet of whiskers from his face.

Skin-Care Products

To choose the right products to buy, you need to know what type of skin you have. To test for dry skin, wash and dry your face as you normally do. If you skin feels tight and dry immediately after you towel off, you have dry skin. To detect oily skin, check your face in the late afternoon; oil or surface shine is the giveaway. Many of the products below come in versions for dry, normal, or oily skin. Here are some products to consider.

Face moisturizers. These creams provide sun protection and help maintain the elasticity of your skin. Some have a sunscreen and vitamins A or E in the ingredients. If you have oily skin, try an oil-free product.

Face scrubs. These are cleansers that contain abrasive particles that help remove old or dead skin cells. Apply a scrub to wet skin, work it over your face in circles, then rinse it off thoroughly. Don't rub it in too forcefully, however, or you may cause abrasions on your face.

Aftershave products. Look for an aftershave balm rather than the traditional lotion that can make your neck feel like hot chile peppers have been implanted in it. Balms, like lotions, usually contain alcohol or witch hazel. But unlike lotions, their other ingredients include emollients and moisturizers that moisten and soothe your face.

Eye Care

Whether it's a woman or a prospective employer who is sizing you up, your eyes are one of the first things they notice. If your eyes look as dreary as January in Juneau, you're not going to make a good first impression. Here are some eyesores you can make better.

Bags under the eyes. Truth is, baggy eyes take a long time to develop and are hard to erase once you have them. Sometimes, they are caused by fat accumulations, so your weight may be an issue. Other times, the skin around your eyes is thin; basic skin care, as in keeping your face moist and protected from sun, may help.

We can offer you this short-term solution, though: Put some bags on those bags. Place two cool, moist tea bags over your closed eyes for 15 minutes. The tannin in the tea leaves helps pull your skin taut and reduces puffiness. In addition, the cold reduces swelling. Or try two slices of chilled cucumber. This actually works.

Lines around the eyes. Squint enough, and you'll get well-creased facial lines.

WHEN IT'S PAINFUL TO PUCKER

Vicious winds and sun, indoor heating, and dry winter days can all contribute to chapped lips that crack, bleed, and hurt. That's because lips lack the natural oils and pigments that the rest of your skin uses to protect itself. To zap chapped lips, use a lip balm with an SPF of 25 or higher when you're outside. This will protect you from both the elements and the sun.

The only problem with lip balm is that the little tubes are easily lost. The solution is to buy a half-dozen tubes at a time and scatter them among several handy locations: in your car, in your winter jacket, by the bathroom sink, by the back door. Keep an extra two for backup.

To avoid squinting, stop furrowing your brow in an attempt to look smart or fierce. But most important, wear shades when you're not in the shade. The benefits of sunglasses are more than cosmetic. Sunglasses also protect you from cataracts, macular degeneration, and other eye disorders.

When you go shopping for shades, buy a pair that blocks 75 to 90 percent of visible light and 99 percent or more of ultraviolet, or UV, rays. This information should be on the label. Look for glasses with large lenses that cover your entire eyes, preferably with gray lenses for minimal color distortion. Sunglasses with the seal of the American Optometric Association Seal of Acceptance meet these guidelines.

Acne

It can be pretty depressing when you have more pimples than your 15-year-old son. Adult acne affects millions of Americans, but there are numerous ways to control those outbreaks.

- Wash your face once a day with a mild, 2.5 percent form of benzoyl peroxide wash. This over-the-counter medication kills bacteria that cause acne.
- If your skin isn't dry, don't use a moisturizer. It'll just clog up your pores and cause acne.
- Avoid touching your face with your hands. The bacteria and acne-causing oils on your hands can cause you to break out.

- Change towels and pillowcases more often—as much as a few times a week. This helps keep blemish-causing bacteria off your face.
- Get stressed less. Stress triggers zit attacks. Don't pile on more work and responsibilities than you can handle. Find some quiet time for yourself.

Chin Appearance

We can't promise you a chiseled chin, but if you have too much or too little, there are steps you can take to achieve a firmer appearance.

Weak chin. To counteract the image of weakness that a lack of chin unfairly connotes, don't wear collarless shirts. Collars suggest authority. Strive to wear collars that contrast in color with the clothes that surround them. The classic combination of a dark blue suit, a white shirt, and a burgundy tie beautifully downplays a small chin.

Double chin. If your chin has a twin, you probably have more of everything else too. Unless you're genetically predisposed to a double chin, you need to lose weight, Bub. Weight loss is a complex subject, but here's a simple way to get started. About 10 percent of your metabolism is devoted to digesting the food you eat. The more often you eat, the higher you ramp up this part of your metabolism. Eat many small meals a day—every 3 hours or so, even if you're not all that hungry.

Losing weight takes time, of course. While you're waiting for the pounds to melt, dress in ways that deemphasize your chin. Try a dark blue or black cotton-knit turtleneck, tucking it under about an inch at the top. Never wear a shirt that's too tight in the neck. Keep your hair closely cropped and combed back at the sides. Longer hair draws attention to a double chin.

If you smoke or spend a lot of time in the sun, stop it. Both can hasten your skin's loss of elasticity. Vitamin C creams and alpha hydroxy acids can help retain your skin's youthfulness. Apply them to clean skin, morning and evening, following the directions on the label.

You also can do exercises to firm up your chin. Lie on your back on the floor with your head up and repeatedly touch your chin to your chest. Do two or three sets of 8 to 15 repetitions, two or three times a week. A variation that will work the sides of your chin is to lie on your side and touch your chin to your raised shoulder. Do two or three sets of 8 to 15 repetitions, then switch sides and repeat. These exercises also help you tone the turkey-neck effect you may get once you do lose weight.

Facial Shape

Some facial features are harder to compensate for, but even in these cases there are a few things you can do.

Jowls. Dark colors make you appear thinner, so wear them. In casual wear, dark polo shirts and mock turtlenecks will help.

Thin face. If you can, go with a fuller hairstyle. Wear thicker shirts such as flannel ones, if you can get away with it at the office, and wear houndstooth and tweed jackets. These fabrics draw attention away from your face, creating the illusion that your face is wider.

Large nose. Fuller hair around the sides of your face, wider shoulders in your suits and sport coats, and layered clothing such as a T-shirt, an open-collared shirt, and a jacket or sport coat will all make everything around your face appear somewhat larger. The idea is to draw visual attention downward and outward.

Get a Haircut

The Day's Task

Tell the missus that you'll be an hour late coming home tonight—you're bringing her a surprise.

Even if you have a regular barber or stylist, ask a few guys—preferably guys who don't look like their hair has been cut with hedge trimmers—who cuts their hair and whether they're satisfied. Then, call one of the recommended haircutters and set up an appointment for after work. When you get there, ask for a simple trim.

A good haircutter should ask you questions about how you've been wearing your hair and whether you're happy with the way it looks. If he doesn't ask questions, speak up before the first scissors snip and elaborate on your simple-trim request. Tell him how long you like your hair and what style you have in mind.

After the cut, pick up chocolates, flowers, or champagne for your wife and give her two surprises: the gift and a more presentable you.

Not sure what hairstyle would look best on you? Of course not. Hair is something we rarely give a thought to until it's gone. But caring for your coif, however much or little of it you may have, is important. Granted, a good haircut won't add years to your life, but it can make you look and feel younger and more vital than your years. Similarly, poor hair care makes you look and feel like an aging slob, a wizened old guy with unattractive kinks of hair shooting from his head, his ears, his collar. Here are some guidelines for helping your hair do its, er, part in your overall Longevity Program.

The Right Barber for Your Pate

"Guys don't want to waste time on their hair," says Michael diCesare, an Emmy Award–winning stylist in New York City who does hair for the guests on *The Late Show with David Letterman*. "Get a cut every 4 to 6 weeks to provide style with minimum effort."

There are a few ways to tell if your barber is worth a return visit. First, he isn't content with your instructions to "take a little off" or "cut it short." These aren't specific enough for him to do a good job. A good stylist will probe deeper. Because men often don't have the vocabulary to effectively talk about hair, the best communication is often through photos, either ones you've brought in (that's a hint) or ones in a book the barber keeps for just such occasions. Another topic of conversation should be the hair products you use. The cut might be different if you use styling gel every morning, for example.

A barber should concentrate on your hair, not on his probing questions about your work or your love life or the ball game on television. You should not feel compelled to have a conversation while the cutting is going on, although it doesn't hurt either. Just make sure he's not overly distracted.

Next, he should take care of the smaller details, such as trimming your eyebrows and ear hair as well as the fuzz on the back of your neck.

Finally, he should ask how you want to finish your hair: Do you want some gel or spray, or do you want your hair left dry? There's nothing quite as frustrating as walking out of the barbershop with your hair plastered to your skull even though you wear it dry and loose the rest of your life.

You almost certainly will look good in the minutes after a cut has been completed. The trick is looking good the next day. How can you tell if your barber earned his keep? A good haircut is one that responds well after you wash it. It should take no more than 3 minutes to style and should fall right in place for you, diCesare says. In other words, a good cut precludes cowlicks. "A good haircut in itself is all you need to eliminate a cowlick. A stylist should never correct a cowlick by cutting into it," diCesare says.

The Right Style for Your Face

Picking the right style is often a function of the shape of your face. If you don't know the shape of your face, ask the stylist, then bear in mind these guidelines.

Round or oval face. Avoid a round do, à la Art Garfunkel. Round on round creates a halo effect, so unless you're looking to capitalize on the craze over angels, avoid it.

Go for a cut with straight lines to balance out the roundness of your face. Have your barber or stylist taper your hair very close in through the sides. Then, as your

HAIR-CARE WARES

So many hair products, so little time to learn what the devil they are. Briefly, we explain.

Clarifying shampoo. Use this to clean away buildup from other hair products.

Conditioner. Apply to wet hair after shampooing, then rinse out. It adds moisture, shine, protein, and more while taking out the tangles.

Gel. This goop holds hair in place. It's good for styling short hair. If you apply it to wet hair, it dries hard, leaving a wet look. Apply it to dry hair, and it takes off the fluff and is less noticeable. "I've been styling hair for more than 15 years, and the one thing that has been apparent all along is that men love gel," says New York City stylist Michael diCesare. "It's masculine, it's quick, and it's easy—a real guy thing."

Glosser, shiner, polisher, laminator, or glass. These are potions filled with silicone or oil that you rub onto your hair to smooth it and make it gleam. A few drops will do.

Moisturizing products. These include shampoos, conditioners, and other treatments that soften dry, brittle hair. Many of them contain glycerin, which helps hair grab and retain moisture.

Mousse. This foaming conditioner helps hold hair in place. Its works best on wavy, longer hair.

Spritz or spray gel. These lighter, liquefied gels are sprayed onto hair as a mist to keep it in place. They're good for all hair textures and can be applied to wet or dry hair.

Thickeners, volumizers, or bodybuilders. These can be ingredients found in shampoos and conditioners. They're also available as stand-alone products that infuse hair with proteins or coat it with polymers or waxes to make it seem thicker.

head gradually rounds, he should leave a bit more length on top, creating a square shape. Sideburns can also help balance a round face. Keep them closely trimmed.

If you have thinning hair, avoid styles that have too much length on top, but still try for this look. Just have it cut a little closer on top and even closer on the sides. Too much hair on the sides draws attention to the lack of hair on top.

Long face. Get a cut with a little volume on the sides and maybe a little hair showing at the nape of your neck. Have your hair cut very close at your ears, then gradually add length up past your temples. It should be cut fairly short on top. The overall effect will add volume to the sides of your face instead of more length. If your hair is too full on top, it will accentuate the length of your face—just what you don't want.

Don't grow your hair long if you have a long face, and don't grow long sideburns. Both will increase—you guessed it—the long look of your face.

Square face. The lucky guys with square faces have the most latitude in how they style their hair. Almost any cut that isn't square will do. If your hair is thinning, be sure it gets proportionately shorter as you work your way down from the top. Medium length sideburns are best. They showcase your strong jaw without overdoing it.

Hair and Race

Men of color have hair that's just as distinctive as they are. Here are some tips on the best ways to have your hair cut.

- African-Americans should be especially diligent about shampooing with a conditioner that will keep their hair well-oiled. That's because the curl pattern of the hairs makes it hard for natural oils secreted by the hair follicle to slide out along the hair shafts to the ends. You should also get your hair cut in sections with scissors and comb, rather than with a clipper, so that the ends can be cut. Otherwise, your hair may look dull and frizzy.
- Asian men generally have thick, coarse hair that should be cut and thinned out every month or so to keep it looking good and healthy. Conditioning also is important because this type of hair tends to be dry.
- Latino men should wear their hair longer because it's so straight. There is little, if anything, you can do with it when it's too short.

Hair Today, Gone Tomorrow

All this talk about hairstyles and hair products may seem a wee bit depressing if your hair is disappearing faster than the Amazon rainforest. One option that has become increasingly popular is to shave your head. It doesn't seem to have

TIPPING THE BARBER

It's become an expensive but worthwhile rule of life: When a person provides you with high-quality service, you reward them with a gratuity. It applies to waitresses, porters, taxi drivers, repairmen, and hairstylists as well. "A good rule of thumb is to tip your stylist the same as you would a waiter, 15 to 20 percent, depending on service," says New York City stylist Michael diCesare. Why the largesse? For one thing, much of the price of your haircut goes to the shop, not the stylist. A tip says that you value their professionalism and think they deserve a good living for what they do. It is also a great way to guarantee that your next cut will be every bit as good, if not better. Believe us, they will remember, even if 6 weeks go by.

hurt Michael Jordan or Jesse Ventura. Here's how to give your head a close shave.

Shave with the same razor and shaving cream or gel you use on your face. Shave in the direction in which your hair grows. Hair on the back of your head grows downward; hair on the top of your head tends to grow toward the back and to the sides.

When you're finished shaving and drying off your head, apply a little moisturizer to replace the natural oils that you scraped off along with the hair. To keep your head as smooth as a cue ball, shave every day with an electric razor.

Get an Attitude

The Day's Task

You will learn a lot about yourself today, merely by seeing if the task at hand is difficult or easy. Here's the drill.

As you go about your day, practice the art of the perfect hello with every friend, coworker, and acquaintance you encounter. There should be four parts to your greeting (do them simultaneously).

1. **Smile at the person.**
2. **Look the person in the eye.**
3. **Use his or her name in your greeting, even if it's just "Hello, Bubba."**
4. **Speak loudly and clearly.**

This works even when you're passing someone in a hall. If the person wants to stop and talk, then do so: stop, face them straight on, continuing to follow the steps above and standing with your arms at your sides or your hands crossed at your waist (but not across your chest). Be the one to cut off the conversation, with a polite and smiling "Please excuse me. I do need to run, but let's continue this soon" or some such polite but honest and confident comment.

Maintain this friendly, confident demeanor for all of your waking hours. No matter how tired, ornery, stressed, or confused you may be inside, appear to be pleased and in control. No complaining today.

We cannot say with certainty that having a confident, bold personality will add years to your life. What we can tell you is that health has many components—physical, mental, even spiritual—that blend together into an impossibly complex concoction that defines your well-being. Being happy, of course, is a big factor in your long-term well-being. And part of being happy is having a winning, unique attitude.

And so, on this day, we want you to focus on the intangible part of your style: your presence, your persona, your public face. We'll throw out some small bits of advice and some big-picture thoughts for you to ponder. Consider this an important day in this 12-week program. This is more than just grooming and clothes, friend. This is who you are.

The Confidence Factor

Ask any image consultant worth his fancy fountain pen, and he'll tell you that confidence is a cornerstone of style. It doesn't matter what fabric hangs from your shoulders or whether your shoes are so shiny that they signal distant planes. If you don't believe in yourself, your accoutrements are superfluous. "A power suit will never save you if you're coming off as a Milquetoast," says Ken Karpinski, an image consultant in Sterling, Virginia.

Don't mistake confidence for arrogance. We are not recommending that you be overbearing or obnoxious. Confidence can—and often should—be quiet, not loud. You don't have to be Muhammad Ali, telling the world that you are the greatest. Ali, after all, was one of the true originals of the 20th century. He could get away with it just because he was Ali. Look at how phony and pathetic most other athletes come across when they mimic his act.

True confidence comes from knowing what you're capable of doing. And it can be conveyed in many ways, most of them without uttering a word.

"Confidence is many things to many people, but you can't go wrong knowing the basics: good posture, a firm handshake, excellent eye contact, intellect, a sense of humor, and a pleasant speaking voice," says Louise Elerding of the Association of Image Consultants International in Glendale, California.

The Role of Individuality

When we talk about stylish, confident men, we invariably talk about men who have a strong sense of who they are. Being your own man comes from deep within. It's not a designer label, a hairstyle, or a cologne. It's not an external affectation, like a cigar, a derby, or a pair of suspenders.

"Being your own man is an attitude. It's a sense of self, an expression of your soul," says David Wolfe, a trend forecaster with the Donegal Group in New York City. "Most men don't give this much thought; they seem to have more interesting things to do. Instead, they'll follow someone else's lead."

We face tremendous pressures—some subtle, some blatantly obvious—to conform. But even in the most buttoned-down, rigid settings, there is room for you to be your own man. Here are some ways to not only maintain your individuality but also assert it.

Do what gives you pleasure. Being your own man means not letting others dictate how you act, what you wear, or where you spend your time. A man of style knows the fads and generally ignores them. If he likes tea more than coffee, he orders tea when everyone else orders cappuccino.

He also doesn't take up tennis because the boss loves to play or drink microbrew beer to impress his buddies. Instead, he does what he likes, unabashedly, whether it be cooking, hang gliding, volunteering at the local library, or running ultramarathons.

Surround yourself with people you like. Do you think that the janitor is a great guy? Then be his friend, with pride. In the civilized world, there is no caste system. A man who is true to himself doesn't let social conventions or peer pressure dictate his acquaintances or friends. The truly wise man has friends of many ages, backgrounds, educations, and beliefs. The commonality is that they all spark his mind or soul in some way that he values.

Don't mistake contrariness for uniqueness. Merely having the opposite opinion doesn't make you an individual. These days, it is almost trendy to be cynical, to challenge all authority, to question everything, and to tear down people and institutions. Sometimes it is valid and even fun to do, a type of mental gymnastics; sometimes it's just obnoxious. The bottom line is that a man with positive energy is a greater force than a man with negative energy. Want to be your own man? Make the world a better place not just by tearing down the bad but by offering some good, both in words and actions.

Be modest. Being your own man often means that you have hobbies, achievements, even friends that are unique. You should be proud of this. But don't brag. Nothing will make you seem more common than touting all the things that you did over the weekend. A man of style carries himself with dignity and humility; he does what he does not to impress others but to make himself happy.

Don't be mucho macho. "Confident individuals are not hampered by a masculine image anymore," says Leon Hall of the Fashion Association of New York City. This extends from appearance (wearing an earring or shorts, for example) to expressing emotions (letting a tear drop when Ingrid Bergman gets on the plane, leaving Humphrey Bogart behind in *Casablanca*) to being one of the guys (telling your pals to can it when they start describing what they would like to do to that new "babe" in accounting).

Grace in Every Situation

It's important to cultivate who you are on the inside before you worry too much about how you appear on the outside. That said, let's shift to some specific advice on how to carry yourself with confidence and style in several situations.

Entering a crowded room. Whether it's at a cocktail party, a bustling convention center, or a crowded restaurant, the way you move through a room can convey a sense of elegance and style, even to those who see you from afar. "Some people walk into a room. Other people enter it," says Princess Jenkins of Majestic Images International in New York City. "Most of us have walked into a room and walked past three people we knew without saying hello, because we didn't notice them. That's because we walked into the room, we didn't enter it."

To make a grand entrance, Jenkins suggests the following tips.

- Pause after you walk through the door.
- Quickly survey the room with your eyes, acknowledging whom you know at the far end first.
- As you walk toward familiar faces, scan nearby, nodding and acknowledging people close to you, offering warm greetings and engaging in chitchat.
- Continue working the room until you catch up with the people you know at the far end. By then, you will have made a favorable impression on those you chatted with as well as those who just observed you.

Making introductions. Excel at introductions. You'd be surprised how many people bungle an otherwise easy opportunity to look genteel. Here's a formula to follow for flawless intros.

Graciously interrupt your current conversation, using the name of the person to whom you're talking. Introduce the newcomer first, by his or her first and last name, and include some personal details. Then, as the newcomer and the person you were talking with shake hands, introduce the latter, using the same approach. For example, "Excuse me, Tom, I'd like you to meet Bill Smith. Bill's an attorney at Blindem and Bilkem." [Shake] "Bill, Tom Jones. He's a professor at Whassamatta U."

Making small talk. Whether it's a wedding, a business meeting, or a backyard barbeque, every get-together involves small talk. If you're not good at it, scan the newspaper before you leave home. It'll give you something to lead with.

The best way to make small talk is to ask questions. People love to talk about themselves, their careers, their families, their opinions. Don't go for profound or provocative initial questions. Try simple queries about their careers or their connection to the party's host. When they finish replying, ask a good follow-up question, something that shows that you were listening and interested. "Don't try too hard, though, or you could come off as patronizing or insincere. People want sincerity, not schmooze," cautions Jeff Livingston, Ph.D., an information analyst at Cisco Systems in Research Triangle Park, North Carolina.

Handling cultural situations. When in a new cultural situation, be a student. Observe how those around you are eating, interacting, and speaking. Don't try to dazzle your hosts with endless monologues; let others do the talking until you have a good understanding of the rules of the conversation. Even then, understand that you are an outsider; just because others are being boisterous doesn't mean that you can be loud and lewd too. Speak frugally and respectfully.

Most cross-cultural events involve eating. You'll make a strong impression, good or bad, with how you handle yourself at the table. Fortunately, this is an area in which you can practice on a regular basis. Most every city has a diversity of ethnic restaurants; use these to learn the foods and eating styles of the cultures that you likely will be encountering in the future. Learn to use chopsticks. Try the various soups and appetizers. Fear no food. Having a well-developed, worldly palate is not only a clear sign of a stylish, confident man but also enormously enjoyable.

Finally, don't be provincial. In cross-cultural encounters, you'll annoy people if you constantly tell stories about how things are in your own part of the world. Stop yourself from comparing food, rituals, and roles to the ones to which you are accustomed. Your goal is to fit into the situation. Constantly pointing out that you are an outsider precludes this. It also appears arrogant and small-minded.

10 Ways to Prevent Wrinkles

1 **Halt the progress of existing wrinkles.** The number one reason that your skin got wrinkled is that you spent too much time in the sun as a kid. In fact, most sun damage, or photoaging, occurs in the first 10 to 12 years of your life, says George J. Hruza, M.D., associate professor of dermatology at Washington University School of Medicine in St. Louis.

There's not much you can do about that now. But what you can do is keep your wrinkles from deepening. To do that, you need to wear sunscreen with an SPF of at least 15 and apply it at least 15 minutes before you head outside. Reapply it any time you get wet, sweat a lot, or have been the sun for more than 2 hours.

2 **Try an over-the-counter antiwrinkle cream that contains retinoids, suggests Dr. Hruza.** Retinoids, which are derived from vitamin A, increase cell turnover speed. The result is that you get newer, fresher skin faster. "It's best to start using these products once a day, at night, and let your skin get used to them," Dr. Hruza adds. "Also, they make your skin more sensitive to light, so this is another reason to wear sunscreen."

3 **Consider using a cream containing coenzyme Q_{10}.** This nutrient, also called co-Q_{10}, is produced in your body and provides life-sustaining energy to all organs. Researchers found that when 20 volunteers applied a 0.3 percent co-Q_{10} cream once daily to the skin around their eye areas, fine lines and wrinkles decreased by 27 percent within 6 months. The cream tested in this study was Nivea Visage Q10 Wrinkle Control Creme. Other creams have the same amount of co-Q_{10} in a moisturizing base, plus added vitamins.

4 **Another lotion to consider is topical vitamin C.** Vitamin C helps your skin in two ways, explains Lorraine Faxon Meisner, Ph.D., professor of preventive medicine at the University of Wisconsin Medical School and coinventor of Cellex-C, the first antiwrinkle cream to use vitamin C. First, it's needed to make collagen throughout your body, and collagen is needed to support skin. Second, it's a free radical scavenger, helping your skin fight sun damage.

Still, you can't just squeeze an orange on your face and expect results. You need a formulation that penetrates the skin. Products like Cellex-C are sold through dermatologists, plastic surgeons, and licensed skin-care professionals.

5 **Other potions that are great for skin are lotions with alpha hydroxy acids.** These are natural exfoliators (dead-skin removers) made from one of three types of cleansing acid. They reduce wrinkles, but you have to be patient. It'll take a few months. Look for products that contain 8 percent or more glycolic acid. Use them once a day.

6 **Believe it or not, daily shaving might be good for preventing facial wrinkles.** "Men have a higher turnover of dead skin cells because their faces are pushed and pulled when they shave," says Dr. Hruza. "Some people theorize that's one of the reasons that men get wrinkles later in life than women do."

7 **Wear sunglasses whenever you are outdoors.** Squinting in bright sunlight causes wrinkles around the eyes, says David H. McDaniel, M.D., assistant professor of clinical dermatology and plastic surgery at Eastern Virginia Medical School of the Medical College of Hampton Roads in Norfolk. If you wear dark sunglasses, you reduce sun glare and reduce squinting. "I have seen people's fine squint lines disappear within 6 to 8 months once they start wearing dark sunglasses," Dr. McDaniel says.

8 **Keep your weight steady.** Bouncing up and down on the scale dial can create wrinkles too, says Dr. McDaniel. The constant stretching and slackening of skin that occurs when your weight fluctuates wreaks havoc, especially with the skin on your face. The best thing to do if you're on a weight-loss plan is to slim down slowly. It's not only healthier to do it this way but you'll also form fewer wrinkles.

9 **Spit out those cigarettes.** Dermatologists can always pick the smokers out of a crowd, even if the latter don't have cigarettes in their mouths. Smoking constricts capillaries in the face, depriving the skin of blood and decreasing the oxygen supply to the tissues there. Also, pursing your lips around a butt eventually gives you telltale wrinkles above your top lip.

10 **Finally, forget the suntan and stay pale.** Considering that every year more than 10,000 Americans die from skin cancer, you really want to protect your skin as much as possible, with hats, sunglasses, clothes, and, of course, sunblock. "Suntans aren't considered a sign of health anymore," says Vail Reese, M.D., a dermatologist in San Francisco. "In fact, if you look at many of the male and female movie stars of today, most of them are downright pale."

10 Ways to Deal With Hair Loss

1 **Go get a haircut.** We're not joking. "Men who are losing their hair tend to wear their hair the way they did when they were younger—to cling to a style that's just not working anymore," says Vaughn Acord, a senior hairstylist at Bumble and Bumble Hair Salon in New York City. "You have to face the problem and work with what you have." His recommendation is to go short, especially if you have a receding hairline.

2 **Belly up to the sushi bar.** Eating a traditionally American steak-and-potatoes diet can not only plug up your arteries but also might lead to hair plugs. After reviewing 30 years of hair loss and heart disease data collected from more than 2,000 American men, researchers at the University of Texas and Boston University found that those with the least hair also had the highest risks of dying from heart disease. The connection is likely due to nitric oxide, a naturally occurring chemical that prevents blood clots and dilates blood vessels. It also seems to foster hair growth and erections. When atherosclerosis damages the linings of blood vessels, it causes them to produce less nitric oxide, which some physicians think might lead to hair loss.

Eating a low-fat diet and plenty of fish (which is rich in heart-healthy omega-3 fatty acids) and exercising three times a week won't just keep you thinner and alive longer, it might also stop you from looking like Yul Brynner.

3 **Give up cigarettes.** By the time smokers turn 40, many sport the withered hair follicles of much older men. Smoking may play the same role in hair loss as it does in heart disease, says Peter Proctor, M.D., a dermatologist and research pharmacologist in Houston. Tobacco smoke damages the lining of blood vessels, leading them to produce less nitric oxide, and this might short-circuit hair growth. Smoking also diminishes bloodflow to the scalp and causes premature aging in hair follicles. Kick the habit for your hair's sake, if for no other reason.

4 **Tell your boss to back off.** If hair loss is in your genes, everyday stress can accelerate the process, says Dr. Proctor. Stress increases the production of androgen, the male sex hormones destined to kill your hair follicles.

Reducing your stress levels is key (and you'll find some ways to do that in Week 4 of this book). Stress management won't cause the lost hair to grow back, but it may keep you from prematurely losing any more.

5 **Wear a hat when in the sun.** A sunburned scalp is the price of going hatless, especially when you're already thinning on top. But that bad burn causes more than pain; it can make your wispy pate even more sparse.

Sunburns irritate your skin, which responds by creating a natural inflammatory compound called superoxide. This stuff also happens to be the messenger that tells your hair follicle to begin a shedding phase, explains Dr. Proctor. Even when your hair does grow back, it'll be thinner than before.

Wear a spray-on sunblock with an SPF of 30 or greater. Even better, throw on a cap. You'll be glad you did.

6 **Be on guard for skin disorders along your scalp.** Conditions like psoriasis (which causes red, scaly patches on your scalp) and seborrheic dermatitis (an inflammation of the scalp's oil glands) can flare up from time to time, leaving your scalp bumpy, flaky, and itchy. If it happens to you, get to a dermatologist pronto. "Any type of skin disorder on your scalp can make balding worse," says Dr. Proctor.

7 **Pass on unusually strict weight-loss plans.** Fad diets and products that claim to help you get slim fast have an undeniable appeal. But some of the weight you drop might be hair. "The physical stress of a strict diet can cause you to shed hair," says Wilma F. Bergfeld, M.D., head of clinical research in the department of dermatology at the Cleveland Clinic. "And some of the hair might not regrow."

Calorie-sparse diets (fewer than 1,000 calories per day) and big weight fluctuations may also cause genetic hair loss to start sooner, Dr. Bergfeld adds. Never go on a diet that causes you to lose more than a couple of pounds a week, or you might have to buy a hat along with those size-32 pants.

8 **Consider using the herb sage to help battle baldness.** Sage has had a long-standing reputation as a hair preserver. In the old days, people often used sage extracts in hair rinses and shampoos. The herb allegedly had the ability to prevent hair loss and maintain color. Since this use of sage is unlikely to be harmful, add a few teaspoons of sage tincture to your shampoo, suggests James Duke, Ph.D., author of *The Green Pharmacy*.

9 **Check your drugs.** "Certain prescription drugs can cause hair loss," says Peter Panagotacos, M.D., a dermatologist in San Francisco. One of the most likely culprits is isotretinoin (Accutane), an anti-acne medication derived from vitamin A. Other suspects are the calcium blockers used to treat high blood pressure and many cholesterol-lowering drugs. When your doctor prescribes a drug, ask if hair loss is a possible side effect. If it is, pay attention to whether or not you lose more of your mane. Or see if the doc can prescribe a similar drug that won't have that effect.

10 **Try using a hair-thickening shampoo.** Such a shampoo coats your hair with protein and seals in moisture, increasing the diameter of each hair by as much as 50 percent. Unfortunately, it's not cumulative—the effect lasts about a day, or until you shampoo again.

WEEK 9

EAT TO AGE-PROOF YOUR BODY

Analyze Your Food Intake

The Day's Task

Today's task is pretty involved, but we think you will find it most interesting and revealing. It will require an hour or two near the end of the day, plus a few random moments spread throughout the day. To do it most easily, you will need to log on to the Internet later tonight. A calculator will be helpful too.

Here's what to do. When you get dressed this morning, put a folded sheet of blank paper and a pen into your hip or shirt pocket. As the day goes by, write down on that sheet everything that you eat or drink. Do the writing immediately after consumption; don't wait to do it later. Your notes should include amounts. Don't write just "potato chips" but rather "two 1-ounce bags of potato chips."

Eat what you ordinarily do (we hope that it is healthy fare that is based on what we taught you in Week 1). You defeat the purpose if you alter your diet just for today in order to test well. When all your eating is done, isolate yourself with your computer and calculator, and analyze your diet.

Here, we're going to show you ways to assess the quality of your food intake.

Before you can take this on, though, you need to do one thing: sort your list of the food you've eaten today. Put the following headings at the top of a clean page of paper. Under each, write foods you ate that fall into that category. We give you some examples to help you sort.

- Fruits/veggies (include salads)
- Starches (bread, potatoes, rice)
- Entrées (lasagna, pork chops, bacon and eggs, sandwiches)
- Beverages (any drink other than water, tea, or coffee)
- Junk food (chocolate, potato chips, desserts, candy)
- Condiments (butters, jellies, sauces)

Look over everything to just get a feel for how your diet is breaking down. Is there a lengthy line under junk food? Is your fruit-and-veggie list nearly nonexistent? You can tell a lot from just this quick glance.

When you're finished doing that, it's time to ferret out the details. You may want to do this exercise again in a few months, by the way, to see if you have indeed improved your diet.

Calories

Fire up your computer and log on to the Internet. There are a bunch of great calorie counter Web sites out there. Do a search under "calorie counter" and you'll see what we mean. One that we like is from the Calorie Control Council site at www.caloriecontrol.org. All you do is type in the name of the food you ate, and you get a reading. On your day's food inventory, write down next to each food the number of calories it contains and come up with a daily total. You might be surprised at the number of calories you've unknowingly being stowing away.

The question then is, how many should you be taking in? If you're a regular, active man, you need about 2,500 calories per day to meet your energy requirements. If you are active and large, that could go up to 3,200 calories. If you are small and inert, that could go down to 2,000 or so.

Of those calories, roughly 70 percent get burned by basic bodily functions such as digestion, breathing, sleeping, and heart activity. The rest are burnt by physical activity, even if it is just typing or walking to your car. Obviously, the more active you are, the more calories you burn.

It takes 3,500 calories to make a pound of fat. If you shave off a measly 230 calories a day, you'll lose about 2 pounds a month. For the record, 230 calories is roughly equal to a large handful of potato chips or two 16-ounce bottles of sweetened iced tea—hardly a great sacrifice.

Healthy Mix

Here's where you go back to elementary school to relearn the Food Guide Pyramid. Again, do a search on "food guide pyramid" on the Web, or you can go right to the horse's mouth at the U.S. Department of Agriculture's Web site at www.usda.gov and find the pyramid there by seraching with that phrase. Compare your actual day to the day recommended by the USDA.

At the top of the pyramid are fats, oils, and sweets. Did you use them sparingly? That means you don't have to have them every day. Did you get 2 to 3 servings from the dairy group? How about 2 to 3 servings from meat or meat substitutes? Then there are the 3 to 5 servings of veggies and the 2 to 4 fruits. Finally, the bulk of your day's diet should have come from 6 to 11 servings from the grain group. How close did your day come?

If you're wondering what constitutes a serving, here's a crash course.

- A 1-ounce sausage link is the same size as a shotgun shell.
- A 1-ounce cube of cheese is the same size as four dice.
- Three ounces of meat is the size of a deck of cards.
- A half-cup of ice cream is like a tennis ball.
- Eight ounces of lasagna is comparable to two hockey pucks.
- A teaspoon of butter is the size of your thumbnail.
- A tablespoon of salad dressing would fit into half of a golf ball.
- One to 2 ounces of nuts, pretzels, or cereal can fit in your cupped hand.

Fat

Though you need roughly 2,500 calories to get through the day, no more than one-quarter of those calories should come from fat. Here's how you can figure out where the lard is. Go back to your Internet calorie counter. Beside each calorie count there should be a number showing you how many grams of fat are in that particular food. If there's not, find a better calorie counter.

Go ahead and add up the total number of grams of fat you put away today. Let's say that you're the above-mentioned average guy. At 2,500 calories a day, no more than 625 (or one-quarter) should have come from fat. A gram of fat equals 9 calories, so do the math. Your fat total should have come to no more than 69.4 grams. If you pounded down more than that, have a look over your food list to see what the high-fat culprits are.

Go ahead and turn your computer off. The rest of the analyses are easier.

Fiber

Fiber is the Drano of the intestinal world (you'll read all about it on Day 6 of this week). It not only keeps you regular but it's also an essential disease fighter. Getting 25 to 35 grams of fiber every day may lower your risk of cancer, heart disease, stroke, obesity, diabetes, and diverticulitis. Unfortunately, most people get only about half of the fiber they need. You don't have to get nitpicky about counting grams here; just take a good look at your list to see if it looks like you get enough fiber.

Most of your dietary fiber comes from the bottom of the food pyramid. Fruits and veggies each have about 1.5 grams per serving, while whole grains give you 2.5 grams per serving. Toss down a serving of baked beans or lentils, and you'll get a whopping 5 grams.

If you notice few fruits and veggies and lots of white bread and rice on your list, you're not getting enough fiber. It's easy to add it to your diet; start the day with a bran muffin or bran cereal. Get your full allotment of fruits and vegetables, and order brown rice and whole-grain toast with your meals.

Impulse Eating

Here's the thing that gets many guys right in the gut. We eat pretty well, all things considered. Most meals, we get our apples and oranges in, we watch our fat intakes, and we don't go crazy on the portion sizes.

But then peanut-butter-and-jelly sandwiches call our names at midnight. A slow saunter past the snack machine results in a bag of chips. We rush in to pay for our gas and wander out with chili dogs.

Take a final look over today's list. Put a red check mark beside each thing you ate that could be considered an impulse snack. Include obvious ones like candy bars and corn chips. But also add in the second helping you took to keep you busy while your wife was noodling with her first plateful. Look for too many high-calorie sodas; look for strange patterns in timing (did you consume many of your calories late in the evening?).

Pull out all those check-marked items and total their calorie counts. These were the foods that you ate when you weren't really hungry. These were the times when you were mindlessly filling the tube. This is food that you can cut out without feeling deprived. The key is to become mindful. In the days to come, ask yourself if you really want those things that you've identified as your impulse eats. If you do, have them. If you don't, leave them in the machine.

Go Meatless

The Day's Task

Easy, big guy. It's just for a day. And you're going to eat so well that you won't even miss that animal flesh. You may even want to do it again.

What's more, you don't even have to think because we got all your meatless meals planned out for you. Here's what you'll eat today (be sure to wash it all down with lots of water).

Breakfast. Have the same thing you ate way back on Week 1, Day 2. Remember, that was cereal with fat-free milk and fruit on top, a big glass of orange juice, whole-wheat toast with a little low-fat cream cheese, and coffee.

Mid-morning snack. Have some whole-wheat crackers with cheese and some grape juice.

Lunch. Try a bean burrito with a salad and some fruit.

Mid-afternoon snack. Enjoy half of a peanut butter sandwich on whole-grain bread, with an apple.

Dinner. Chow down on the same spread you ate on Day 3 of Week 1, but hold the shrimp. Either make the pasta with vegetables alone or substitute a vegetable lasagna. To refresh your memory, the rest of the meal consists of a green salad, a whole-wheat baguette with Italian cheese, a glass of red wine, and a dessert of fresh mango or berries with frozen yogurt.

Not such a leap, is it? For 2 months now, you've deemphasized meat, making carbohydrates the focus of your meals. All you're doing today is deemphasizing it a little more—to the point of oblivion.

Your meatless menu doesn't even qualify you as Vegetarian for a Day, in strictly literal terms. The milk and cheese are, after all, animal foods. That makes you an ovo-lactovegetarian, the kind who allows himself egg and dairy products, but no meat or fish. True vegetarians, who eat no animal foods whatsoever, are often called vegans.

Call them what you will, there are some 12 million vegetarians of one kind or another in the United States. And though there are lots of reasons why all those people choose that path, your concern today is the same as it's been from the beginning of this program: health and longevity. Here's what you begin to accomplish by forsaking meat for a day.

You increase your life expectancy. Replacing some of the meat in your diet with soy products or beans and other legumes can increase your life expectancy by up to 13 percent. And you don't have to entirely give up meat to see a benefit.

You slow the aging process. Vegetarians tend to eat more fruits, vegetables, and grains than meat eaters do, so they tend to get more antioxidants in their diets. Furthermore, they avoid the red meat that creates free radicals that can damage cells and tissues and speed up aging.

You improve your all-around health. "The closer you get to a plant-based diet, the healthier you'll be," says T. Colin Campbell, M.D., professor of nutritional biochemistry at Cornell University in Ithaca, New York.

You help yourself stay trim. Since vegetarian diets are usually lower in calories and higher in fiber than carnivorous diets, vegetarians are less likely to be overweight. Their svelte profiles aren't good just for vanity's sake. They could also explain why vegetarians have lower blood pressures and lower incidence of diabetes than meat eaters.

You lower your risk of heart disease. The low-fat, low-cholesterol nature of a vegetarian diet usually means lower blood-cholesterol counts. Remember, dietary cholesterol comes only from animal foods. Meat is also the top source of saturated fat, which your body converts to cholesterol. In a study of 500 high-fat-food eaters, researchers in California recently confirmed that 12 days of a strict vegetarian diet caused significant drops in total cholesterol levels and blood pressure, two major risk factors for heart disease.

You lower your risk of colon cancer. Men who eat beef, pork, or lamb as a main dish five or six times a week are more than twice as likely to develop colon cancer as men who eat red meat less than once a week. Colon cancer is infrequent in countries where meat is rarely eaten. And it's less frequent among Americans who eat vegetarian diets.

You lower your risk of diabetes. In a study conducted at Georgetown University in Washington, D.C., researchers had one group consume a plant-based diet with no meat, eggs, or dairy products. After 3 months, the group's fasting blood sugar levels (that is, their levels after they hadn't eaten in 8 to 10 hours) had fallen 59 percent more than the levels of those in a group who got 30 percent of their calories from fat. This suggests that vegans are less likely than meat eaters to be diabetic.

Retreat from Meat

We're not insisting that you become a full-time vegetarian. We are suggesting that you go vegetarian for 1 day a week. It's a minimal sacrifice. You probably do it some days already without knowing it. We're sure you can get through today's menu without a problem. Try repeating it next week. See if you could start a routine that, say, Thursdays are no-meat days.

The secret to meatless eating is variety. If a vegetarian diet meant nothing but brussels sprouts and broccoli day in and day out, you'd be a regular at the Hungry Heifer before the week was up. But there's no reason to be bored, since there's more variety outside the meat world than inside it.

Probably the most popular meatless dinner for men is spaghetti and tomato sauce with a salad and garlic bread. Start there, getting creative with the sauce. Then move to new ingredients. Besides the whole panoply of fruits and vegetables, you can focus on grains, from brown rice to oatmeal to whole-grain breads and cereals to alternative pastas. From there, you have beans and nuts and soy products and seeds. And in our version of meatless eating, all the dairy products are available to you, including cheeses from around the world.

Soy is one of your top allies in meatless eating. It's not only an excellent alternative source of protein but also a heart-helping food in its own right. Oriental soy forms like tofu and tempeh have a well-deserved reputation for blandness, but that can be an asset since they readily absorb flavors from sauces and seasonings. There are lots of other kinds of soy products on the market these days, including meat substitutes that run the gamut from veggie burgers to soy chorizo.

Soy aside, one question that usually comes up with the idea of meatless eating is, what about protein? Even that assuming you don't eat protein-rich dairy products like eggs and cheese, you can easily meet your protein requirements with a consistent variety of beans, whole grains, peas, nuts, and seeds.

Finally, while a veggie diet usually leads to lower fat intake, there's nothing automatic about it, especially if you allow yourself dairy foods. Cheese, ice cream, mayonnaise, and coconut oil are all ovo-lacto-vegetarian and very high in fat. So look for low-fat or nonfat dairy products, fat-free mayonnaise, and even low-fat tofu. And bake, broil, or steam your food; don't deep-fry it.

Try Some Heart-Healthy Foods

The Day's Task

Get that negative image out of your mind. Heart-healthy doesn't mean rabbit food. Nature wants you to like food that's good for your heart. So do we.

Truth is, you're going to *love* today's meal plan. Hey, there are even two bottles of beer in it for you.

Feel better now? Your goal for the day is to eat all of the following to see how easy and pleasant it is to eat food that'll keep your pump going long enough to see the Cubs win back-to-back World Series. We're not saying that this is all you can eat today. Just make sure our suggested foods are included in the following meals.

Breakfast. Drink an 8-ounce glass of orange juice, plus two cups of green or black tea instead of coffee.

Mid-morning snack. Munch an apple.

Lunch. Have chili and beans with plenty of garlic, and some grapes.

Mid-afternoon snack. Eat half of a peanut butter sandwich on whole-grain bread, with an iced tea.

Dinner. Try salmon with onions, a cup of leafy greens, and two dark beers.

There's a key difference between this meal plan and yesterday's meatless menu. Yesterday, you concentrated on *avoiding* one kind of food that's definitely not a heart pleaser, animal meat. Today, though, you're *loading up* on the kinds of foods that help your heart take a licking and keep on ticking.

You're doing this because what you eat matters when it comes to preventing heart disease. The road to heart disease starts with a diet high in fatty, protein-rich foods and low in fruits and vegetables. Those bad eating habits raise the levels of harmful LDL (low-density lipoprotein) cholesterol and triglycerides, both of which are fatty substances circulating in your blood that can clog or harden your arteries, encourage plaque growth there, and promote clotting. All of that makes a heart attack much more likely.

On the other hand, the right diet can help prevent and even reverse some forms of heart disease. What's the right diet for your heart? Pretty much the same diet that delivers all-around health and longevity. That means lots of variety. It means an emphasis on fruits and vegetables, with all their heart-helping fiber and antioxidant phytochemicals. It means plenty of grains for more fiber. And it means limited fat.

The Heart-Healthy All-Star Food Roster

Besides an all-around good diet, there are specific heart-healthy foods that you can shoot for. You're eating a number of them today, and there are plenty more. From now on, do your heart a favor by making sure you eat or drink several of the following every day.

Orange juice and oranges. Here's one more reason to suck down all you can of this primo vitamin C source. Vitamin C prevents heart disease by reducing cholesterol, repairing damaged artery walls, and preventing LDL cholesterol from oxidizing. If you prefer eating oranges, peel them and eat the sections instead of cutting them up. That way, you'll eat more of that white stringy stuff on the outside. It has lots of the fiber called pectin in it.

Tea. Drinking green or black tea can lower your levels of homocysteine, the amino acid that's associated with heart disease when there's too much of it circulating. That's because teas contain folate, the B vitamin that is thought to lower homocysteine levels. But tea, especially green tea, is also loaded with phytochemical antioxidants. We don't need to tell you again about all the good things antioxidants do for your heart. But we can tell you that green or black tea has approximately half the caffeine content of coffee, so you can drink more of it.

Apples and apple juice. These are another fruit with lots of polyphenols. Because of those active little antioxidants, eating apples or drinking apple juice regularly can reduce oxidation of harmful LDL cholesterol by as much as 38 percent. That's good because less-oxidized cholesterol is less-dangerous cholesterol. Don't peel your apples. The skins are filled with a fiber called pectin that grabs hold of cholesterol floating around your body and takes it out of your system.

Legumes. This category to include everything from kidney beans and lentils to black-eyed peas. Legumes are loaded with cholesterol-lowering fiber. And eating lots of fiber is one of the best things you can do for your heart and most of the rest of your body. Any kind of legume is a good source of folate, which also lowers cholesterol.

Tomatoes and tomato products. You already know that these help keep your prostate a decent size and may lower your risk of prostate cancer. But in Europe, men with the highest tissue levels of lycopene, the chief beneficial compound in tomatoes, were only half as likely to suffer heart attacks as men with the lowest levels. So keep eating tomato sauce and tomato paste, and keep drinking tomato juice or vegetable juice cocktails.

Garlic. This is one of the greatest heart foods on Earth. A clove a day in your food will do wonders. Since almost all those vegetables you're eating taste better with some garlic mixed in (as do countless other dishes), you'll be way ahead of the game. If you don't like garlic, try to learn. If you still don't like it, go back to Week 3, Day 5 and reconsider taking it in no-taste capsule form. It's that good.

Here's what garlic does to keep your heart healthy. It helps to lower high blood pressure and high cholesterol levels. It reduces the risk of platelets sticking together and clotting your blood. It fights clogged arteries (atherosclerosis). All of these problems that garlic prevents can easily lead to serious heart disease and heart attacks.

Grape juice and grapes. Grape juice offers the same heart-enhancing natural chemicals (such as polyphenols or flavonoids) that red wine does. Concord grape juice has more antioxidants than other types; grape "drinks" are not much more than grape-flavored water with lots of sugar and probably don't have any. Choose accordingly. Also, eat plenty of fresh grapes.

Nuts. Yes, nuts are full of fat, and fat is not something you eat a lot of for your heart's sake. But take nuts off the taboo list and put them on your eat-with-moderation list. Studies show that people who eat nuts four or five times a week have far less heart disease then people who don't. This may be because nuts like walnuts, or even natural peanut butter (the kind without the trans fats or hydrogenated fats), consist overwhelmingly of the more benign monounsaturated or polyunsaturated fats. So you can get a nice jolt of heart-healthy stuff like vitamin E, magnesium, and omega-3 fatty acids without too much of the saturated fat that converts to cholesterol in your body. But even the good fats are fats, so watch your intake to avoid finding yourself noshing down 1,000 calories in a quick 10 minutes.

Dark beer. One or two bottles of dark beer a day will give you the anti-clotting, vitamin-like flavonoids that may help keep your arteries clear, research suggests. There are lots of these antioxidant phytochemicals in hops, the ingredient that gives beer a bitter taste. Why must the beer be dark beer? It seems the brewing process used for paler beers usually filters out many of the flavonoids. Why two? Because three is too many, at least for heart health. Too much of any alcohol can raise your blood pressure, which is the opposite of what you want to do to prevent heart disease. So if you're going to drink for your heart, stick to one or two dark 12 ouncers a day.

Fish. Yes, vegetarians have less heart disease. But one of the best heart-protecting foods falls into the meat category. It's meat from the sea: fish.

Eating a lot of fish may prevent heart disease by, among other things, lowering your levels of triglycerides. In a study of more than 20,000 male physicians in Boston, those who ate fish once a week had 52 percent lower risks of having sudden fatal heart attacks than those who didn't have seafood weekly.

Fish is a great heart protector because, in general, it has much less total fat than most meats. It also has less saturated fat, so it's clearly a better choice for keeping your cholesterol levels down.

But the best thing about fish may be the fat that it does have. Fatty, cold-water fish like salmon are loaded with those omega-3 fatty acids we've already talked about. Other fish, like swordfish or whitefish, are also healthier for your heart than red meat. But for the omega-3's, you need salmon, herring, mackerel, tuna, or similar fatty fish. Canned tuna or salmon will do fine.

There are also nonfish sources of omega-3 fatty acids, including whole grains, beans, and soybeans. Then, of course, there are the new fish-oil pasta sauces. Yep, you heard that right. If you check the health food stores or natural food supermarkets, you may find a variety of pasta sauces that include omega-3's without any fish taste. For example, Millina's Finest organic pasta sauces get you 0.6 gram of omega-3's per half-cup. Flavors include marinara, tomato and basil, and garlic.

Red wine. We've mentioned red wine before as a surprisingly heart-healthy treat, but it's such good news that we'll tell you about it again. An American Cancer Society study showed that people who drank a small amount of any kind of alcohol daily had 30 to 40 percent lower risks of heart disease. But red wine helps in another way as well because, like beer, it offers antioxidant phytochemicals. Again, if you go beyond two glasses, you do more harm than good. And of course, you need to choose between beer and wine on any one day.

Time Your Eating for Maximum Energy

The Day's Task

Today, you're going to do some strategic eating. That is, you're going to concentrate on eating the right foods at the right times for maximum performance in whatever you plan to do.

We hope you've been reading ahead—this is much easier if you start the night before. If not, do it first thing this morning while the coffee is brewing. Your first step is to make a schedule of everything you're going to be doing throughout the day. Emphasize those activities that will require the most physical exertion or mental concentration. Do you have a 10:30 A.M. meeting or presentation? Write it down. Is there a particularly grueling work task waiting for you in mid-afternoon? Note it. A scheduled exercise session? Enter it. An evening out? Log it in.

Next, schedule your meals and snacks. Notice which meals come before which tasks. Plan and prepare very specific foods to give you the most energy or mental alertness exactly when you're going to need it. That probably means packing your own lunch and snacks and adjusting the times when you eat them. It'll be worth it.

How do you know what to include in your meals for maximum energy? How do you know when to eat them? Read on.

You've heard plenty from us about eating to take advantage of nutrients that slow aging, fight disease, and make you feel better. But there's another reason why you eat. In fact, it's the most important reason why you eat. Food is for energy. Food is literally fuel for your body to burn.

Most people think of food not much differently than they think of gas for their cars. When the tanks approach empty, we refill them, reaching automatically for the regular unleaded nozzles. And so it is with our bodies: When we feel hungry, we fill up our stores without much attention to the grade of the fuel.

But science shows that certain kinds of foods provide certain kinds of energy in certain kinds of ways. There is enormous power in this notion. It means you can eat strategically. You can plan your meals with an eye to what kind of energy you'll need after eating them. And you can time your meals based on when you'll need that energy.

Think of it in terms of that car analogy. Imagine that there were one grade of gas that specifically helped your car perform better on the freeway and an entirely different formulation just for driving in the city and others for going fast or doing lots of ascending and descending. Being a guy, you'd likely rotate among the different gasoline types based on the type of driving you were going to do on a particular day.

Well, we have that opportunity with our own bodies, and hardly anyone knows it.

Forward-Looking Eating

Here's a short physiology lesson. When you eat, the food is broken down into (among other things) a form of sugar called glucose, which is absorbed into your bloodstream. As your blood sugar level rises after a meal, it triggers the release of insulin, a hormone that helps glucose enter cells, where it's used for energy.

The simple carbohydrates in sugary foods turn into glucose very quickly, causing a rapid increase in your blood sugar level followed by a rapid dip. So sweets often give you a quick burst of energy that soon gives way to fatigue.

Complex carbs like whole-wheat bread, grains, and vegetables are metabolized more slowly in your body. As a result, they keep your blood sugar level relatively stable over a longer period of time, providing you with a steadier energy supply. Factors that influence the endurance of the energy derived from carbohydrates include how much fiber you get with them and whether you eat protein or fat along with the carbs.

So controlling your blood sugar level by choosing certain kinds of foods is a great tool for synchronizing your eating with your energy needs. But there's more to it than that. Some foods trigger the release of hormones that hone your alertness. Others increase hormones that calm.

For example, the simple carbohydrates in a sugary doughnut not only send your blood sugar level on a spike-and-dip ride but also bring about an increase in serotonin, a neurotransmitter in your brain that induces sleep. Soon, your sugar buzz is gone and you're drowsier than Dan Quayle at an art-film festival.

Let's look at how you can use foods as tools to help you perform at your best.

Muscle Up Your Morning

If you're not a morning person, your makeshift calendar may start with the exertion of just dragging your butt in to work. As if that weren't taxing enough, we have a hunch that on your day's schedule you've included some work-related activity to be done right around mid-morning. Sadistic supervisors seem to have decided that 10:30 A.M. is the perfect time to torture workers with interminable meetings or unaccomplishable tasks. But mid-morning is just the time when you tend to start to fade.

This is where breakfast and a mid-morning snack can help you out in a way that you'll really feel.

Breakfast. Your glucose levels are usually lowest when you first wake up in the morning. After all, you probably haven't eaten in 8 or more hours. So you might crave sweets, the quickest route to higher blood sugar levels. Not that you'd eat three bowls of chocolate-covered-sugarcane cereal. You're an adult. You'd go for three donuts and a cup of coffee instead.

The quick burst of energy from a sweet breakfast will leave you dragging by the time you get to work. Instead, eat a breakfast that combines complex carbohydrates, lots of fiber, some protein, and a little fat. Your body digests these more slowly, providing a steadier source of fuel that will get you through the morning. Try low-fat granola with fruit and yogurt, and whole-grain toast with low-fat cream cheese. Or browse back to the model breakfast of Week 1, Day 2.

Mid-morning snack. That early meeting may start at 10:30, but it sure won't end at 10:45. Time your mid-morning mini-meal so the last bite goes down just as you walk in the door of the conference room. That will keep you sharp for the duration and also make it easier to ignore those awful snacks that somebody always puts out at meetings.

Protein is the strategic food in this situation. Sharp thinking skills, word retrieval, and mental quickness depend on it. Protein boosts your level of tyrosine, the amino acid that is converted to dopamine and norepinephrine—chemicals that leap from nerve ending to nerve ending inside your brain when you're thinking. So forget the candy bar, chocolate-covered granola bar, doughnut and coffee, or can of cola with jelly beans. Instead, go for one of the following suggestions:

- Try one-half of a peanut butter sandwich on whole-wheat bread, with an apple.
- A tuna fish sandwich on whole-wheat bread, with fruit juice, is not exactly standard morning fare. But we're talking about mental alertness, not tradition.
- Turn to two slices of low-fat turkey lunchmeat with six fat-free whole-wheat crackers and some apple-cranberry juice.

Break Out of That Slump

Now for those mid-day tasks that you wrote down. They come right at a time when we mere humans have a biological tendency to slump. We're still programmed to take siestas after lunch, but only little kids, octogenarians, and very powerful executives have the luxury of power naps. The rest of us need to power eat.

Lunch. If you're planning on taking off after lunch and lying on the beach until Monday, eat whatever you want. But if you have things to do after your lunch break, eat protein such as low-calorie meats and cheeses, poultry, seafood, or nonfat dairy products. An all-carb lunch like pasta and salad may seem energetic, but it will flatten you like a truck accident. Again, protein's tyrosin synthesizes more of your brain's alertness chemicals.

Just make sure you don't overdo the fat with the protein. Avoid creamy soups, fast-food hamburgers, and cheesy potatoes. And take it easy on the portions. Eating a big meal diverts blood to your digestive system and away from your brain.

Mid-afternoon snack. Struggling toward the end of the workday to meet some deadline? Lots of running around to do after the whistle blows? You can plan and time your mid-afternoon snack for just when you need it, sometime during that long stretch between the end of lunch and the beginning of dinner.

Guys less energy savvy than you turn to candy bars or other sugar bombs at around 3:30 in the afternoon. That's a bad idea, unless you want to be a clock-watcher for the rest of your never-ending workday. Better options feature complex carbohydrates with protein for brainpower and steady energy. Try some of these.

- Consider yogurt with rice cakes, low-fat crackers, or whole-grain bread; reduced-sodium instant soups; or even a handful of unsalted dry-roasted peanuts or cashews.
- A more offbeat option is one whole-wheat pita bread broken into pieces and dipped in ¼ cup of hummus. Have an apple with it.
- A fruitier choice is diced kiwifruit mixed with 6 ounces of low-fat strawberry yogurt and three graham crackers.

- Fruitier still is 6 ounces of low-fat vanilla yogurt sprinkled with ⅓ cup of low-fat granola and 2 tablespoons of dried cranberries, raisins, chopped dates, and other dried fruit.
- A very different strategy that might work for you in the afternoon is a carbohydrate/caffeine combination. Eat four fig bars or three gingersnaps with a cup of coffee, hot chocolate, or diet cola no later than 4:30 P.M. for a long-lasting mental-energy boost. Caffeine boosts your mental energy, and the serotonin released by the carbohydrates helps you settle down and refocus on your tasks for the rest of the day.

Evenings Out and In

Too often, a night out kicks off with an energy-sapping dinner that redirects your thoughts from doing the town to dozing on the king-size. Here are some hints for retaining vigor in the evening.

- Stay away from steak, fatty sour cream, buttered vegetables, pasta with cream sauce, and turkey with stuffing, gravy, and the works. Remember, high-fat foods weigh you down and tire you out.
- Choose an entrée like broiled salmon with brown rice and steamed vegetables, grilled chicken with a baked potato and grilled vegetables, or vegetarian chili; a tossed green salad with low-fat dressing; and a slice of whole-wheat bread. For dessert, order one-quarter of a honeydew melon or a half-cup of fresh blueberries.

On the other hand, if you plan to relax in the evening and calm yourself for sleep, take one of these routes to slumberland instead.

- This is the time for your carb-loaded dinner of pasta, vegetables, and grains. It's thought that carbohydrates eaten alone make more of the amino acid tryptophan, which leads to more serotonin, leaving you less stressed, less anxious, and more relaxed.
- Keep it modest. If you have your biggest meal at night, you make your body work hard to digest it right when you're trying to shut down for the night and go to sleep.
- Experiment with a late-night calming snack for a good night's rest and an energetic next day. Put several drops of almond extract in 8 ounces of warm fat-free milk and drink it with two fig bars. Or have a half of a toasted English muffin topped with all-fruit jam.

Eating for Exercise

A workout might change the dynamic of your eating-for-energy strategy. Eating the right foods at the right times not only gives you the energy you need for better exercise endurance but also helps you recover more quickly too.

- If you work out in the morning, eat breakfast first. Fill your breakfast bowl with an all-bran cereal and have it with yogurt and an apple 30 minutes before you exercise. It's been shown that such a slow-carb meal helps cyclers pedal 59 percent longer than those who eat fast-acting carbohydrates like cornflakes.
- If you exercise at lunchtime, make your mid-morning snack higher in carbohydrates than you otherwise would. If you exercise after work, up the carbohydrate content of your mid-afternoon snack. Carbohydrates that are consumed an hour or so before exercise directly serve as energy to burn for your workout.
- Fruit is the perfect workout food. Most fruits are rich sources of carbohydrates. Fruits are also high in a form of sugar called fructose that your body processes more slowly than the sugar in other carbohydrate-rich foods. As a result, fruit sugars give your muscles a steady stream of carbohydrate energy for the duration of your exercise session.
- Try to eat your next meal soon after you finish your workout. Exercise lowers your blood sugar, so enjoying a balanced meal afterward will help stabilize your glucose level and keep you going for the rest of the day. If you work out around lunchtime, wait until afterward to eat lunch. A turkey sandwich with fruit is a good choice. If you work out after breakfast, you might want to have your mid-morning snack a little bit earlier than usual.
- Energy bars may not be much better workout foods than well-planned snacks are, but they're handy and a better choice than candy bars. They're not all the same, so if you want your energy bar to fuel your workout, look for one that's mostly carbohydrates. For example, the apple-cherry flavor Clif bar packs 52 grams of carbs, with just 4 grams of protein and 2 of fat.
- Protein drinks don't boost your energy, no matter when you drink them. Their purpose is to make sure you have enough essential amino acids, the ones your body doesn't make but uses to create muscle mass. Unless you're planning on qualifying for one of those bodybuilding shows on ESPN2, you probably get enough of those amino acids in your diet.

Diversify Your Palate

The Day's Task

This is going to be an interesting day. It's going to be adventurous, perhaps challenging, most assuredly not dull. Your assignment could very well change your life. It will definitely improve your health.

Intrigued? Let's get to it: At every meal today, eat one food that you have never eaten before. This includes your mid-morning and mid-afternoon snacks.

Yup, you counted right. You're going to eat at least five new foods. What's more, you're going to make sure that the newcomers are low in fat and that they fit in comfortably with your commitment to health and longevity.

Skeptical? Here's some help to get you started. When you restocked your refrigerator and pantry on the first day of the first week of your Longevity Program, we suggested some condiments that go beyond ketchup and mustard. Remember? Chile-garlic paste. Black bean sauce. Hoisin sauce. Oyster sauce. Plum sauce. Have you tried all of them yet? We thought not. How about the oil-packed sun-dried tomatoes? Hmmm. . . .

How experienced are you with tropical fruits? Are you still a kiwifruit virgin? At snack time today, eat one instead of an apple.

Have you had entrées cooked with flaxseed oil? How about walnut oil? No? Then they qualify since they're healthy (in moderation) and they're new.

Or scan your spice rack for a seasoning that you've never thought much about. Basil? Rosemary? Cumin? Sure, they've probably been included in dishes that somebody else has served you. But we're not sticklers. If you don't remember a food, count it as new.

You haven't even put it into action yet, but today's task has probably made you think about what you usually eat. If you're typical, it's a lot of the same old, same old—pretty much the same breakfast every morning, the same pool of three or four dinner choices, even the same restaurants when you eat out.

That's boring. And it's not conducive to healthy eating. You need to diversify your palate, for a number of reasons.

- Variety lets you introduce the most healthful foods into your eating patterns. If you eat only what you've always eaten, you can't make room for the foods that will help you live longer and better.
- Variety keeps you enthused about good food. Your longevity quest calls for eating a lot more fruits, vegetables, grains, and beans than you were probably used to eating. The key to success here is to keep those foods ever-exciting and ever-new. Choosing from a broad range of foods not only keeps you healthy but also fights boredom. Never will you say, "Oh, no, not *that* again."
- Variety is where the nutrients are. To grab the full benefits of fruits and vegetables, you have to become a man of varied tastes. Each fruit and vegetable has its own stable of disease-preventing powerhouses. But no single one has them all. By casting a wide net, you're bound to take in plenty of different nutrients. By sticking to only a few foods, you're missing out on most of the good stuff.
- Variety means never having to say you're sorry. The fast-food joint down on the corner looks irresistible when nothing in your house looks appetizing. If you keep lots of different options in your kitchen at all times, you're never more than a few minutes away from a good healthy meal.

Today's exercise aside, you don't always have to add new foods to your diet to get variety. Sometimes just tweaking your favorite dishes a bit can make them new and healthy. For instance, if you love tacos or burritos, try them with chicken or beans instead of beef or pork. Have your chili with turkey or make it vegetarian.

And in your ongoing effort to reconcile your carnivorous instincts with your new low-fat lifestyle, try a species switch. As noted, fish instead of red meat is always a good idea. But also, search for ostrich or buffalo meat. Each tastes like beef but has the fat content of chicken.

As you work your way through nine servings of fruits and vegetables a day, let color be your diversifying guide. If you mix them up among orange, yellow, green, and red, you'll snag a wider selection of anti-aging vitamins, minerals, and plant chemicals like beta-carotene and lycopene.

NOTHING BUT THE BEST

Truth is, once you decide to seek culinary variety, you'll discover that it's the easiest thing in the world to find. We're going to show you how easy it is to mix up your meals at home by providing you with some lists of the very best foods for your health. They're the best because they're lean, full of fiber, or full of anti-aging antioxidants that eliminate dangerous free radicals that age you every second you're alive. Most offer all three.

We're not talking about anything too exotic. All of these foods are readily available at any decent supermarket. The point is, even if you choose only the very best foods—those below—there's still so much variety available that if you want to, you can go weeks without repeating a food.

Vegetables

Artichokes
Asparagus
Avocado
Baked potatoes
Beets
Bell peppers
Broccoli
Broccoli sprouts
Brussels sprouts
Cabbage
Carrots
Cauliflower
Celery
Corn
Cucumbers
Eggplant
Garlic
Kale
Leafy green lettuce
Mitake mushrooms
Onions
Portobello mushrooms
Red lettuce
Romaine lettuce
Shiitake mushrooms
Spinach
String beans
Sweet potatoes
Tomatoes
Tomato paste
Tomato sauce
Vegetable juice
White mushrooms
Zucchini

Fruits

Apple juice
Apples
Bananas
Blackberries
Blueberries
Cantaloupes
Cherries
Citrus fruits and juices
Concord grape juice

Getting Familiar with Foreign Food

You can broaden your dietary horizon by trying different ethnic foods. May we order for you? Here, broken down by nationality, are some of the healthiest choices at the kinds of international restaurants easily found almost anywhere in the United States.

French. *Bouillabaisse* (pronounced boo-yuh-BAYZ) is red seafood stew that's

Cranberry juice	Orange juice	Prunes
Grapefruit juice	Oranges	Raisins
Grapes	Papayas	Raspberries
Honeydew melons	Peaches	Strawberries
Kiwifruit	Pears	Watermelons
Mangoes	Pink grapefruit	
Nectarines	Plum	

Grains

Bran	Oatmeal	Whole-grain cereal
Brown rice	Pasta	Whole-wheat bread
Buckwheat pancakes	Pumpernickel bread	Whole-wheat pasta
Graham crackers	Rye bread	

Beans, Other Legumes, and Soy Products

Black beans	Lima beans	Soy milk
Kidney beans	Pinto beans	Veggie burgers
Light tofu	Peas	

Eggs, Meats, Fish, and Dairy Products

Egg whites	Low-fat yogurt	Sardines
Fat-free milk	Mackerel	Shellfish
Fat-free ricotta cheese	Oysters	Skinless white-meat chicken
Freshwater fish	Salmon	Turkey breast

Other

Almonds	Olive oil	Sunflower seeds
Black tea	Red wine	Walnuts
Green tea	Salsa	Water

usually generous in shellfish and fish per cup. You get lots of heart-healthy omega-3 fatty acids with only about 10 grams of fat and 340 calories per cup.

Coulis (koo-LEE) may be the only sauce in the French cookbook that's lean and still delicious. It's thick and smooth, and it's usually made from vegetables but sometimes from fruits.

En papillote (pronounced on pah-pee-YOHT) is anything baked or steamed in parchment paper. Go for fish, and you're probably eating the healthiest thing on the menu. But is it still good? Hey, it's French. It has to be good, by law.

Also go for consommé, salade niçoise, any grilled seafood or chicken, or sorbet.

Italian. *Puttanesca sauce* is one of the healthiest dishes on any Italian menu, with a mere 10 grams of fat and plenty of prostate-saving, heart-healthy lycopene. It's a piquant tomato sauce with capers, olives, and anchovies that is generally served over pasta. The word puttanesca is pronounced poot-tah-NEHS-kah and is derived from the Italian word for prostitute. It was inspired by the theory that the aroma of the sauce was as enticing as a lady of the evening.

Bruschetta (broo-SKEH-tah) is a good appetizer choice if you stick to one or two of these 140-calorie slices of crispy garlic bread topped with tomatoes and basil. Each has 6 grams of fat, more if you don't tell the waiter to maker sure it isn't overdrenched in olive oil.

Also go for minestrone, breads, pasta with marinara sauce, seafood dishes, chicken cacciatore, gelato, or Italian ice.

Japanese. *Sashimi* can be just about any kind of fresh raw fish served with daikon (Japanese radish), wasabi (Japanese horseradish), ginger, or soy sauce. It's virtually fat-free, and there are only about 44 calories per serving.

Or try *sushi*, cuts of raw fish served on rolls of rice, often wrapped in dry seaweed. It's hard to stop at just a few, but the low fat content (0.3 gram per serving) leaves you as lean as your wallet will be.

Sunomono is typically raw or cooked vegetables tossed with a sweet-and-sour vinaigrette. It's virtually fat-free, so eat all you want.

Also go for miso soup, grilled fish, vegetarian sushi, teriyaki chicken or vegetables, or soba or udon noodles.

Mexican. *Mole* (MOH-lay) is a rich, dark sauce made from mild chile peppers, onions, and chocolate that's a tasty and healthy choice if you get it served over chicken or turkey and make sure the skin has been removed. *Seviche* is another low-fat taste treat (2 grams per serving). It's diced raw fish "cooked" (actually, marinated) in citrus juice.

Also go for salsa, chicken fajitas (hold the sour cream), vegetarian chili, and mesquite-grilled chicken or fish.

Maximize Your Fiber

The Day's Task

Your goal for today is to eat 35 grams of fiber. That's considered a high fiber intake, and it's enough to do you a world of good. But it's an easy goal to attain.

Here's how you're going to eat 35 grams of fiber today.

Breakfast. **Eat a bowl of General Mills Fiber One cereal mixed with a cup of seedless raisins and accompanied by an oat bran muffin.**

Mid-morning snack. **Just like on the third day of this week, munch an apple.**

Lunch. **Have a green salad that includes a sliced-up medium avocado.**

That's it. You're already well over 35 grams. We told you it was easy.

We suspect that there may be a question you've been wanting to ask since the first week. Maybe we're wrong. Maybe you already know the answer. But most guys who take the plunge into healthy, feel-good eating can't help asking the one unavoidable, irresistible question that gnaws incessantly at their consciousness: What the hell is fiber?

That's an excellent question. Here's the answer. Fiber is the part of plant-based food that you don't digest. It just passes on through. It's not a nutrient; it's a transportation specialist. Fiber may not sound like something that makes the difference between a long-and-healthy life and a not-so-long-and-healthy life. But it is. That's why today you're training yourself to get lots of it.

There are two forms of fiber: *insoluble* fiber, which bulks up your stool and speeds it through your intestines; and *soluble* fiber, which slows down your body's absorption of food.

That still doesn't sound like much, does it? But the salutary effects of zipping waste through your gut are legion. That's why getting enough insoluble fiber—a sure bet with your 35 grams of total fiber—is the best thing you can do for your digestive system. Bulkier, faster-moving stool relieves or prevents all kinds of intestinal problems, including constipation, hemorrhoids, irritable bowel syndrome, and perhaps even gallstones. More important, some studies suggest that insoluble fiber may reduce your risk of colon and other cancers.

The work of soluble fiber is just as noble. It slows the absorption of carbohydrates into your bloodstream. As you learned on Day 4 of this week, that helps spread out their energy benefits over time. But it also slows the absorption of cholesterol. Indeed, it soaks up that artery-hardening substance and carries it out of your digestive system. That can't be anything but good.

Maximize your fiber, and you'll also find that it's much easier to keep your weight down to where it should be. If you eat 35 grams of fiber a day, that, in effect, replaces 30 to 180 calories a day because fiber slows down your digestion, so you feel full longer and are less likely to overeat. Over the course of a year, that translates to as much as 19 fewer pounds gained.

We have two important warnings about increasing your fiber intake. First, an overly rapid boost in dietary fiber can cause you to feel bloated, gassy, and uncomfortable. So let your body get used to your high-fiber diet. To be cautious, increase your daily fiber intake by just 5 grams. After a week, go for another 5 grams. In a month, you'll probably be at the levels you need for long-term benefit.

Our second warning is that if you eat lots of fiber but don't increase your water intake, it can make you constipated. So shoot for eight big glasses of water per day to help keep the fiber moving smoothly through your digestive tract.

Fiber Foods

All those fruits and vegetables you've been eating are a big reason why you'll probably slam-dunk today's task. Eating lots of different fruits and vegetables gives you plenty of both kinds of fiber.

Whole grains, especially bran, are also full of fiber, which is why we've been pushing them at you since Week 1, Day 1. Wheat bran is a great source of insoluble fiber, while oat bran is perhaps the best source of soluble fiber. So mix 'em up. And while the bran form is best, any kind of whole wheat is good, as is any kind of whole-grain oat, including rolled oats and even Cheerios.

Just make sure the label has words like "whole-grain" or "whole-wheat flour." Or, of course, "bran." "Multigrain" isn't enough. It just means there's more than one grain, none of which is necessarily a whole grain. You also want brown rice, bulgur, or quinoa instead of white rice and whole-wheat pasta instead of the white kind.

BULKING UP

Okay, let's get down to some numbers. If you've been following the Longevity Program so far, you're probably eating plenty of high-fiber foods. And there's a good chance that you're already getting your 35 grams of daily fiber.

But let's run down the list to be sure. Here are some of the best fiber sources. Let this table serve as a general guide as you estimate your total grams of fiber for the day.

FOOD	FIBER (g)
Legumes	
½ cup lentils	7.8
½ cup black beans	7.5
½ cup kidney beans	6.5
½ cup chickpeas	6.2
½ cup navy beans	5.8
½ cup lima beans	4.5
½ cup peas	4.4
Grains and Cereals	
1 oz General Mills Fiber One	12.3
1 oz Kellogg's All-Bran	9.2
1 oz Post 100% Bran	7.8
½ cup bulgur	4.0
½ cup oatmeal	3.9
1 oz Post Raisin Bran	3.8
½ cup whole-wheat spaghetti	3.2
½ cup pearled barley	2.9

FOOD	FIBER (g)
Vegetables	
1 cup acorn squash	9.0
1 artichoke	6.0
1 potato with skin	5.0
1 sweet potato	3.4
Fruits	
1 avocado	12.0
1 cup raspberries	8.0
3 dried figs	6.9
1 guava	4.9
3 dried pear halves	4.3
1 mango	4.0
1 orange	3.0
1 apple	3.0

By the way, remember that we're talking about only the plant kingdom here. Animal-based food is fiberless. So substituting beans for meat in your taco or burrito is a good example of a smart fiber-boosting and fat-reducing strategy.

Fiber supplements are another option. If for some reason you just can't get enough fiber from food, there's plenty of it in psyllium products such as Metamucil, Fiber-Sol, or Konsyl. Follow the label instructions. Start with small amounts and increase gradually to avoid diarrhea and flatulence.

10 Ways to Prevent Diabetes

1 Maintain a healthy weight. Diabetes has no cure. Once you have it, it's yours for life. But at least 75 percent of all new cases of diabetes type 2, the kind you're most likely to get, can be prevented, says JoAnn Manson, M.D., an epidemiologist and endocrinologist at Harvard Medical School.

The number one way to prevent the disease is to avoid becoming overweight. Here's why. In diabetes type 2, your body's cells become resistant to the insulin that moves sugar out of your bloodstream. When this happens, blood sugar builds up to corrosive levels while your body starves because its cells are not getting the necessary fuel. Excess fat compounds things by making your cells even more insulin-resistant.

Maintaining a healthy weight is vital in diabetes prevention, so many of the nine tips that follow are designed to help you stay trim.

2 Eat less fat. A high-fat diet sets you up for obesity, but it also reduces your cells' sensitivity to insulin. Make yourself a calorie budget and spend it this way: 60 percent on carbohydrates, 15 percent on protein, and no more than 25 percent on fat. One quick way to reduce the amount of fat in your foods is to lose the cheese from sandwiches, burgers, casseroles, and pasta.

3 Eat 25 to 35 grams of fiber each day. Without a doubt, consuming more fiber can help prevent diabetes, says Jorge Salmeron, M.D., Ph.D., of the Social Security Institute of Mexico City. First, the more fiber you eat, the less fat you tend to consume. Second, soluble fiber delays the movement of food into the small intestine. This slows postmeal surges in blood sugar.

One way to increase the amount of fiber in your diet is to eat more complex carbohydrates: fruits, vegetables, and whole grains. Go easy on the simple carbohydrates: refined foods like white pasta, rice, and bread; cakes; cookies; and pastries. Eating that stuff could double your risk of developing diabetes because it tends to elevate blood sugar much more than fiber-rich complex carbs do.

4 Eat at least five fruits and vegetables a day. Eating more fruits and vegetables could help prevent diabetes, says Earl Ford, M.D., of the Centers for Disease Control and Prevention. In one study, Dr. Ford found that people with normal glucose levels had the highest levels of carotenoids, compounds found abundantly in sweet potatoes, tomatoes, cantaloupe, carrots, oranges, and broccoli. Fruits and vegetables are also treasure troves of other nutrients that fight diabetes, such as antioxidants and flavonoids.

5 **Eat fatty fish like salmon each day.** Preliminary evidence suggests that a daily dose of fatty fish, including salmon, sardines, mackerel, and halibut, may do as much good for in fighting diabetes as losing weight does. Researchers found that people who ate salmon every day had 50 percent lower chances of having glucose intolerance, a common precursor to diabetes, than people who ate that fish less often.

6 **Take 400 IU of vitamin D each day.** When researchers in Sweden measured levels of vitamin D in 34 men, they found that the more vitamin D in the blood, the better the insulin was at delivering glucose to the muscles, thus minimizing diabetes risk. Your body produces vitamin D when your skin is exposed to sunlight. But that's not enough. Take a daily supplement, says Robert E. C. Wildman, R.D., Ph.D., professor of human nutrition at the University of Delaware in Newark.

7 **Take vitamin E too.** In one study, men with the lowest blood levels of vitamin E were four times more likely to get diabetes than men with the highest levels. Experts think vitamin E may prevent diabetes by helping insulin move sugar from the blood into the cells. Take 400 IU of vitamin E each day, says Iswarlal Jialal, M.D., professor of clinical nutrition at the University of Texas Southwestern Medical Center at Dallas Southwestern Medical School. Because vitamin E is a blood thinner, consult your doctor before beginning supplementation in any amount if you are already taking aspirin or blood-thinning medication, such as warfarin (Coumadin), or if you're at high risk for stroke.

8 **Make room for magnesium.** You should be getting 350 milligrams of magnesium each day, says Steve Austin, N.D., a naturopathic physician at the Center for Natural Medicine in Portland, Oregon. Researchers found that the more magnesium in your diet, the less likely you are to get diabetes. You'll find this mineral in fortified cereals, spinach, black-eyed peas, and beans.

9 **Take 200 micrograms of chromium picolinate two or three times per day.** Do this only if you've been diagnosed with glucose intolerance, says Richard A. Anderson, Ph.D., USDA chromium expert. Chromium helps make your cells receptive to insulin. Some studies show it helps normalize glucose and insulin levels.

10 **Add motion to your life.** Physical exercise combined with a modified diet appears to be the best combination for reducing the risk of diabetes, says Andrea Kriska, Ph.D., associate professor in the department of epidemiology in the School of Public Health at the University of Pittsburgh. Try to get in 2½ to 3 hours of exercise each week, she says. You'll reduce your body's resistance to insulin and also help yourself maintain a healthy weight.

10 Ways to Prevent Ulcers and Ulcer Pain

1 **Eat half an onion each and every day.** Scientists believe that onions can help reduce your risk of an ulcer, an open wound in the lining of your stomach or small intestine. Sulfur compounds in the pungent vegetable may attack the *H. pylori* bacterium that causes about 80 percent of ulcers. So try to get onions into your diet whenever you can.

To help deal with the ensuing onion breath, keep tins or containers of breath mints in several strategic spots: in your car, next to your computer, by the kitchen door, in your briefcase, in your desk drawer. Don't carry them around in your pockets; they make funny rattling noises as you walk and get coated with pocket funk.

2 **Choose your painkillers wisely.**The only significant causes of ulcers besides *H. pylori* are nonsteroidal anti-inflammatory drugs (NSAIDs), like aspirin and ibuprofen. If you don't have the bacteria in your stomach, these drugs increase your risk of ulcers; and if you do carry the bacteria, which about half the U.S. population does, NSAIDs increase your risk even further.

An alternative to NSAIDs is a new class of pain-relief drugs known as COX-2 specific inhibitors. Celecoxib (Celebrex) and rofecoxib (Vioxx) are now available by prescription. "While they may not be the first choice for minor problems, they are reported to have fewer gastrointestinal side effects than the NSAIDs," says Kenneth A. Goldberg, M.D., of the Male Health Center.

When aches and pains flare up, try products containing acetaminophen instead, recommends David A. Peura, M.D., associate chief of the division of gastroenterology and hepatology at the University of Virginia in Charlottesville.

3 **Stop smoking.** Make room for ulcers on the lengthy list of ailments linked to smoking. If you're predisposed to having an ulcer, smoking will increase your risk of getting one, says Lawrence S. Friedman, M.D., associate professor of medicine at Harvard Medical School. Also, smokers are more likely to suffer serious ulcer complications like perforation. So if you smoke, your stomach would thank you to quit. And if you're already a non-smoker, it and all your other organs would shake your hand if they could.

4 **Don't drink.** Alcohol can damage the lining of your stomach. Drinking after you have an ulcer is even worse—it will exacerbate the damage.

5 **Fill up with fiber.** Some evidence points to a high-fiber diet as a way to prevent ulcers, Dr. Friedman says. One study found that people who ate an

average of 30 grams of fiber a day cut by half their risk of duodenal ulcers, which are found in the first part of the small intestine. Because of its many health improvements, you should get plenty of fiber in your diet, regardless of the possible ulcer-preventing benefits. High-fiber foods include dried pears, apples, and peaches as well as many beans, such as lima beans, kidney beans, navy beans, and black beans, and cereals and muffins high in bran.

6 **Occasionally use licorice to keep away ulcers.** We're referring to the herb licorice, with the scientific name *glycyrrhiza glabra*, not the candy, which usually doesn't have any real licorice in it.

Licorice, available at health-food stores, contains several anti-ulcer compounds. Use it as an ingredient in tea, recommends James Duke, Ph.D., author of *The Green Pharmacy*. However, long-term use (daily for more than 4 to 6 weeks) or taking too much at once (more than three cups of tea per day) may be bad for your heart or kidneys, raise your blood pressure, or increase water retention. To avoid side effects, you can take a processed form called DGL, or deglycyrrhizinated licorice, also available in health food stores.

7 **Eat smaller, more frequent meals.** Eating triggers your stomach to secrete acid to digest the food, which is good. But excess acid can irritate the stomach lining, and overeating can cause that to occur. So evolve away from three big feasts a day and develop instead an eating habit that includes five or six small meals per day. That will keep your acid levels friendlier to your stomach, says Roger L. Gebhard, M.D., of the University of Minnesota.

8 **If you have an ulcer, refrain from consuming citrus.** Highly acidic citrus foods and juices can aggravate your symptoms, says Marie L. Borum, M.D., of the George Washington University Medical Center.

9 **Leave the dairy in the fridge.** The age-old recommendation of milk and other dairy products for ulcer pain has fallen by the wayside, Dr. Gebhard says. Avoid them while you have an ulcer, since they contain proteins that stimulate acid secretion.

10 **Integrate fresh ginger into your eating habits.** Ginger contains 11 compounds with anti-ulcer effects, according to Dr. Duke. You can take ginger a variety of ways: in 500-milligram capsules; in a cup of tea made with ½ to 1 teaspoon grated fresh ginger in a cup of hot water, sweetened with honey if desired; or as a piece of candied ginger measuring about 1 square inch and ¼-inch thick. *Note:* Ginger may increase bile secretion, so if you have gallstones, do not use therapeutic amounts of the dried root or powder without guidance from a health-care practitioner.

WEEK 10

EXERCISE TO GET STRONG

Set Up a Home Workout Area

The Day's Task

Today, you are going to create or improve upon your home gym. Pick a spot somewhere in your greater domain where you can make the necessary space and where you will enjoy working out. You need room for a weight bench and weights, and you need room to get seriously physically active. You'll be doing both weight training and aerobic exercise for optimum health.

In theory, for the past 2 months you've been doing some form of aerobic exercise at least twice a week, mostly an outdoor form, but an indoor form as well on cold or rainy days. Have you gotten into a routine? Have you chosen your aerobic workout of choice? We ask because the size and location of your home workout space will be defined in good part by your aerobic exercise preferences.

With that in mind, get a tape measure, a pad of paper to list anything you have to buy, and a toolbox in case you need to hang anything on the walls. Finally, get your wallet ready; you might have to spend a few bucks here. Equipped and ready? Read on.

In the 1999 Oscar-winning movie *American Beauty*, the character played by Kevin Spacey, undergoing a sudden midlife transformation, turns his garage into his own private exercise hangout, complete with psychedelic posters on the wall, lots of space for lounging around, and a stereo blasting classic rock tunes. And of course, he has a weight bench and other strength-training equipment right in the middle. He loves it in there.

If you saw the movie and were like most guys watching it, you secretly thought, "Nice setup." And that's the lesson of this chapter. Not to be like the guy in the movie—you don't want to end up like him. But that you, too, deserve an exercise space that you actually want to be in, that is personal, comfortable, and uniquely yours. In this 10th week of the Longevity Pro-

FREE WEIGHTS ON A BUDGET

If at first you can't afford to spring for dumbbells and a barbell, get the dumbbells. Here's why.

- Dumbbells give you more freedom of movement. For example, if doing biceps curls with your palms up hurts your elbows, you can turn your hands as you lower the weights so that you end with your palms facing your body. This takes some of the stress off your elbows. With a barbell, your wrists, elbows, and shoulders are locked into one position.
- Both sides of your body get the same workout with dumbbells since you hold the same amount of weight in each hand. With a barbell, both hands hold one weight, so your stronger side may do more work.
- Dumbbells are more versatile; you can do more exercises with them.

gram, you start lifting weights. We'll outline the benefits tomorrow. Before you can get to the benefits, you have to get to the "doing," and it takes a workout space to do it.

Start by picking the right size space. Here are some dimensions to keep in mind. A weight bench, weights, and room to work with them require an area approximately 9 feet by 9 feet. More is better. Some of that is simply clear floor space, which you'll use for stretching, floor exercises like crunches, aerobic exercise like jumping jacks or rope skipping, and warmup and cooldown periods. If you're installing an aerobic exercise machine of some kind, allow additional space for it. And while you have the measuring tape out, measure the widths of the doors, halls, and so on to make sure you (with the help of a couple of gorillas) can get your exercise gear where it's going.

Next, call a good sporting goods/fitness store that delivers, and order the following, if you do not already have them.

- Rubber floor padding that's the right size to cover your workout area
- One Olympic-style 7-foot-long weight bar
- One easy curl bar: 20 to 25 pounds
- Two collars that use spring tension to lock the weights onto the bar
- Weight plates: four 5-pound plates, four 10s, two 25s, two 35s, and two 45s to

start; if you're already an intermediate or advanced lifter, you'll know what other ones to buy for your current level

- Dumbbells: six pairs if you want to be thorough; get 10-, 15-, 20-, 25-, 30-, and 35-pound sets
- A good quality, sturdy weight bench that will incline (cheap ones are flimsy)

Sure, you'll shell out some bucks. But this basic weight set is going to cost you less than a year's membership in a decent health club. Plus, the hours at Club Casa are much, much better; there's never a crowd or lines; and there's no dress code. One of the benefits of working out at home is that you can feel right at home.

Work a bit on the environment. Make your home gym pleasant and inviting. Think spa, not high school locker room. Paint the walls, if necessary. Take in a fan or a heater. Add lighting—nice lighting, not bare bulbs—and play music, if you like. If you want a good, healthy, long life, you're going to spend some time in your gym. Make it a place that you look forward to visiting. As we said earlier, think of this as not just a gym but a sanctuary or retreat. Realize that this is *your* space, not your kids', not your wife's.

Some accoutrements that you might add, as your wallet allows, include a dumbbell rack and a weight tree, for storage and keeping the area neat, and a nice mirror. It's okay to admire your muscles in the mirror, but the real reason we want you to have one is so you can check your form as you do each exercise.

Aerobic Machines

As we pointed out in Week 2, you can jump rope, do calisthenics, and engage in a number of other activities at home to get an aerobic workout that will provide you with those all-important cardio benefits. But perhaps you'd prefer a practical machine to get your pump pumping. Here are the particulars on several potential purchases.

Treadmill. Buy one with a motor. The nonmotorized ones just don't cut it. They're hard to use whether you walk or run. You want a treadmill with at least a 1.5 horsepower motor. Be sure that horsepower number is rated on the label for "continuous duty." Cheaper models use a "peak power" rating that overstates the power available over a sustained period.

A top-notch treadmill will have a welded frame of aircraft-quality aluminum or heavy steel (12-gauge or less) for stability. Look for a model that is at least 50 inches long and 18 inches wide, or else you may find yourself struggling to stay on it. You should be able to raise and lower the tread elevation while you're walking or running on it.

Stationary bike. The bike has to work against you somehow, or you'll make the wheel spin faster than you are pedaling, creating a coasting effect. A model with a weighted flywheel that's driven by a belt is effective as long as the wheel has a weight of 25 to 50 pounds. A bikes with caliper brakes, on the other hand, will feel awkward and tend to wear out relatively quickly.

Another option is a bike with air resistance caused by fanlike aerodynamics of the wheel. The fan blades create a breeze that gets stronger the harder you work. The faster you pedal, the greater the resistance. Or choose a bike with magnetic resistance. With this, a thin flywheel passes between two magnets that electronically move closer or farther apart to change the resistance. This is the most expensive type of stationary bike.

The most important qualities to look for in a bike are comfort and solid construction. Your bike should not shimmy when you're pedaling, and it shouldn't give you a pain in the butt or back. The saddle and handlebar should be adjustable but firmly held in place with a pin that drives all the way through the seat tube and seatpost, then locks into place.

As with other exercise equipment, you can get a stationary bike with a variety of bells and whistles—electronic displays that provide such data as calories burned, heart rate, and revolutions per minute. Those options are completely up to you and your wallet.

Stairclimber. There are two types of these machines: steppers, which work just your lower body, and climbers, which provide handles to grasp so that your motion is similar to that of scaling a ladder.

There also are two types of foot platforms. With one, the pedals move in tandem so that when one foot goes down, the opposite pedal goes up automatically. It feels balanced and is easy to learn. With the other type, each pedal moves independently of the other. This takes a bit more getting used to, but once you adapt, it feels quite natural. Try them both and decide which you prefer.

On a less-expensive stairclimber, resistance comes from pushing the pedals against pressure from a hydraulic or pneumatic cylinder. A hydraulic cylinder is usually filled with oil, which keeps it lubricated and free of maintenance woes. A pneumatic cylinder is a bit more troublesome because inner friction and heat tend to wear it down.

INFOMERCIAL INFO

We've all seen infomercials hawking exercise equipment. Tempting, aren't they? Guys with rock-hard bodies and gals with . . . well, rock-hard bodies . . . promise us that we can add muscle or lose fat by buying and using their inexpensive product.

Don't bother.

Consider the ab devices. You can work your abs just as effectively by doing crunches, without the gizmos, for free.

Indeed, a study conducted by the department of kinesiology at California State University, Northridge, on behalf of the American Council on Exercise tested 19 volunteers on the four best-selling abdominal trainers. The study concluded there were no statistically significant differences in muscle activity for the basic crunch, oblique crunch, and reverse curl done with the ab contraptions when compared with the same exercises performed without the gizmos.

Don't be tempted by discount superstore and shopping channel "bargain" gym equipment either. Most of it is cheaply and imprecisely made. The object of this whole program is longevity and quality of life. That extends to exercise equipment as well. Good quality equipment that is cared for well will be long-lived.

A higher-end model forgoes cylinders altogether in favor of cables or chains that wrap around a flywheel. This provides a quieter and smoother workout. As with other exercise equipment, you will pay more for an elaborate graphic display that provides data on your workout.

Whatever stairclimber you buy should have pedals that are wide enough that your feet feel stable and secure, and the motion should feel smooth and steady.

Strength-Training Session Number 1

The Day's Task

Today, you begin your strength-training program, with a focus on your upper body. Allow 55 minutes. And you must eat first. Thirty minutes to an hour before your workout, eat a bagel or a jam-filled cereal bar. This primes your body chemistry for muscle building. Wear comfortable clothing, such as a loose T-shirt, shorts, and cross-trainer athletic shoes. Here's the routine.

1. **Warm up for 3 minutes. Walk on a treadmill, ride a stationary bike, jump rope, do jumping jacks, or jog in place.**
2. **Stretch for 2 minutes. As you stretch, mentally prepare for the workout. Imagine moving from one exercise to the next, performing each exercise using proper form.**
3. **Perform weight lifting exercises that work your chest, shoulders, back, and arms in that order. You should do three sets of each exercise. (If you're brand new to weight training, you can do just one set of each exercise.) Perform 8 to 12 repetitions in each set.**

   To pick the right amount of weight, experiment. Find a weight for each exercise with which you can just manage to make the minimum number of repetitions. (Soon, as you quickly build strength and endurance, add weight. Do that when you find it easy to perform the maximum number of repetitions.)
4. **Rest for 1 minute between sets.**

We're going to explain why you need to do strength training. But to keep your momentum going, we're first going to continue with the specifics of

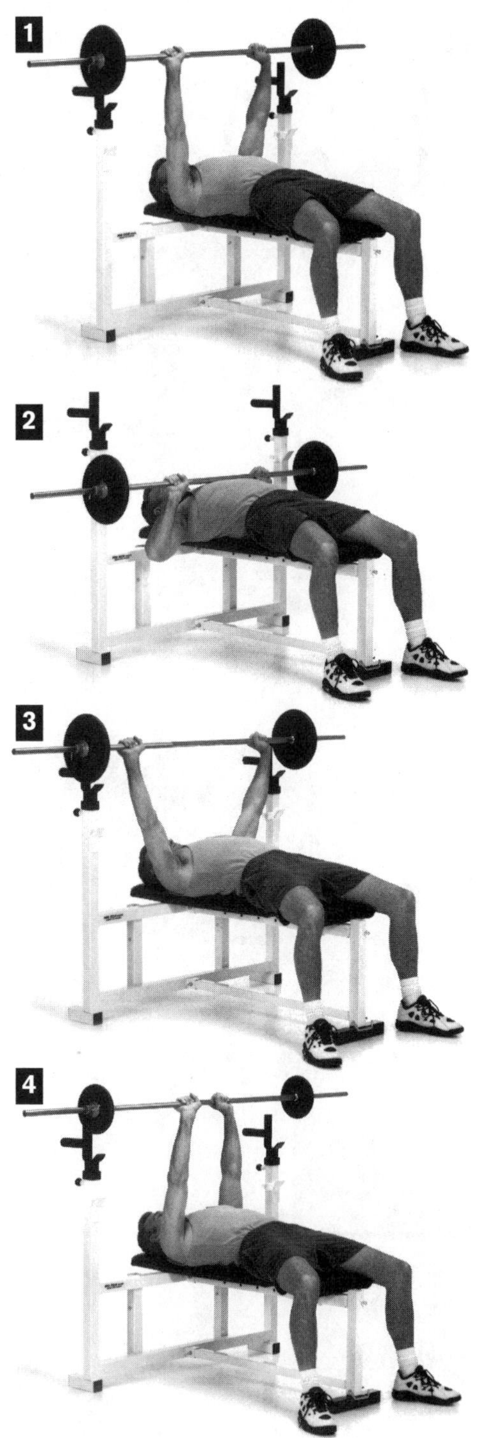

the strength-training program. Do the exercises in this order to work your bigger muscle groups first.

Chest

Even if you've never picked up a barbell in your life, you've probably heard of the following exercise. It's your key to a broad chest and the pectoral power that will make you proud.

Bench press. (1) Lie on your weight bench with a barbell above your chest. Grasp the bar with a medium grip, hands about shoulder-width apart or slightly wider. Your palms should face your legs, and your feet should rest flat on the floor. Keep your back straight and against the bench.

(2) Lower the bar to your chest at nipple level. Your elbows should point out while the rest of your body remains in position. Don't arch your back or bounce the bar off your chest. Then repeat.

To work the pectoral muscles in your chest at different angles, vary your routine with wide-grip (3) and narrow-grip (4) presses. Or perform an inclined bench press (see photos 5 and 6 on page 324) maintaining the same form as above.

Shoulders

Big shoulders connote power and raw masculinity. They consist of front, side,

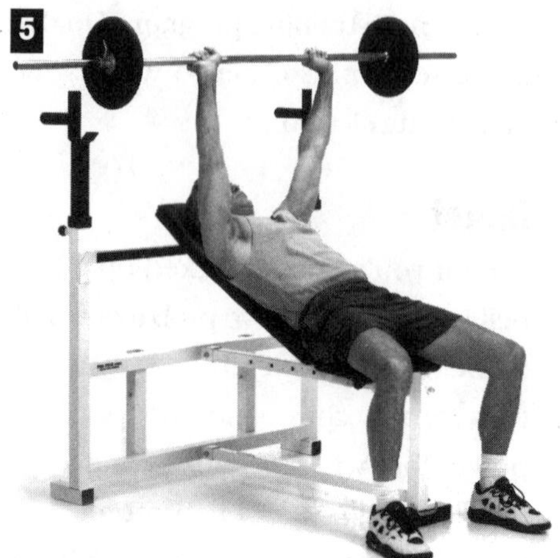

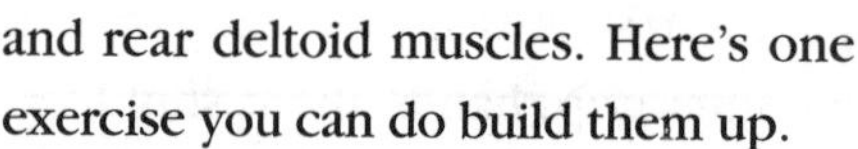

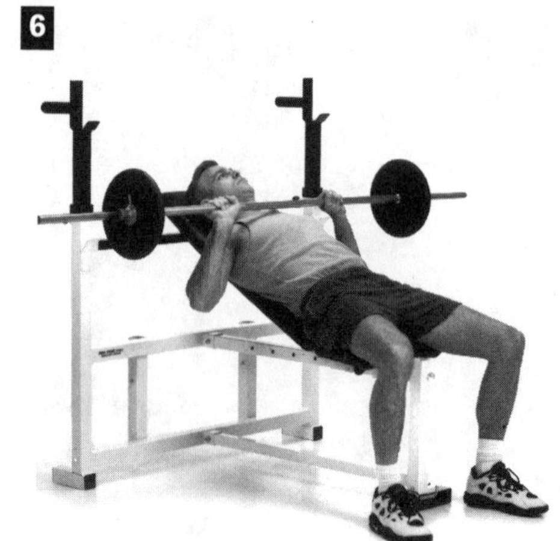

and rear deltoid muscles. Here's one exercise you can do build them up.

Alternating press with dumbbells. (7) Straddle your weight bench with your legs slightly parted. Keep your feet flat on the floor. Grasp two dumbbells, holding them shoulder-width apart at shoulder level, with your palms facing each other. Keep your shoulders back, your chest out, and a slight forward lean in your lower back. Keep your elbows unlocked.

(8) Raise the right dumbbell until your arm is straight, but don't lock your elbow. Lower to the starting position, then repeat with your left arm.

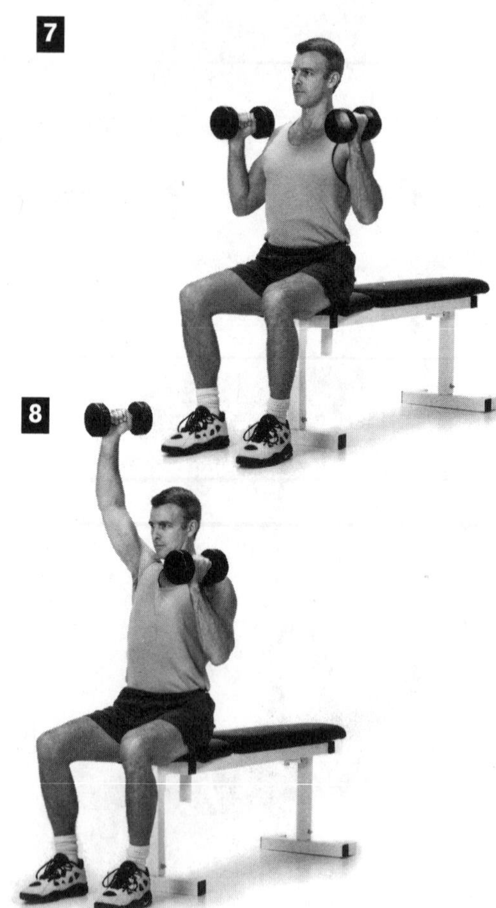

Back

If you want to feel old and worn out even at a young age, ignore your back muscles. As many as four out of five men suffer back pain at times, and the problem often begins with weak back muscles. Besides lessening your likelihood of pain and injury, building your back muscles adds power and lets you stand straighter. You need to work both your upper back and lower back.

One-arm dumbbell row. This exercise works your upper back.

(9) Stand partly over your weight bench with your body weight resting on your bent right leg and your right hand, both of which should be on the center of the padded portion of the bench. With your left foot firmly on the floor, hold a dumbbell in your left hand with your palm facing your body. Keep your back straight and your eyes looking toward the floor. Extend your left arm down toward the floor, elbow unlocked.

(10) Pull the dumbbell up and in toward your torso. Raise it as high as you can, bringing it in toward your lower chest muscles. Your left elbow should point up toward the ceiling as you lift. Lower to the starting position and repeat.

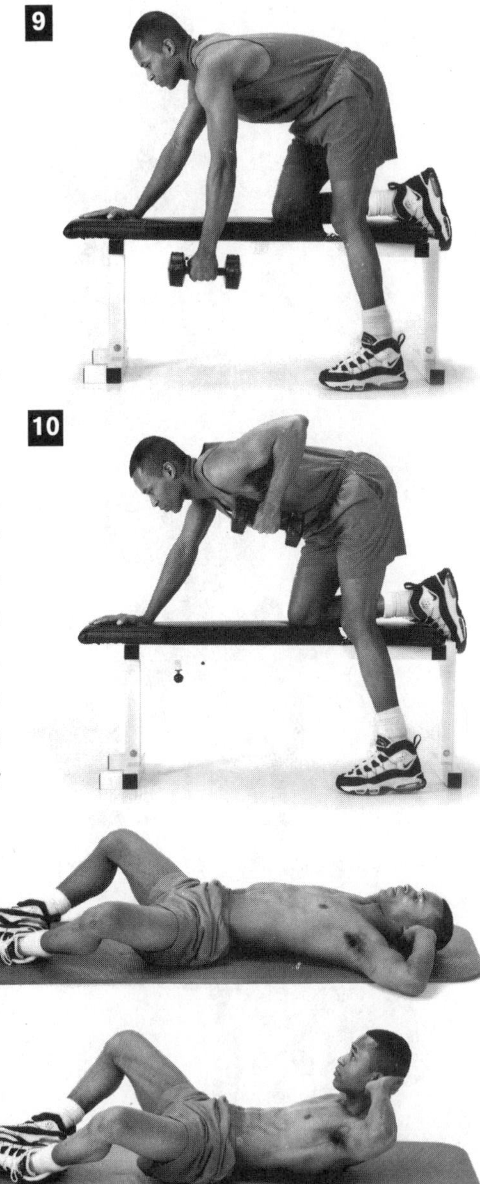

Frog-leg crunch. This exercise works your lower back.

(11) Lie flat on your back with your knees spread and the soles of your feet together. Your knees should be as close to the floor as you can comfortably get them. Rest your fingertips lightly on the sides of your head and put your elbows out to the sides, or fold your arms across your chest.

(12) Keeping the rest of your body in place, lift your shoulder blades and upper back off the floor. At the same time, slightly curl your pelvis up and in, but

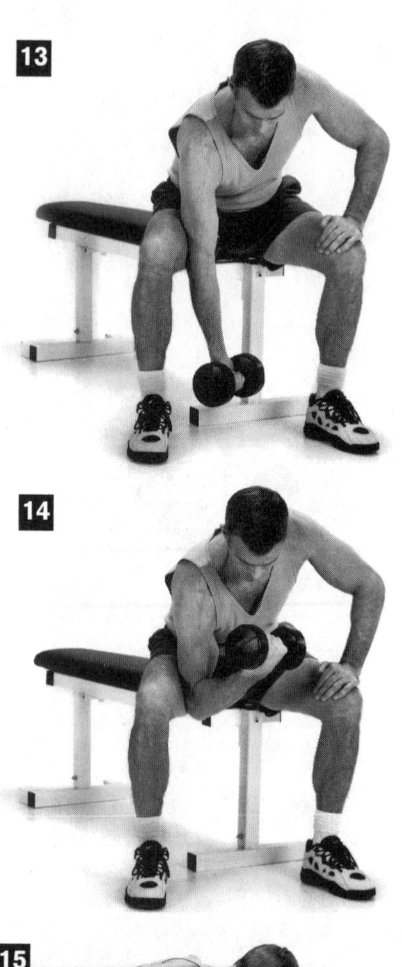

13

14

15

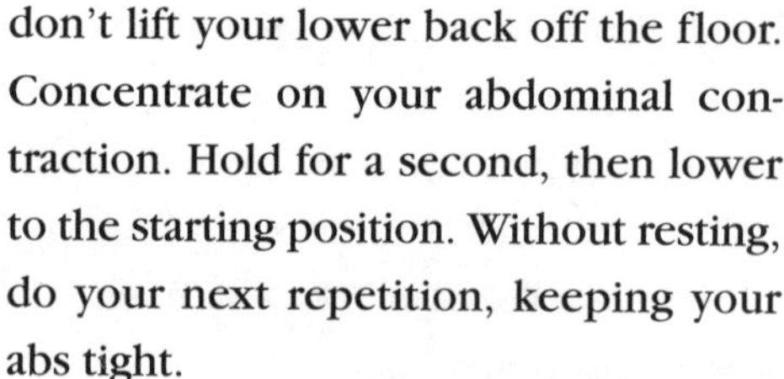

don't lift your lower back off the floor. Concentrate on your abdominal contraction. Hold for a second, then lower to the starting position. Without resting, do your next repetition, keeping your abs tight.

The beauty of all this exercise and most others is that they actually work several muscle groups. While frog-leg crunches buttress your back, they also harden your abs. Meanwhile, the bench press builds you not only a bigger chest but also triceps and shoulders.

Arms

Most guys don't need a lot of encouragement to develop their arms. Do arm exercises last. You use your arms in other exercises, such as the chest and shoulder routines. If you work your arms first, they may be too worn out to work the other muscle groups.

Concentration curl. This works your biceps.

(13) Sitting at the end of your weight bench with your feet shoulder-width apart, lean forward and put your right arm between your legs. Your elbow and upper arm should rest against your thigh. Extend your right arm, holding a dumbbell with your palm facing up. Rest your left hand on your left thigh.

(14) Slowly lift the dumbbell to your right shoulder. Brace your elbow against your thigh and lean on your left hand if

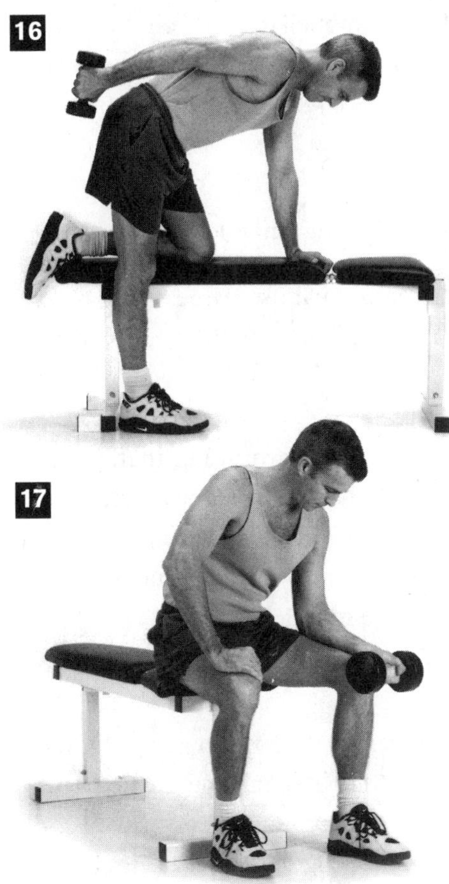

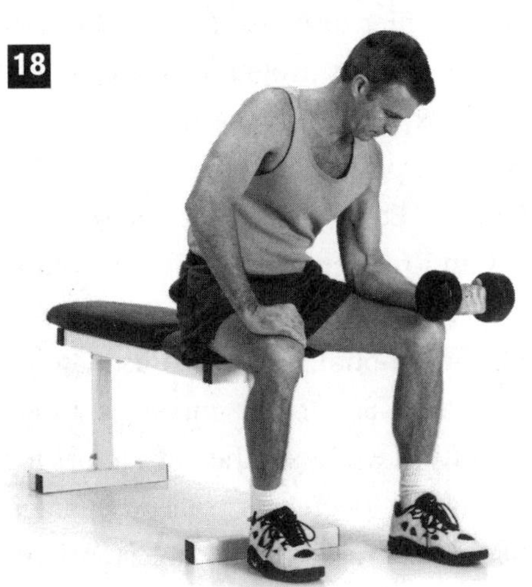

you need support. Lower to the starting position, then repeat with your left arm.

Dumbbell kickback. This is for your triceps.

(15) Stand partly over your weight bench with your body weight resting on your bent left leg and your left hand, both of which should be on the center of the padded portion of the bench. With your right foot firmly on the floor, hold a dumbbell in your right hand with your palm facing your body. Your right elbow should point up toward the ceiling. Keep your back straight and your eyes looking toward the floor.

(16) Straighten your arm out behind you, extending the dumbbell away from your body. Keep extending until you feel your triceps fully contract, then bend your arm and lower to the starting position. Repeat with your left arm.

Forearm curl. Would you believe that this exercise is for your forearms?

(17) Sit on your weight bench with your legs a little more than hip-width apart. Hold a dumbbell in your left hand with your palm up. Lean your left forearm on your left thigh, with the back of your wrist positioned just slightly over your knee for maximum mobility. Allow your left wrist to bend back naturally as the dumbbell pulls it down. Rest your right hand on your right thigh. Keep your body upright, slightly leaning on your left leg for support.

(18) Using only your left wrist and

keeping the rest of your arm stationary, curl the dumbbell toward your body as far as it will go. Hold for a second, then lower to the starting position. Repeat with your right arm.

Weight Routine Wrap-Up

Finish your strength-training session with the following activities.

- Cool down with 2 minutes of any aerobic exercise that uses large, major muscle groups in a rhythmic, continuous fashion, such as pumping the pedals on a stationary bike.
- Do 1 minute of light stretches.
- Shower, giving yourself 10 minutes of soothing, lukewarm water therapy. Consider this a treat and enjoy it. Relax your mind. This is not an appropriate time to worry about the world outside. This is a wonderful, private time to de-stress.
- Eat a cereal bar. Do this within 15 minutes of ending your workout. This gives you a boost precisely when needed to maximize muscle building.

Why Muscles Matter

Exercise offers an aesthetic benefit: nicer appearance. It also offers major physical benefits that contribute to longevity and quality of life. Building muscle helps ward off and even reverse the effects of degenerative diseases such as arthritis. People with arthritis who are placed on strength-training programs increase their range of motion and lose weight, researchers have found.

In fact, exercise combats most degenerative, killer diseases. Fitness through exercise is a proven disease-risk reducer. A regular fitness program should be the cornerstone of every man's anti-disease strategy, experts say.

"The numbers clearly show that people who are physically active have less disease—particularly heart disease," says Kerry Stewart, Ed.D., a clinical exercise physiologist and director of cardiac rehabilitation and prevention at Johns Hopkins Bayview Medical Center in Baltimore. Since heart disease is the number one killer of Americans, that's no insignificant piece of information. Exercise works its wonders directly and indirectly. Directly, according to Dr. Stewart, it improves things like heart function and body metabolism. Indirectly, it works on the risk factors for disease. For example, exercise lowers blood pressure, decreases your percentage of body fat, and improves your ratio of "good" cholesterol to "bad" cholesterol. All of those things are major factors in heart disease.

DON'T GET STUCK

You must vary your workout. This not only keeps you from getting bored but also tricks your muscles into responding with new growth. If you don't vary your routine, you'll hit a plateau at which you won't see any more muscle gains.

Mix in a few new exercises. Alternate the amount of weight and the number of reps you do in your core routine. Use lighter weight and more reps, for instance. That is a strategy for building endurance. Or try heavier weight and fewer reps. That is a strategy for gaining brute strength. Just never go to a weight that's so heavy that you sacrifice form or jerk or swing the weights to heft them.

But fitness fights more than just heart disease. It's the treatment of choice for diabetes as well as your best bet to avoid that ailment. And only recently has exercise's cancer-fighting value come to light, most notably for men as a risk reducer for colon and prostate cancers.

Exercise not only keeps you alive but also keeps your life worth living. "Most of what people think of as 'growing older' isn't. It's disuse," says Walter M. Bortz II, M.D., clinical associate professor of medicine at Stanford University School of Medicine and author of *Dare to Be 100*. That, he says, is why it's so important to recognize the power of exercise.

Various studies have shown that weight training helps you maintain strength and flexibility; balance; and even bone strength and density, clarity of mind, and positive outlook well into your senior years. The key is to stay with the program. If you stop for one reason or another, start again, at any age, to reap age-defying benefits.

Those far-off, future benefits are well worth the effort. But you also gain see-it-now, feel-it-now results. You lose fat. For every pound of muscle you gain, your resting metabolic rate goes up 50 calories a day. That means you burn fat more efficiently, whether at rest or at play.

Another benefit of working with weights is that you increase your testosterone levels, which can boost your sex drive. That certainly makes you feel better. In one study, researchers found a 10 percent increase in testosterone levels in just 12 weeks. And in wonderful and convenient full-circle logic, the higher your testosterone level, the more muscle you amass.

Maximize Your Recovery

The Day's Task

Today's task is the easiest of the entire 12-week program. We want you to do . . . nothing. Or more accurately, do nothing strenuous with your upper body. Don't lift weights, don't rearrange any furniture, don't play baseball. You can still lift a bag of groceries or take out the trash—working out yesterday is not an excuse to shirk family duties today. But the important thing is to not stress the muscle groups that you exercised yesterday. Doing so will set you back in your efforts to gain muscle and strength.

We didn't want to alarm you yesterday, so we didn't tell you that when you lift weights, you rip apart your muscles, making little microscopic tears. It sounds rough but, in actuality, it's how sports medicine researchers believe muscles are built. You break down your muscles with resistance and deplete their fuel, then they grow back bigger and stronger as they replenish. How much bigger and stronger they get depends upon the type of muscle, your genetics, and your testosterone level. Guys with higher testosterone levels amass more muscle.

So ripping apart your muscles and letting them rebuild is part of the process. That's why you must rest. You must give your muscles time to rebuild.

How long should you rest between workouts? Forty-eight hours is the general rule, but the truth is that it depends. The amount of recovery time you need is determined by how intensely you train. Lifting 100 pounds in a bench press and doing 20 repetitions will not require as much recovery time as lifting 150 pounds and performing 6 repetitions. The heavier the load, the more extensive the damage to muscle fibers and the longer it will take to repair them.

Rest, Assured

Getting enough rest between workouts is pretty easy. If you work all your upper-body muscle groups one day and your lower-body muscle groups the next, you can exercise every day and still give each muscle group a proper rest. You could work upper body on Monday, lower body on Tuesday, upper body on Wednesday, and so forth.

If you choose instead to do a total-body workout each time you exercise, you can work out only 3 or 4 days a week. If you are new to weight training, regardless of which schedule you choose, you may need more recovery time than we've suggested. Listen to your body.

It's not enough to simply go 48 hours without exercising the same muscle. If you crawl home from bars in the wee hours or spend all night engrossed in a Three Stooges TV marathon, you probably will be fatigued. During sleep, your body battles many of the fatigue and stress toxins, including those produced by strenuous exercise. And during the first 90 minutes of deep sleep, your body releases the greatest quantities of growth hormone that helps you build muscle. So sound sleep is sensible.

Here are some other ways you can ensure that you don't overtrain your muscles.

- If you're brand new to weight training, start off doing just one set of each exercise with the heaviest weight you can handle. Researchers concluded that the results that beginners got from doing one set were comparable to the results they got by doing three.
- Alternate heavy and light workouts during the week. If you pump a lot of iron in your upper-body exercises on Monday, go lighter on Wednesday then back to heavier weights on Friday.
- Don't perform more than three exercises on your larger muscle groups—upper legs, back, and chest—during any one training session. And do no more than one or two exercises per smaller muscle groups—biceps and calves, for example—in a single workout.
- As you grow stronger, you'll want to add more weight to your exercise routines. Add no more than 5 to 10 percent of the weight you're already using, however, and don't increase the weight until you're able to do at least six repetitions with it.

Too Much of a Good Thing

If you overtrain, your body will tell you. Here are some ways that it will communicate this to you.

- You are chronically tired and have trouble sleeping.
- You're irritable, moody, or depressed more than usual.
- You're more often sick with colds and flu, or you're more prone to infections.
- Your resting pulse rate is higher than normal. Take your pulse in the morning before you get out of bed, counting the number of heartbeats in 1 minute. If your pulse rises by the same amount each week for a period of several weeks, you may be overtraining.
- Your blood pressure has risen.

Strength-Training Session Number 2

The Day's Task

Today, you will work your lower body. The basics from Day 2 apply in terms of what to eat, what to wear, and how to warm up, stretch, cool down, and shower. Allow 50 minutes. Do three sets (or one set, if you're a beginner) of 8 to 12 repetitions. Exercise your calf muscles last; they're the smallest.

Ever notice that American sports are dominated by arm activities? Baseball is mostly arms that are throwing and hitting. Basketball is all about shooting. And if you go outside with a buddy and a football, you spend most of your time passing around the pigskin. We're guessing that the lack of an arm component is one reason why soccer has never fully caught on in the States.

Likewise, in most gyms, guys tend toward upper-body strength training. But there are many compelling reasons why you should put at least equal emphasis on lower-body strengthening.

Your legs are your body's foundation. You need good legs to bend, pull, push, shove, and lift, not to mention to walk, run, and jump.

Strong legs can save your back. A lot of back pain comes from using your arm and shoulder muscles instead of your legs when lifting heavy objects. When lifting, support should come from the hamstrings and quadriceps in your thighs.

Strong legs can save your knees. If your leg muscles are developed, you'll be better able to withstand shocks that otherwise would travel directly to your knees.

RECOVERY SOUP

Eating right after a strenuous workout can help you efficiently rebuild damage to muscle tissues, which is necessary to grow bigger muscles. Your body needs protein—a key muscle-building component—and carbohydrates to replenish stores of glycogen, the muscle fuel that's lost during exercise. Here's a soup that has both, plus calcium, magnesium, and potassium to protect against muscle cramping.

12 **ounces ground sirloin**
2½ **cups reduced-sodium beef broth**
1½ **teaspoons dried Italian seasoning**
¼ **teaspoon onion powder**
Pinch of garlic powder
½ **cup elbow macaroni**
1 **can (16 ounces) reduced-sodium stewed tomatoes**
1 **can (16 ounces) kidney beans, rinsed and drained**

Warm a skillet over medium-high heat. Add the ground sirloin and cook, stirring frequently, for about 5 minutes, or until no longer pink. Remove to paper towels to drain. Transfer to a large saucepan over medium-high heat. Stir in the broth, Italian seasoning, onion powder, and garlic powder. Cover and bring to a boil. Stir in the macaroni and return to a boil. Reduce the heat to medium and simmer for 8 minutes, or until the macaroni is tender. Stir in the tomatoes (with juice) and beans. Simmer until the beans are heated through.

Makes 4 servings
Per serving (2 cups): 298 calories, 36 g protein, 35 g carbohydrates, 3 g fat, 6 g fiber

Strong legs burn more calories. Large muscles burn a lot more calories than small ones. Since your legs contain the biggest muscles in your body, making them bigger and stronger can increase the number of calories you burn.

Strong legs give you the endurance and power you need for a wide range of activities, from playing tennis to mowing the lawn. "Great," you say, "I'm doing leg exercises so I can mow the lawn more often." Not really. If you enjoy playing a game of hoops or softball or almost any other sport, you need strong legs. Your legs and hips generate the power, speed, and explosiveness that you need to perform well. Developed leg muscles are vital in almost any athletic undertaking.

This program will develop your lower body well. Eat your pre-workout, high-carb snack, do your warmup, and dive in! These leg builders can be done with either dumbbells or a barbell. (Leg-extension and leg-curl machines in gyms also provide good leg workouts.) If you're a novice weight lifter and want to be particularly careful, start off without using weights. Make sure that you are comfortable going through the full range of motion before you pick up the dumbbells.

Quadriceps

These are the large muscles on the fronts of your thighs. Whether you're running, jumping, or pushing, your quads are crucial.

Dumbbell lunge. (1) Stand upright with a dumbbell in each hand. Your arms should be fully extended at your sides, with your palms facing toward your body. Your feet should be about hip-width apart.

(2) With your right leg, step farther forward than you would in a normal step. Your right leg should be bent at close to a 90-degree angle. Your knee should not go beyond your toes. Your left leg should be bent at the knee. Your left foot should remain in the same position, although it's okay if your heel rises slightly. Your upper body should remain upright and slightly forward. Return to the starting position and repeat. Once you've done 8 to 12 repetitions, switch to lunging with your left leg; or alternate legs with each rep, if you prefer.

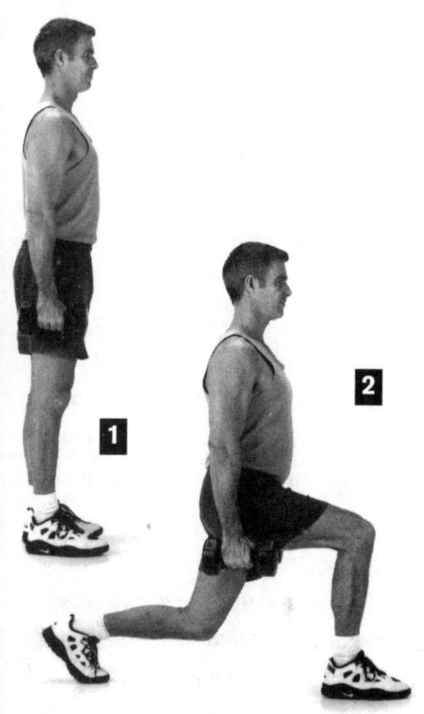

Squat. This exercise works your hamstrings as well as your quads. From a squatting position, grasp a barbell with your palms facing forward.

(See photo 3 on page 336.) Place

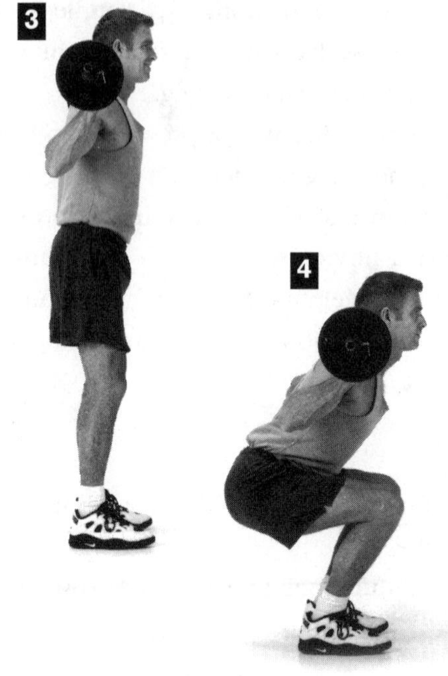

the barbell behind your neck. It should be even across your upper shoulder muscles. Stand up straight with your feet hip-width apart and your toes forward and slightly out. Bend your knees slightly, and lean slightly forward.

(4) Squat down as though you were about to sit in a chair. Your thighs should be nearly parallel to the floor. Keep your feet flat. Rise to the starting position and repeat.

Hamstrings

Your hamstrings are at the backs of your thighs, opposite your quadriceps. If you develop one of these groups and neglect the other, you create an imbalance. That can lead to a painful pulls or tears.

Stiff-legged deadlift. This exercise will also strengthen your lower back and buttocks in addition to your hamstrings.

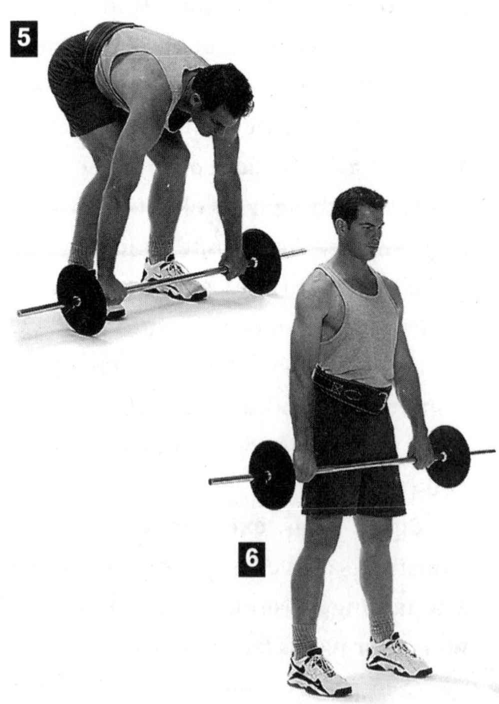

(5) Stand with your feet shoulder-width apart, with a barbell on the floor in front of you. The bar should be over your feet and close to your shins. Keeping your back straight, your head up, and your shoulders directly over or a little ahead of the bar, squat down and grasp the bar with your palms facing in and your arms extended and positioned just outside your knees. This is the starting position.

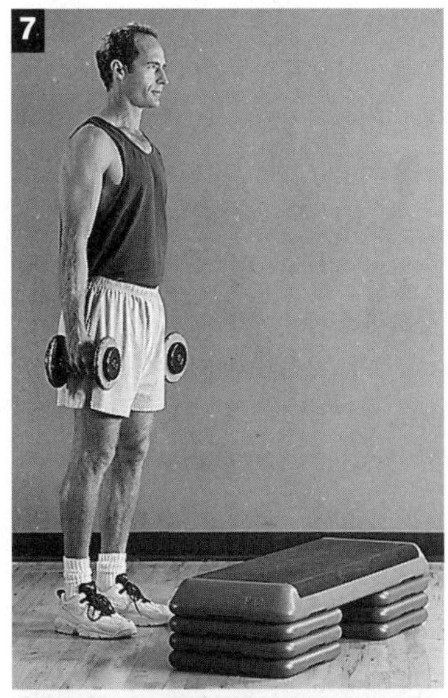
7

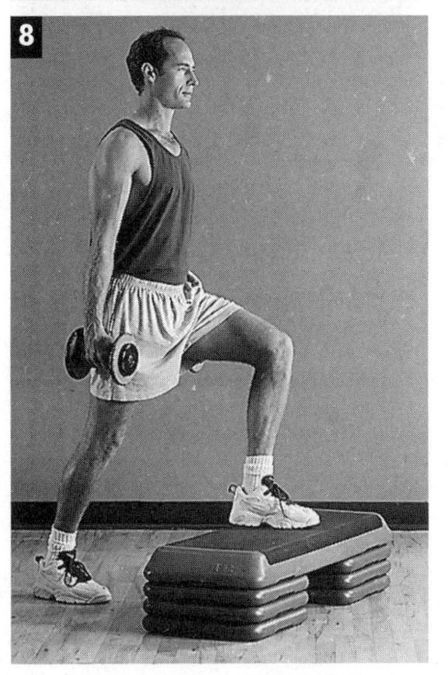
8

(6) Using your thighs and back and keeping your arms extended and your back straight, stand up, raising the bar straight up off the floor.

Once upright, lower the barbell back to the starting position. Repeat.

Stepup. Like the squat, this is a dual-purpose exercise. It will make your quadriceps stronger and work smaller lower-body muscles while giving you a bit of an aerobic workout.

(7) Hold a dumbbell in each hand, with your arms at your sides and your palms facing toward your body. Stand upright about 1 foot away from a sturdy box or platform that is 12 to 18 inches high or aerobic steps of that height. Keep your shoulders back and your chest out.

(8) Keeping the dumbbells at your sides and your upper body straight, step forward with your left foot, placing it on the center of the box. Complete the stepup by bringing your right foot next to your left.

Step backward with your left foot so that your left leg is about where you started. Step down with your right foot to return to the starting position. Repeat, this time leading with your right foot.

Calves

Calves are one of the hardest muscle groups in the body to develop. They enable you to stand on your tiptoes, walk, jump, and sprint.

One-leg heel raise. (See photo 9 on page 338.) Stand on your right leg with your heel off the edge of a stable platform that is 6 to 10 inches high (a stair will do). Your knees should be slightly bent and your toes should point straight ahead. Let your right heel drop down as far as it will comfortably go. Tuck your left foot behind the calf of your right leg. Hold a dumbbell in your right hand, with your

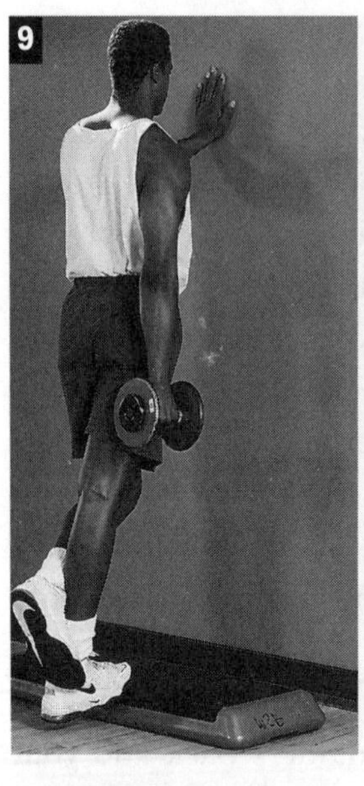
9

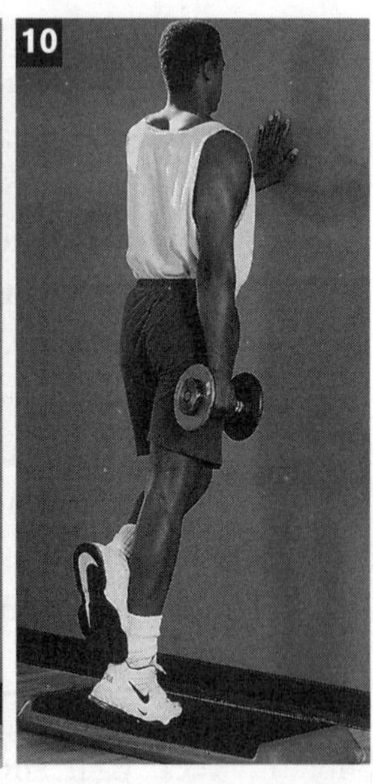
10

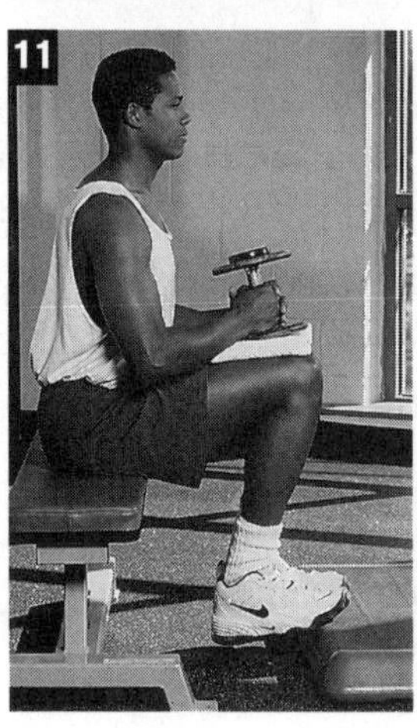
11

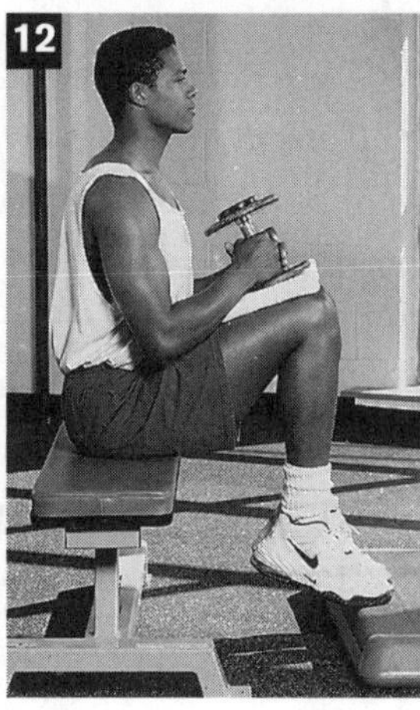
12

palm facing toward your body. Put your left hand on a chair, wall, or other support for balance.

(10) Slowly rise up as high as possible on the ball of your right foot. Hold for a second, then slowly lower to the starting position. Repeat.

After completing the set, repeat, this time supporting your weight with your left leg.

Seated heel raise. This exercise puts particular stress on the lower part of your calf, called the soleus muscle.

(11) Sit up straight on the side of your weight bench. Rest the balls of your feet on a 6- to 8-inch platform, such as an aerobics step. Let your heels drop down as far as they will comfortably go. Keep your knees together and bent at a 45-degree angle. Hold a dumbbell with both hands, resting it vertically on a folded towel on your thighs. Or balance a barbell across your thighs, if you prefer.

(12) Push up as high as possible on the balls of your feet. Hold for a second, then lower to the starting position. Repeat.

The Ultimate Abs Regimen

The Day's Task

Today's workout takes about 30 minutes. We suggest doing it first thing in the morning since your sleep clothes are probably appropriate for this type of exercise. You can then proceed with the rest of the day with minimal hassle.

You need to choose between an old-fashioned workout focused on crunches and a program that is much more varied and unusual but takes more gear. If you pick the latter, you'll need a football or pillow, a basketball, a barbell, a broomstick, and your weight bench or a piece of sturdy furniture. For the former, you'll need just a broomstick and two dumbbells. Close the door to keep out people and other major distractions. Stretch for a few minutes to help you wake up and keep you flexible.

You're ready to exercise. Follow either of the two abdominal workouts in this chapter. Afterward, do some more light stretching for 1 minute. Then carry on with your day, soldier.

Abs have almost become a parody (but don't blame us at *Men's Health* Books—we pick our cover models because of their *attitudes*). The lingo is everywhere: six-pack abs; washboard abs; abs that are cut, ripped, shredded, or chiseled; abs of steel, platinum, or titanium. A perfect torso has become the ultimate symbol of male health and strength in magazines, on television, in advertisements, and in movies. Forget arms or chests or shoulders; guys fixate on their guts.

The reason for this is a little deeper than mere vanity. We men are physiologically predisposed to gaining weight around our stomachs as we age. (Women are different. Extra weight usually lands on their butts and legs.) Often, these male stomach rolls start showing up in our thirties or forties, a time when we aren't ready to acknowledge that our bodies might be moving past their prime. So we attack the problem. If a 40-year-old guy has a flat gut, well, damn, he's still alright.

Statistics back this up. One study, seeking to find how people feel about different parts of their bodies, found that about half of men are dissatisfied with their stomachs. So we crunch, we twist, we suck 'em in, we buy pants that are too tight, all to make these bulges go away.

All these strategies ignore an important point: Exercising your abs doesn't make belly flab go away. Only sensible eating and aerobic exercise can do that, by burning off the excess weight. Ab muscles will show definition only if there is minimal fat lying atop them.

This isn't to say that ab exercises are futile—quite the opposite. Strong abs help you in many ways.

They save your back. The muscles in your midsection don't function in isolation. They weave through your torso like a cargo net, even attaching to your spine. So it's not surprising that a majority of all back pain may be related to weak muscles in your belly. Weak abdominal muscles increase stress on your gluteals and hamstrings. That destabilizes your spine and eventually causes back pain.

They help you move farther, faster. Developing your abs can help your speed. That's because when you stride, each leg moves forward at the same time as the opposite arm. The stronger your core muscles are, the more efficiently those two opposite parts work together. That translates into easier long running and more powerful bursts.

They're a sign that you're really, truly in great shape. When you work out, you improve in your arms and legs first. Your abs shape up last. So, having great abs is a real accomplishment. Abs are a guy's nonverbal way of showing strength.

They help ward off hernias. More than a half-million men will undergo hernia surgery this year. Since hernias are caused by aging and weakness of the abdominal muscles, a good way to protect yourself is to tone your abs.

The ABCs of Ab Workouts

Although they're commonly lumped together as "abs," several muscles actually work in concert in your midsection. That's why you need to do several different exercises—to get to them all. The rectus abdominis is the main midsection muscle. It helps you bend forward at the waist. The external and internal obliques

PUNCH UP YOUR CRUNCHES

If normal and raised-leg crunches are too easy for you, here are a few variations.

Weighted crunch. Hold a weight plate or dumbbell across your chest and use progressively heavier weights. Don't do this if you have a history of back problems.

Throw-in-the-towel crunch. Wedge a rolled-up towel under your lower back when you do crunches. This gently curves your back, forcing your abdominal muscles to stretch a little farther at the starting position and contract to a greater degree when you crunch. Also, rest your hands comfortably under your chin as you crunch (placing your right fist inside your left hand). This trick stops you from jutting your head forward, which can cause neck pain.

help your waist twist and bend at the sides. The deepest abdominal muscle, the transversus abdominis, compresses your internal organs. Your spinal erectors straighten and stabilize your lower back.

Before you launch into an abs workout, you need to heed some wisdom. Experts offer the following advice.

Watch your back. Beginners who don't have abdominal strength typically use their back when doing crunches. That not only makes the crunch less effective but also puts strain on your back. The key is to never let your back arch. Keep your lower back pressed flat against the floor.

Mix it up. Crunches are great exercises, but it's best to also do other exercises that involve other muscles in your midsection. This provides a well-rounded workout, plus it works your muscles from different angles, which helps prevent plateaus in your progress.

Rest. You may have heard that you can never exercise your abs too much. That's not true. Your abs need as much recovery time as any other muscle. Do the exercises in today's workouts only two or three times a week.

Abs are a cinch to exercise, as you'll see by these programs designed to tone and shape them. These moves are both portable and versatile.

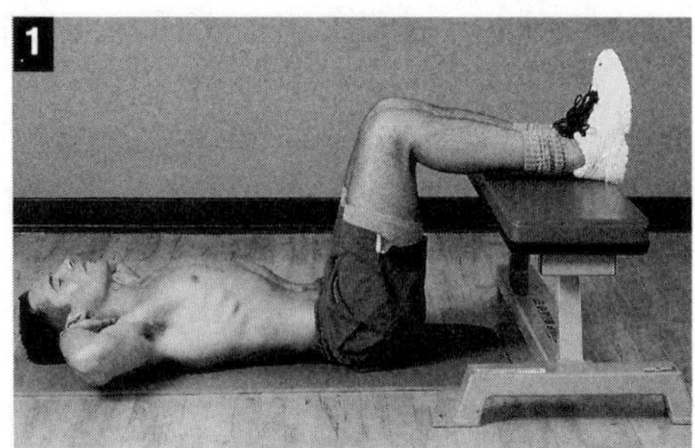

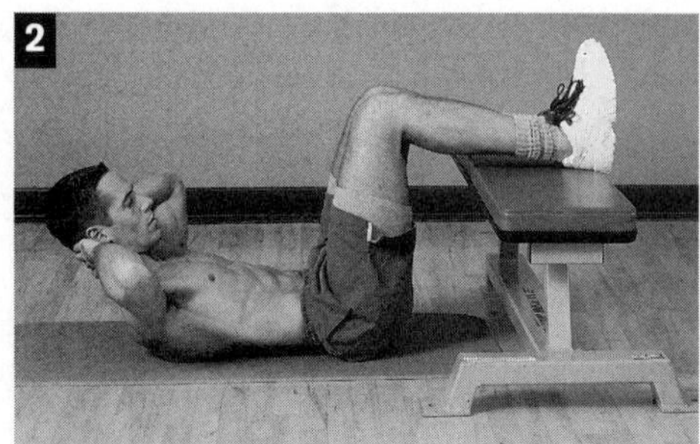

The Traditional Workout

Raised-leg crunch. (1) Lie on your back on the floor and put your lower legs up on your weight bench or a chair. Your hips should be bent at a 90-degree angle. Rest your fingertips lightly on the sides of your head and put your elbows out to the sides.

(2) Tilt your pelvis so that your lower back stays flat on the floor, then curl your upper body up so that your head and shoulders come off the floor.

Hold for a second, then lower to the starting position. Do not relax between repetitions. Do as many as you can, or multiple sets of 10 repetitions.

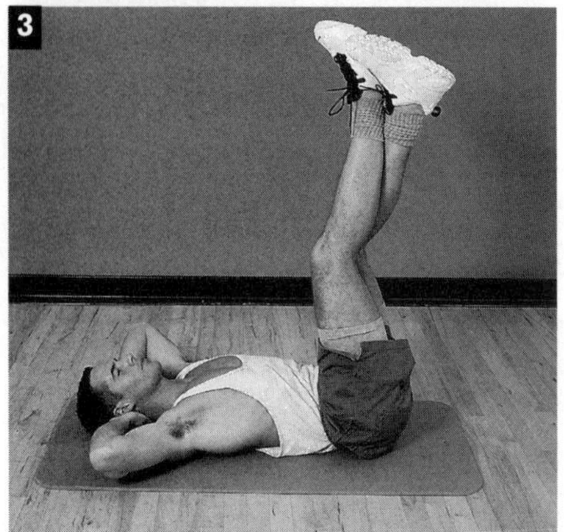

Crossover crunch. (3) Lie on your back on the floor with your legs raised straight up in the air and crossed at the ankles. Rest your fingertips lightly on the sides of your head and put your elbows out to the sides.

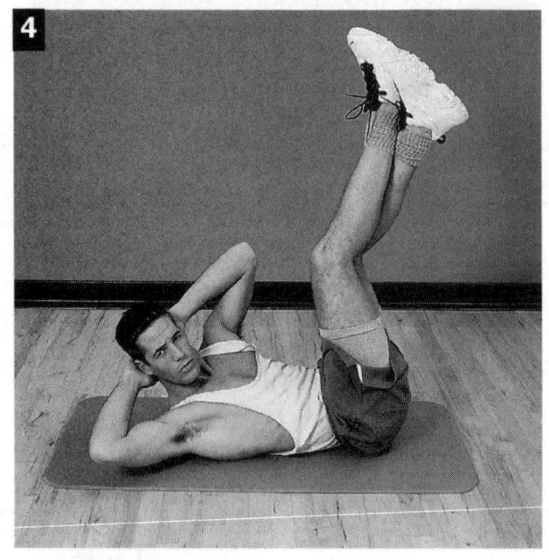

(4) Lift your left shoulder blade off the floor to crunch to your right.

Lower to the starting position, then switch sides. Do 10 to 20 repetitions on each side.

Hip raise. (5) Lie on your back on the floor with your legs raised straight up in

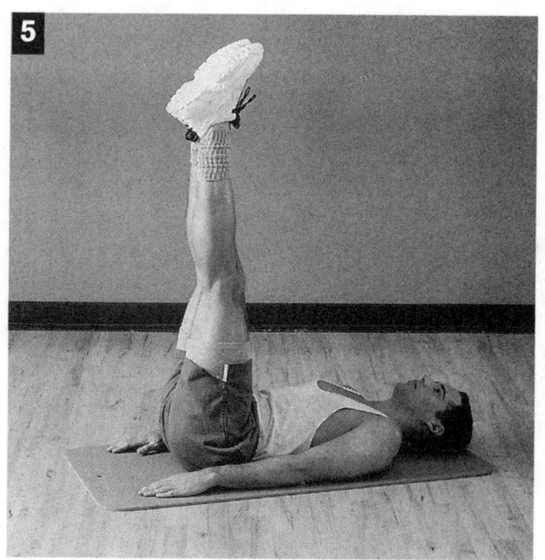

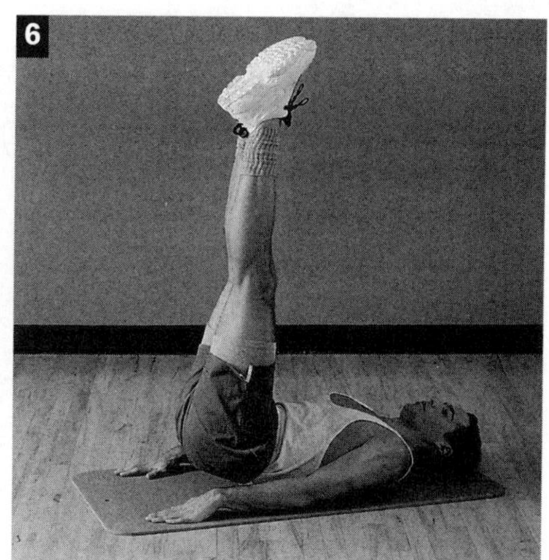

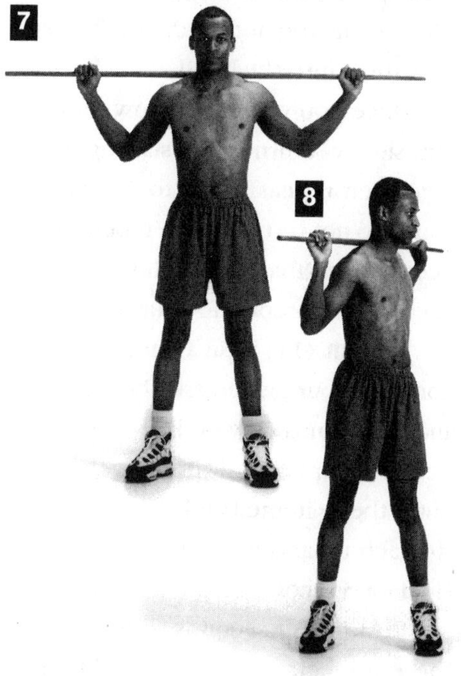

the air. Your knees should be unlocked and your toes should point toward the ceiling. Place your hands at your sides with your palms down.

(6) Using your lower abs and shifting your weight forward toward your shoulders, lift your hips off the floor. Keep your legs in a vertical position throughout the exercise.

Hold for a second, then slowly lower to the starting position. Do 10 repetitions.

Oblique twist. (7) Stand upright with your feet about shoulder-width apart, your hips facing forward, and your knees unlocked. Hold a broomstick with your palms facing forward and place it behind your neck. It should be even across your upper shoulder muscles. Your hands should grasp the ends or outer portions of the broomstick.

(8) Keeping your hips still and facing forward, twist to your left as far as you can go.

Return to the starting position. Pause for a second, then twist to your right.

Keep a slow, steady pace and concentrate on working your obliques. Do 8 to 12 repetitions.

Sidebend with dumbbells. (9) Stand upright with a dumbbell in each hand. Your arms should be fully extended at your sides, with your palms facing toward your body. Your feet should be about shoulder-width apart.

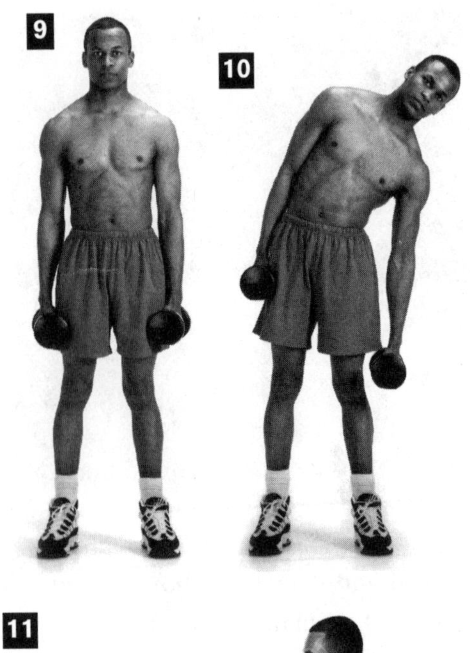

(10) Bend to your left, allowing the dumbbell in your left hand to drop down your leg until you feel your obliques working. Keep your body still and facing forward; don't turn your torso into the bend.

Once you've gone as low as you can, slowly return to the starting position, then repeat. Do 8 to 12 repetitions. Do not rest between repetitions. Keep your abs and obliques contracted. Then, repeat to your right side.

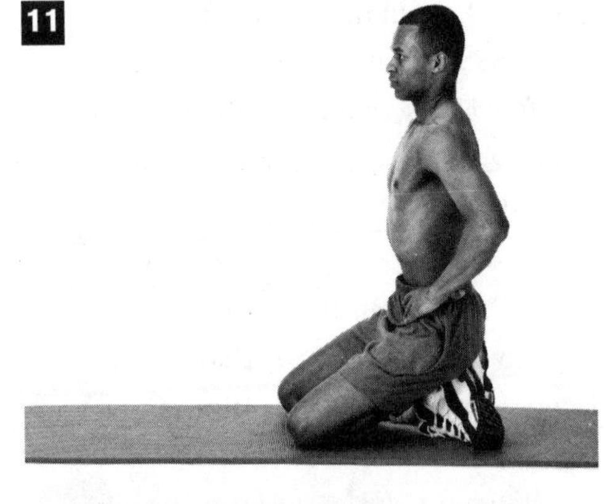

Vacuum. (11) Sit in a kneeling position with your feet crossed behind you and your hands on your hips or thighs. Keep your upper body upright. Breathe out, then immediately suck your stomach up and in as far as it will go. Hold for 5 seconds. Do 10 repetitions.

Rest for 30 seconds, then repeat the entire circuit of the traditional workout.

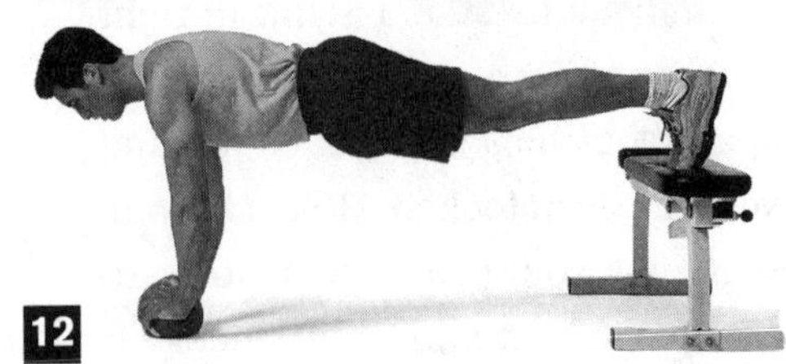

The Avant-Garde Workout

Pushup bridge. (12) Get into the pushup position with your toes resting on top of your weight bench (or a sturdy piece of bench-high furniture) and your hands on top of a football (or pillow). Make sure your body is in a straight line. Look at the floor about a foot in front of the football. Suck in your stomach and hold this position for 20 seconds. Continue breathing without relaxing your stomach muscles. After 20 seconds, rest, then repeat. Eventually, work up to two 60-second sets.

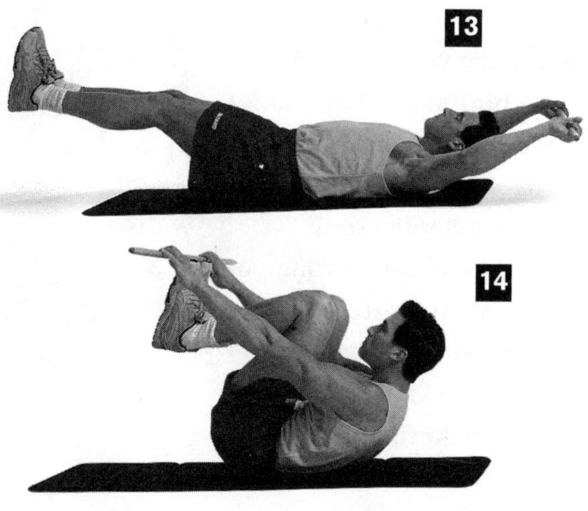

Stick crunch, part 1. (13) Lie on your back on the floor with your feet together and your legs extended and about a foot off the floor. Using both hands, hold a broomstick across your body and parallel with the floor. Raise your arms over your head until they are also about a foot off the floor.

(14) Bring your knees toward your chest and raise your shoulders off the floor. At the same time, circle your arms around, over your head and toward your feet.

Return to the staring position. Do 10 repetitions. Each workout, try to reach a little farther with the broomstick so that eventually you can touch the soles of your feet with it.

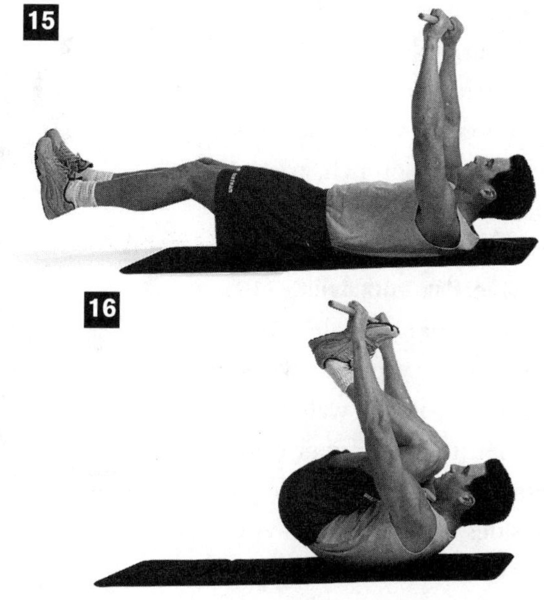

Stick crunch, part 2. (15) Lie on your back on the floor with your feet together and your legs extended and raised about a foot off the floor. Using both hands, hold the broomstick across your body and parallel with the floor. Raise your arms straight up in the air so they're perpendicular to the floor.

(See photo 16 on page 345.) Bring your knees toward your chin. At the same time, push your arms toward your feet a bit so the soles of your feet are under the stick.

Return to the starting position. Do 10 repetitions.

Bent-arm swimmer. (17) Lie on the floor on your stomach with your toes on the floor. Bend your elbows at 90-degree angles and place your hands on either side of your head. Keep your head a few inches off the floor.

(18) Lift your right leg and left arm off the floor, and look to your left at the same time.

Return to the starting position, then switch sides. Do six repetitions on each side. Rest, then do stick crunch, parts 1 and 2, followed by this exercise again. Do three sets of each.

Side flex with twist. (19) Lean on your right side against your weight bench. Wedge your feet against a wall. Cross your left foot over your right. Rest your fingertips lightly on the sides of your head and put your elbows out to the sides.

(20) Rotate your torso to the left, then return to the starting position.

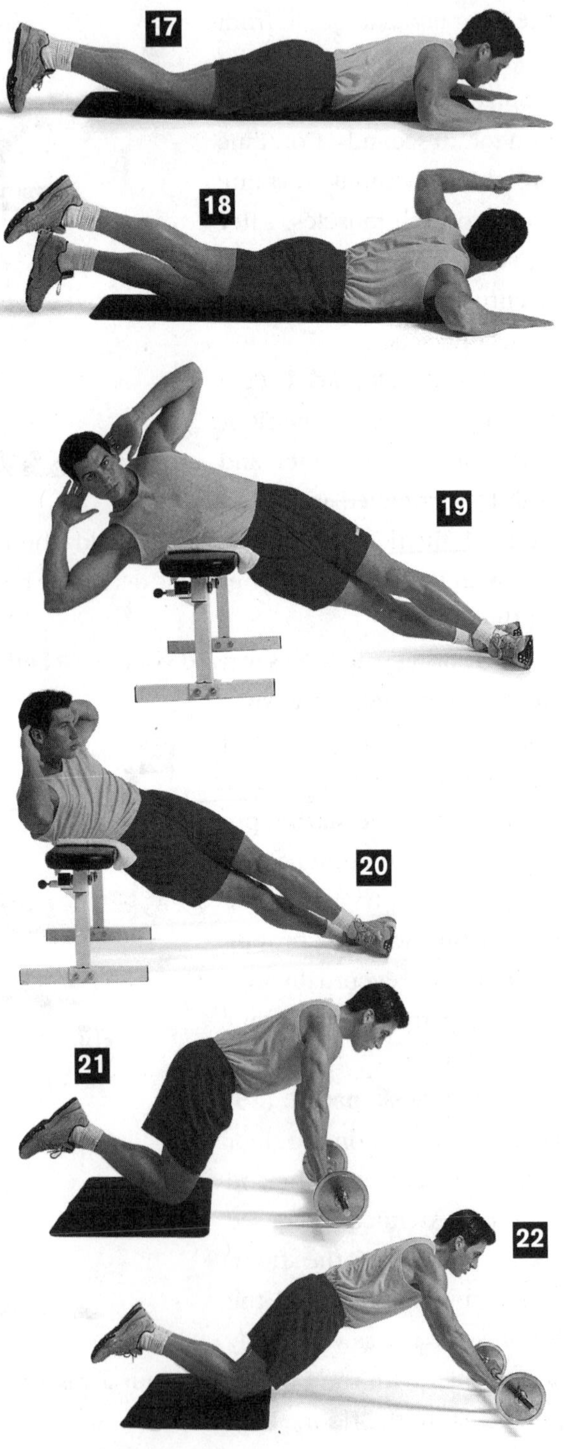
17
18
19
20
21
22

Do 15 repetitions, then switch sides. Do three sets on each side.

Barbell rollout. (21) Grab a barbell. Kneel with only your knees touching the floor. Hold on to the barbell, which should be directly under your chest. Look at the floor a few inches in front of the barbell.

(22) Roll the barbell about a foot forward.

Return to the starting position. Do five repetitions.

Rolling jackknife. (23) Get into the pushup position with a basketball under your legs, just below your knees.

(24) Bring your knees toward your hands, rolling the ball back toward your feet.

Return to the starting position. Do five repetitions, rest, then go back to the barbell rollout. Do three sets of each. In subsequent workouts, build up to 10 repetitions per set.

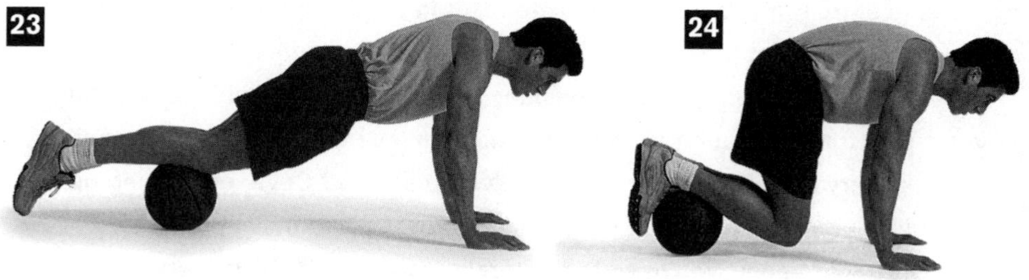

Customize Your Exercise Program

The Day's Task

Today's task requires some research time, maybe even a trip to the library or bookstore. Start at home by grabbing paper and a pencil. On the paper, list the five or so physical activities you do most often. Sports are an easy place to start. Are you on a baseball team or in a golf league or the coach of your kid's soccer team? Then, look at your aerobic routine. Do you run, bike, or swim frequently? Next, consider your work and lifestyle. Do you have a big yard that you spend a lot of time maintaining? Do you load boxes onto a truck every day? Is dancing your weekend pleasure? Cover everything up to and including frequent sex or carrying around an infant all night long.

Once that's done, you need to find a resource that will tell you what specific exercises are appropriate for your activities. We would not be doing our duty if we didn't mention our own *Men's Health Guide to Peak Conditioning*, a book we did a few years back that offers workouts for 35 different sports and lifestyle pursuits (including a complete workout for fathers). But in truth, there are plenty of good resources for weight-training programs for specific activities.

After you've found your resource, pick out three or four exercises that specifically benefit your favorite physical activity, then pick another two or three that cut across your other activities. Integrate these into the upper- and lower-body workouts that you learned earlier this week. In some cases, you might wish to substitute these for other exercises rather than augmenting our workouts.

Today's assignment is called functional fitness. It's an approach to exercise that expounds doing strength training primarily to support your real-life activities.

Underlying the theory is that it is somewhat wasteful of time and energy to build up muscles that you never otherwise use. Sure, big shoulders are impressive. But if you never use your shoulder muscles, why bother working them so hard, other than for pure vanity? Better instead to exercise the muscles that you do use frequently.

We don't completely accept this theory. Vanity is an awfully good motivator, and having a well-rounded strengthening program makes total sense. But we do believe strongly that if you spend a lot of time doing something, it is quite smart to give special attention to the muscles involved in that activity. It's hard to argue against strength training that supports and enhances your daily life.

What follows here are some ideas to get you started. But there are far too many activities for us to be thorough. So plan on digging on your own to get the exercises you need to improve your golf swing, make you a better runner, or merely prevent the onslaught of back pain.

Weekend Athletes

Injuries to hamstrings, those big muscles at the backs of your upper legs, are painful and slow to heal, as many a man discovers. To improve your odds of avoiding this most common of all sports injuries, add the following exercise to your strength-training repertoire.

Hamstring curl (1). Put a weight on your left ankle. Lie on your stomach on the floor with both legs extended. Slowly bend your left knee, moving your foot through an arc until your heel is nearly touching your butt.

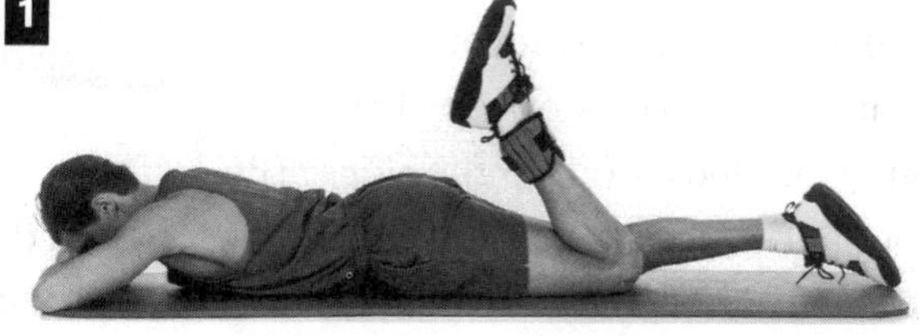

Slowly lower to the starting position. Do two sets of 15 repetitions, resting for 10 seconds in between sets. Then, repeat with your right leg.

Office Workers

Hunkering down over reports and keyboards taxes your lower back. Here's an exercise that will head off back pain. Do it in your office, if you like.

Lower-back stretch (see photo 2 on page 350). Lie on your back on the floor, then bend your legs and tuck them in toward your chest. As you do this, place your hands on the backs of your upper thighs and gently pull them closer to your chest. Hold for 30 seconds. Keep breathing throughout.

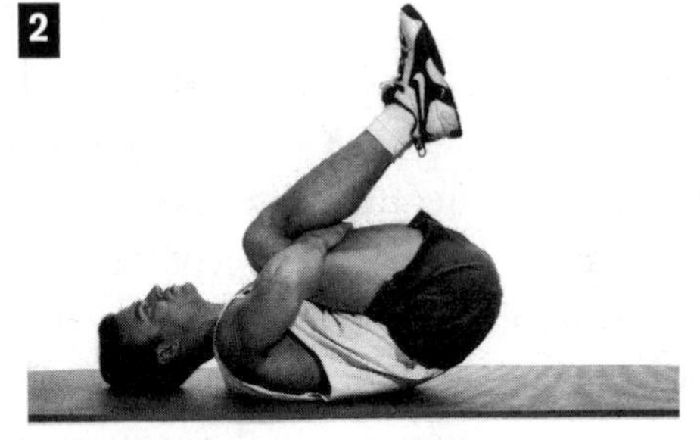

Lead Bellies

When men put on weight, more often than not it's in their guts. Think of Babe Ruth, whose physique was once described as resembling an egg supported by two straws. Or picture George Foreman or Santa.

You can't target fat in any one part of your body and spot reduce by exercising specific muscles in that area. It doesn't work. But crunches are worth doing because they firm up the muscles underneath whatever fat is encircling your belly, making you look better and feel better. They also help support your back and lessen your chances of back injury. Here is a particularly good crunch variation.

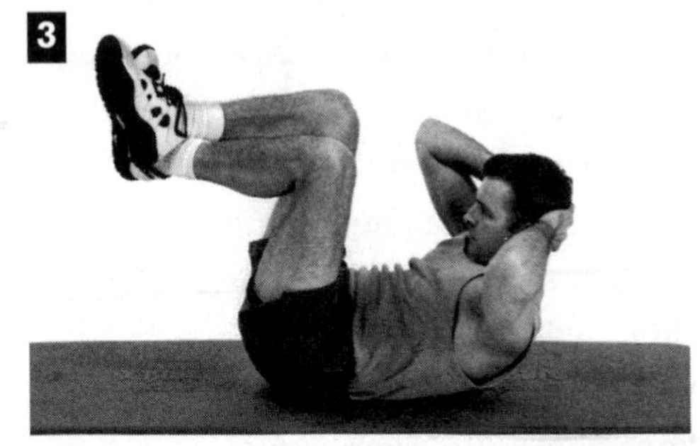

Reverse curl (3). Lie on your back on the floor with your thighs raised perpendicular to the floor and your feet off the ground, hanging loosely by your butt. Your hips should be bent at a 90-degree angle. Rest your fingertips lightly on the sides of your head and put your elbows out to the sides. Tilt your pelvis so that your lower back stays flat on the floor, then curl your body up so that your head and shoulders come off the floor as they would in an ordinary crunch; but also bring your knees toward your chest. Hold for a second, then lower to the starting position. Do not relax between repetitions. Do as many as you can, or multiple sets of 10 repetitions.

To make the exercise more difficult, cross your ankles so that your knees are 1 to 2 feet apart.

Sportsmen

Here are strengthening exercises that are perfect for a dozen popular sports. We provide the common exercise name; if you don't know how to do it, most any fitness Web site or book will be able to provide instructions.

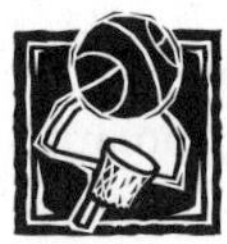

Basketball

You need strong leg muscles for running and jumping strength, plus powerful arms to wrest rebounds away from opponents.

Squat. For leg and hip thrust

Leg curl with ankle weights. To strengthen hamstrings

Narrow-grip bench press. For upper-body thrust

Romanian deadlift. For back extension

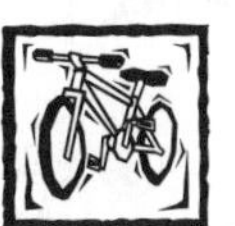

Bicycling

As you would expect, you need strong leg muscles for bicycling, plus some upper-body power to stabilize yourself in the saddle (remember: roughly half of your weight is supported by your arms when you ride).

Seated toe raise and leg curl. To strengthen calf and hamstring muscles

Deadlift. To keep your lower back from hurting

Wrist raise. To give you upper-body strength to keep you as steady as a cowboy in the saddle

Bowling

Overall strength, especially powerful arms and shoulders, can improve your lane prowess.

Alternating dumbbell curls and wrist rollers. For more power throughout your arms

Dumbbell military press. To strengthen shoulders

Lat pulldown. To develop your upper back and provide balanced strength

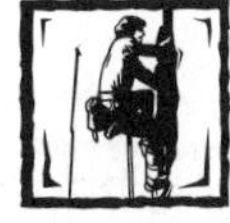

Climbing

This sport requires good overall body strength. You have to be able to pull, push, twist, shove off with your legs, brace yourself, and maintain balance.

Parallel dip. For building triceps strength

Barbell curl. To bolster biceps

Seated row. To strengthen your back

Leg extension. To work your quadriceps

Leg curl. For building your hamstrings

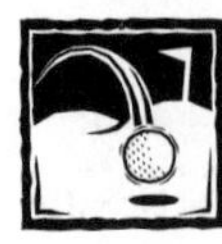

Golf

Powerful legs and shoulders improve your swing, well-developed obliques help you twist your trunk and support your back, and strong forearms and wrists give you greater club control and more accurate shots.

Dumbbell lunge. For hip and leg thrust

Oblique trunk rotation. For strong torso rotation

Upright row. For shoulder development to help you drive the ball farther

Crunch. For a stronger abdomen

Forearm curl. For strong forearms

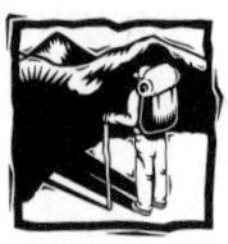

Hiking

Your legs and upper back are most apt to tire if you're carrying a backpack.

Wide-grip row. To work back muscles, rear deltoids in your shoulders, hamstrings, and gluteal muscles

Leg extension. To develop your quadriceps

Leg curl. To develop your hamstrings

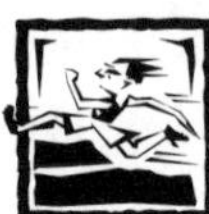

Running

If you do distance running, you need leg muscles that can contract repeatedly over prolonged periods, plus arms, shoulders, and an upper back that won't tire or cramp before you finish.

Lat-machine pulldown. For strengthening your upper back

Stiff-legged deadlift. For your lower back

Bench press. To work your chest and triceps

Barbell curl. To develop your biceps

Sex

You're more apt to be a star performer in this favorite indoor sport if you have a strong chest, arms, and abdominal muscles.

Bench press and pushup. The combonation of these two exercises provides chest power that enables you to support your arms and shoulder muscles, which are especially important in the missionary position

Crunch. Do a variety to work your abdominals and obliques

Soccer

Obviously, you need tremendous leg muscles to excel at soccer, but you also need some upper-body strength.

Squat. For leg and hip thrust

Leg curl with ankle weights. To prevent hamstring injury

Romanian deadlift. For back extension

Military press. For upper-body thrust

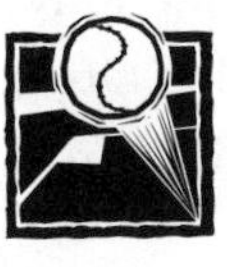

Softball and Baseball

Even a leisurely game of softball requires you to have strong legs for running and powerful forearms and shoulders in order to slam like a slugger.

Bent-over or side lateral raise. For strengthening shoulders

Forearm curl. For stronger forearms

Calf or heel raise. To build up calves

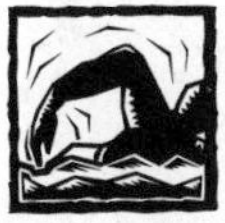

Swimming

You have to work your fins if you want to swim like the fishies. It takes overall body strength in addition to proper technique to excel as a swimmer.

Inclined bench press. For shoulders

Upright row. To build shoulders

Crunch. Do various forms to hit all your abdominals

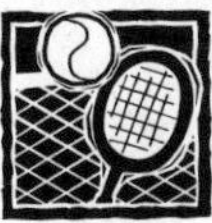

Tennis

If you are to be an ace on the tennis court, it's essential to have strong legs for sudden starts and stops while changing direction, in addition to upper-body strength, especially in your shoulders and forearms.

Squat, lunge, leg extension, and leg curl. To strengthen your quadriceps, hamstrings, and glutes

Barbell curl. For building biceps

Forearm curl. For working your wrists and forearms

Rock of Ages

This book is all about how to have a body and mind at age 50 that you would have been proud of at age 20. That doesn't mean you'll look like a 20-year-old. It means you'll look good and respectably fit. Your fitness needs change as you age. Slowly, inexorably, muscle, bone, and skin break down. This Longevity Program is about ways to fight and, in some cases, overcome that breakdown. Here are some guidelines for customizing your workout decade by decade.

Your twenties. If you're already in pretty good shape, cram your aerobic requirements into a short, very intense session in which you work at 80 to 85 percent of your maximum heart rate, as opposed to the more customary 60 to 70 percent. Keep your body strong and in prime aerobic condition, and it can handle a great (and fun) variety of physical demands. Good exercises for active twentysomethings are the hamstring curls mentioned earlier, straight-leg raises, and shoulder rotations. These help protect your knees and shoulders from injury.

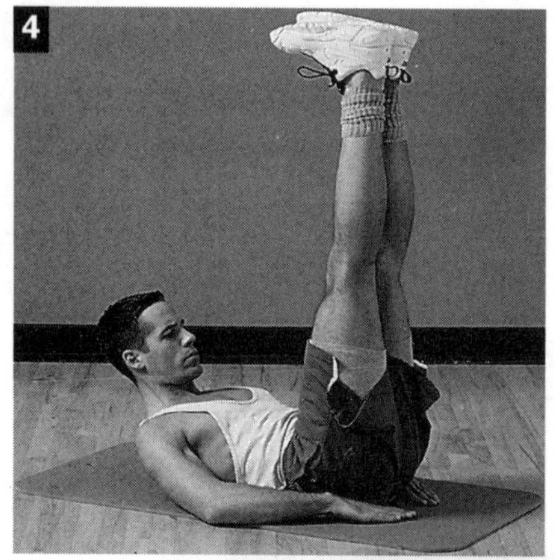

- *Straight-leg raise (4).* Lie on your back on the floor with your hands under your hips, palms down. Press your lower back to the floor. Hold your head up, bringing your chin to your chest, with your shoulder blades off the floor. Extend your legs, knees unlocked and feet flexed, keeping your heels about an inch off the floor.

  Raise your legs until they are perpendicular to your body—or at least as perpendicular as you can get them. Slowly lower them to the starting position to a count of two, keeping control of the downward motion. Do three sets of 10 repetitions, resting for 15 to 30 seconds between sets.

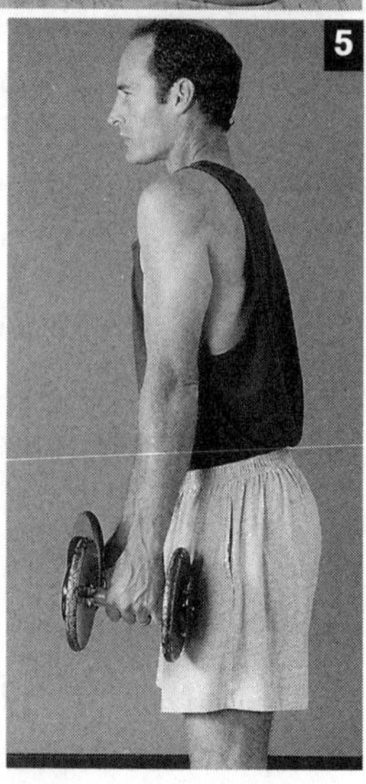

- *Shoulder rotation (5).* Stand upright with a dumbbell in each hand. Your arms should be fully extended at your sides, with your palms facing toward your body. Make sure your shoulders are back and relaxed. Your feet should be about hip-width apart.

  Keeping your head and neck relaxed, slowly shrug your shoulders as high as they will go. In a smooth, flowing motion, rotate your shoulders forward, down, of this circling movement in this direction, then repeat in the opposite direction.

Your thirties. You begin to experience dips in muscle mass, strength, aerobic capacity, and metabolism. Your overall physiological function drops by about 1 percent a year. You'll feel and function better, however, if you stay active. But lighten up and mix it up just a little bit. For instance, if you run 3 days a week, consider replacing 1 day with stairclimbing, biking, or swimming. Reconsider playing aggressive contact sports like football and soccer unless you've already been playing them on a regular basis. This is also a decade in which you begin losing flexibility. Pick up a book on stretching and add stretches for your neck, back, hamstrings, and calves.

Your forties. It's a rare man in his forties who doesn't have to battle the bulge. Your metabolism slows and, if you haven't been systematically working out your muscles, muscle tissue starts to waste away. Both conditions make it easy for you to amass fat and make it harder to lose. Too many men give up. You won't. Heed the following instructions, and you'll burn off extra flab: Start a circuit-training regimen. Lighten the weight for each of your weight-training exercises just enough so that you can increase the repetitions to 15 to 20. Instead of doing multiple sets, proceed immediately to the next station, resting for only about 15 seconds between exercises. Finally, add a second set of crunches to your routine.

Your fifties and up. More than ever, you need to establish and maintain a steady full-body program of weight lifting exercises to keep your bones and muscles from deteriorating. We don't have any special exercises to suggest. But we will suggest modifying some of the tougher exercises in the routines we've previously suggested by shortening the lifts and lowering the weights to guard against injury. You may be young at heart, but your body needs more time to regain the fitness and flexibility levels of years past.

10 Ways to Prevent Foot Pain

1 **Ease your way into new aerobic exercise routines.** Many cases of foot pain occur when you start walking or jogging too far, too soon. We applaud your active lifestyle but remind you to go slowly at first. Likewise, if you've been at it a while, don't notch up the heat too quickly. Add on only a few extra miles each week.

2 **Use your whole foot while on the go.** A surefire way to beat your feet into the dust is to land too far on the insides or outsides of them when you're walking or jogging. This habit can develop for a number of reasons (even a hangnail can cause you to shift your weight as you walk). Check the bottoms of your shoes to see if there's more wear on one side or the other. If there is, pay attention to your stride and consciously correct it until it becomes automatic.

3 **Shop for shoes in the afternoon.** When you buy new shoes, get them in the afternoon when your feet are most swollen, says Douglas Hale, D.P.M., a podiatrist at the Foot and Ankle Center in Seattle. If you pick your shoes early in the day, you may end up with a pair that are too small for your ballooning afternoon feet.

4 **Keep your shoes on at home.** If you're in the habit of shedding your shoes as soon as you walk in the door, you're doing your feet a disservice. Keep your supportive footwear on in the house too.

5 **Stretch your feet each morning.** There are two things that cause most foot pain: plantar fasciitis and fallen arches. Of the two, plantar fasciitis is the more likely. It's an inflammation of the tissue on the underside of your foot. That's why you get shooting pains when you step on your foot, especially in the morning.

Before you get out of bed, stretch and massage your feet, says Marjorie Menacker, D.P.M., a podiatrist with Chesterfield Podiatry Associates in Midlothian, Virginia. While lying on your back, move your feet up and down so that you feel the stretch in your calves. Next, put the heel of one foot under the toes of the other and pull your toes backward with your heel. Hold each stretch for 10 seconds, and repeat each 10 times. Finish off with a foot rub to warm up the tissues.

6 **Determine your foot shape and buy a shoe insert that fits.** Inserts, or orthotics, are available at medical supply shops and pharmacies. To find out

what kind of orthotic you need, step in some water and then on a piece of paper. This should give you a good look at your footprint. If you can see a full footprint, you have flat feet, says Dr. Menacker. If the print has two distinct areas at the toes and heels but no print in the middle, you have a high arch. If the print shows a whole foot with an indent in the area of your arch, you have a moderate arch.

Knowing the shape of your foot will help you choose an orthotic. Also, it's a good piece of information to give to shoe salesmen, who should steer you to the right type of shoe and the proper lacing technique for your foot shape.

7 **Choose the correct firmness when buying an insert.** For a fallen arch, you want firm arch support. If you have plantar fasciitis, look for more a cushiony one, says Richard Braver, D.P.M., a podiatrist and head of the Active Foot and Ankle Care Centers in Englewood and Fair Lawn, New Jersey.

You might need to trim the orthotic down to size. Stand on it to see if the arch in the orthotic matches the arch in your foot. Make sure, too, that your shoe is deep enough to withstand the extra height of the orthotic. If it presses the top of your foot too hard against your shoe, you'll get blisters.

8 **During foot-pain flare-ups, put some ice on your feet for 15 to 20 minutes at a time.** Do this once or twice a day, says Dr. Menacker. Continue for 2 to 3 days in a row to minimize inflammation. Wrap the ice in a dish towel so it doesn't come in direct contact with your feet. Or you can freeze water in a small paper cup and peel off the top edge so the ice sticks out. Massage this in circles over the painful area for 10 minutes. If your foot pain doesn't get better within a couple of weeks, go see a foot doctor. Likewise, if your feet are bruised or if the pain is in your Achilles tendon above your heel, get checked by a doc.

9 **Change exercises so your feet get a break.** If you're a runner experiencing feet problems, switch your mode of exercise to a stationary bike until your feet settle down. Or start swimming instead. Give it a few weeks, then try running a little bit at a time to see if your feet can take it.

10 **Protect your Achilles tendon.** A tight Achilles can force the muscles and tendons under your foot to work too hard, causing pain. To stretch them out, find a wall and stand an arm's length away with your toes pointed toward it. Put your palms against the wall with your arms straight, then slowly bend your elbows to allow yourself to lean against the wall. Keep your feet planted, your heels on the floor. You'll feel the stretch down the backs of your legs.

WEEK 11

REDISCOVER YOUR SENSE OF PURPOSE

Day 1

Put Your Job in Perspective

Day 2

Reconnect with Your Family

Day 3

Remember Who You Were

Day 4

Spend a Few Hours in Nature

Day 5

Acknowledge a Higher Force

Day 6

Buy Into Manhood

Put Your Job in Perspective

The Day's Task

This afternoon, sometime after lunch, stop what you're doing. Roll your chair back from your desk. Or step back from your workstation. Or move away from the deep fryer. You get the idea. Then take a short walk around your place of employment.

Look closely at your coworkers. Watch how intent they are on the tasks at hand. See them scurry to and fro as they rush to get whatever they're doing done. Notice their furrowed brows, their wrung hands, their general sense of being swept along in a workplace wave that carries away anybody who gets caught in it.

It's strange, isn't it?

Back in Week 4, we asked you to take an inventory of the home artifacts you keep in your office and the office work you have lying about at home. The point in that task was to gauge whether too much work was stressing you out and taking over your life.

The message of today's task is in some ways the same. But we want you to go one level deeper and consider not just the short-term implications of your job on your health and time but also the deeper implications of how you let work define who you are. We want you to make a subtle shift in the way you view your job, to step outside it and observe it from a distance.

That's not as easy as it sounds. For a long time, men have been conditioned to identify who they are with what they do. Work is usually the first thing we inquire about when we meet another man. "So what do you do?" You've been asked that plenty of times, we bet.

We take our work way too seriously sometimes, forgetting that we are much more than our job descriptions. When that happens, we turn into those coworkers you're looking at: head down, convinced that the future of the universe hinges on meeting that deadline, invoicing that client, or salting those fries.

That's not to minimize the importance of doing a job well. Few satisfactions rival that of feeling good about a project you've knocked out of the ballpark. But don't get so wrapped up in work that you end up stressed all the time. In a 3-year study of 195 men, reducing work stress lowered blood pressure by 10 points in men with hypertension and 5 points in men without hypertension. Those are the kind of results that come from putting your job in perspective.

To do otherwise is just plain unhealthy. A Japanese study found that men who worked more than 11 hours per day were 2½ times more likely to suffer heart attacks than those who worked 7 to 9 hours. Hey, maybe you have a great job, but is it worth dying over?

Life outside Work

When you remember that there are meaningful matters other than work, interesting things begin to happen.

- Mental energy gets freed up for people instead of for tasks.
- You become more involved with your family. "This doesn't mean that the career isn't important," says Fred E. Stickle, Ph.D., coordinator of counseling programs at Western Kentucky University in Bowling Green. "We're just realizing that it's helpful to hinge some of our self-esteem on a healthy family life."
- And you're not the only one who stands to benefit. Study after study has shown the incredible benefits of a man being involved with his family. Your kids do better all-around. Your wife is happier. And you're happier.

There's another good reason to keep your emotional distance from your job: it makes it easier on you if you get fired. Even in boom times, men get laid off or shunted aside. We said this back in Week 4, but it bears repeating: a job is not a personal thing; it's an impartial business contract that can be canceled at any time, by either side. When you keep your perspective about work, if you and your employer part company, it doesn't feel like a reflection on you as a human being. With that kind of attitude, you'll find smoother sailing as you look for another job.

When you retire, what's going to be important as you look back over the previous 40 years? Is it going to be all the time you spent at work? Will it be the worries you felt as things heated up on the job? Will you recall the vacation time you sacrificed to make sure a project was done just right? Or will you remember the walks in the forest with your kids, the time spent fishing with your dad, the riotous road trip with friends?

A job is a big deal; we realize that. It puts bread on the table and shingles on the roof. But always remember that when the day is done and the clock is punched, it's time to give your full attention to all those things that you're working for, including yourself.

Reconnect with Your Family

The Day's Task

Dig out your camcorder and recharge the batteries. If you don't have a camcorder, borrow one. You really want to get this task down on video.

Next, call your parents and set up an evening with them. Plan to spend at least 2 to 3 uninterrupted hours together. Between now and, set aside an hour or two for yourself. Get out a pad and a pen. You're about to play cub reporter and gather the most important story of your life. You're about to interview your parents.

The key to a good interview is to draw on prepared questions without being afraid to stray from the script if things take an unexpected turn. When one vein of conversation runs out, refer to the next question. In this chapter, we'll give you some questions to get you started.

The reason for the recording device is important: your folks won't be around forever. A video or audio recording is a perfect way to preserve them. You'll be able to sit back and watch the interview whenever you want to spend a few minutes in your parents' company. A recording is also a great way to show your own family—and those still to come—who your parents were, who you are, and, by extension, who they are.

No matter how strong or weak your relationship is, this will only make it better. Trust us, they will be, thoroughly honored and grateful to do this. In fact, consider doing this over 2 nights, one for mom and one for dad.

You know something? You come from somewhere. Stretching back through your parents and on into the dim mists of your family's history, there's a whole line of people who look, act, and think a whole lot like you. This is no small thing.

Whether or not we want to face up to it, each of us is more like his family than he cares to admit. Early in our adult lives, we rebel against this.

Often, when we leave our parents' homes to start our own lives, we can't get far enough away. We set up shop in new towns, make new friends, get our own lives. We get married and have kids, and all of a sudden, our new families (our immediate families, plus our wives' extended relations) fight for the same mental space once filled solely by our parents and siblings.

For lots of people, contact with family gets reduced to occasional phone calls and rushed visits on the holidays. This is regrettable. No matter how much we try to deny it, we are strongly shaped by the families from which we came. If we lose them, we lose ourselves too.

So the purpose of today's task is to reintroduce you to you, via your parents. You'll learn a ton from these people who know you best, who have been watching you from the day you were born.

The very process of doing this will help you in unexpected ways. Researchers have found that sharing stories is not only interesting and gratifying but also emotionally and physically healing. In a one study, people listened to someone recall a meaningful life experience, describe a trip to the store, or read a rule from the building code. For both the speakers and listeners, heart rates and blood pressures were lowest during the life reminiscences.

These physical benefits are short-term. The long-term benefit of reconnecting with your parents, one that is hard to quantify yet impossible to deny, is a sense of belonging and purpose in your life. You have a rich, tangled family history that is uniquely yours. You are part of something bigger, linked together by genetic code and family rituals and shared values and 10,000 shared stories and legends. No matter how stormy life gets, you always have one undeniable anchor: your family. Always keep a thick rope tied to it, and don't let that rope unfurl so far that the anchor no longer provides stability.

A Branch on the Family Tree

You're one of the newest players in a long family history. How do you look back from your vantage point and figure out where you come from? This will depend a lot on how well you conduct your interview. Here are some suggestions of what questions to ask your parents. Feel free to modify the list, make deletions, and add other questions. It is, after all, your family.

- What were my grandparents' full names?
- Where were they born and where did they grow up?

WHAT WE LEARNED FROM YOUR OLD MAN

In 1999, Joe Kita, executive writer for *Men's Health* magazine, published a book called *Wisdom of Our Fathers*. In it, he asked 138 wise old men the questions that he had always wanted to ask his own father. Here's a smattering of the things they told him.

On Work

- "You don't have to be smart to be honest. But you have to be smart to be crooked."
- "Don't take a solid week off from work. The days will rush together, and before you know it, it'll be gone. Instead, take half-days. It'll feel like you cheated and didn't get caught."

On Being a Dad

- "There are two qualities you should look for in your children: a sense of humor and whether they hang in there with a problem. If you see these two things, you needn't worry. They'll turn out okay."

- What are some of your personal memories of them?
- Did they ever tell you about their parents?
- What traditions did they practice that we may have forgotten?
- Where did you fit in birth order among your siblings?
- What were your family duties as children?
- How did you spend holidays and vacations?
- How did you celebrate your birthday?
- Did your family entertain often? Who visited?
- Do you remember any blizzards, floods, tornadoes?
- Who were your playmates and best friend?
- How did you two meet?
- Why did you get married?
- What was it like when your children were born?
- Whom did you admire most when you were young?
- What did you want to be when you grew up?
- What were your dreams? Did you live them?

- "Consider your son to be your apprentice in life. That's the way it used to be. The son was always with the father, either in the shop or in the field. So he learned from an early age what being a man and a father was all about."

On Beating Stress

- "If you can forgive the first guy who messes with you each day, then the second guy is easier."
- "When you're in traffic, let the other guy in ahead of you."

On Loving Women

- "If you find you are not feeling in love anymore, be more loving."
- "Two of the main traits that beautiful women are attracted to in men are power and self-confidence. If you're intimidated by a woman's good looks, she assumes that you're going to be intimidated by the world in general."

- Do you have a philosophy that you'd like to share with your descendants?
- What things in life have given you the most satisfaction or pleasure?
- What has been the greatest advance or invention during your lifetime?
- What do you consider to be your most important achievement and failure?

As you can see, you're going to be going into heavily charged areas as well as more straightforward ones. You may feel odd asking your parents some of these questions. But remember that almost all parents would love to pass down to their children what they know and believe. They'll feel honored when you ask. And you'll develop a whole new appreciation of who they are.

Remember Who You Were

The Day's Task

Maybe you're lucky. Maybe you know exactly where your photo albums are. But you're probably like us—you have photos scattered in a number of drawers, laundry hampers, and bread bags.

Where ever your photos are stored, go get them. Round them all up, concentrating on finding some from each period in your life. Look for baby pictures. Look for the goofy school pictures where the hack photographers always caught you blinking. Look for high school, college, military, wedding, and vacation photos. Try to build a timeline of photos, from your birth to now.

Fix yourself a mug of coffee and fetch a pad of notepaper and a pen. Mark down the various memories that come to mind as you peruse the photos. What were you doing in 1975? Who were you with? What were your plans? For each picture, jot down a quick paragraph listing everything you can remember about that time in your life.

Photographs are incredible things. Although they catch only about $\frac{1}{60}$ of a second in time, the image they capture represents a whole period in your life. With one look at a photo, you can quickly remember what was going on in your life at that moment, what your demons were, what your dreams were, and who you were struggling to be.

But somehow, in the intervening years between then and now, a lot of things got sidetracked. Your hopes of making your mark on this chaotic world got transformed into keeping the lawn cut and the bills paid.

A faint sense of unease strikes mostly late at night when you're lying in bed, trying to sleep. The big questions start: "Did I make the right choice? Is this what I want to be doing? Why do I feel like this?"

Those aren't just good questions, friend; those are essential ones. Those are the ones we want you to ask yourself as you browse through your photos.

Reclaiming Your Youth

It seems like the trappings of youth tend to be forgotten over time. "As we get older, we assume more responsibility," says Glenn E. Good, associate professor of educational and counseling psychology at the University of Missouri at Columbia. Responsibility is a useful and necessary part of life. "We can't all be racing our cars around, half-drunk. Somebody has to stop at the red lights."

That somebody is you. But while you've had to shoulder your share of responsibilities, no way does that mean you have to give up on the things that meant something to you. Quite the opposite, says Bob Beck, associate director of the Baylor Psychiatry Clinic at Baylor College of Medicine in Houston. He suggests spending a few minutes dwelling on your wedding photos and pictures of you and your wife in your early dating days. Those photos are superb reminders of the hopes you had for the future as well as the emotionally powerful times you two spent together. Look over the old plans and wishes that you remembered and wrote down while looking at your photos, and decide which of them still really matter. There may be nothing scarier than looking back on the past and realizing that you never really did what you wanted to do.

Whether your dream is starting a band or opening a bait shop, accomplishing a life goal—living on your own terms—can spell the difference between contentment and regret. But too few of us make such choices consciously. "You can't have it all," says Herb Goldberg, Ph.D., a Los Angeles psychologist and author of *What Men Really Want*. "If you want the mainstream life—money, house, nice car, wife, and children—you can't also have the excitement of freedom."

That's not to say that freedom can't have various faces. We are definitely not advocating that you run off with a comely aerobics instructor. You first need to change your perspective. Instead of focusing on *what* you have done or haven't done, take a look at *how* you lived your life. Looking back on a life lived with integrity is enormously satisfying.

Each person is made unique by the thousands of unique events he has experienced. You are the sum total of all the events that these photos document, and more. So look through your photos with pride. Notice the smiles, the fun, the adventures, the love of family and friends, the places visited, the achievements documented. Admit that life, your life, is good. Or certainly, admit that it's as good as you have allowed it to be.

Once you've made that admission, think deeply to find a way to fulfill the dreams from years past that still mean something to you. Important qualities that

MEMORIES FOR A LIFETIME

If you've ever peeled apart stuck-together photos, you've probably wondered how you can protect your pictures over the long haul. The first thing you need to do is, like a good field medic, triage your photos. Put them into one of the following three categories: (1) nonessential (you couldn't care less about them); (2) nonarchival (you don't want to see 'em wrecked, but they aren't going to be family heirlooms); (3) archival (you want to pass these puppies down to your great-grandkids).

Category 1. Chuck them into a box

Category 2. Separate these photos and display them individually in proper albums. Forget about buying those crappy photo albums at the drugstore. The adhesive and plastic covers will eat your photos alive over time. Find a good quality, acid-free album at a photo supply store. Look on the label for some indication that the album has passed the Photographic Activity Test (PAT). That ensures that the materials in the album won't react with the chemicals in the prints.

Category 3. Store these photos in albums with rag-type mats. They'll cost about twice as much as the acid-free ones, but it's worth it for heirloom photos. Store the albums somewhere cool and dry (around 68°F and 30 to 40 percent relative humidity). A closet might be good. Don't store them in the attic or basement, where the moisture will speed up deterioration. Don't let them be exposed to the solvent fumes in things like paint, cleaning supplies, or stored plywood. Otherwise, your future generations will look on you as one funny-looking guy—or they may not have anything to remember you by at all.

you've developed since those early years are discipline and the ability to see what needs to be done.

If you always wanted to fly, head out this weekend for an introductory flight. If you always wanted to trek across Morocco, start researching what it takes to do that. If you always wanted to write a book, commit just one paragraph to paper every evening. Just get started. The rest will take care of itself.

Spend a Few Hours in Nature

The Day's Task

At lunchtime today, get your brown bag and go outside. Find a park, a patch of green, a walking trail, whatever semblance of nature you can root out. Eat there.

While you're chowing down on a nice healthy lunch, start pondering. Figure out where you can go to really get away from it all for at least a few hours. Is there someplace within driving, hiking, or biking distance where you can sit back, cock an ear, and not hear a single man-made sound?

Sit back and enjoy the day around you. Then make plans to get to your nature spot this weekend.

We're being kind of devious about the lunch thing. Sure, we want you to get a quick taste of nature while you plan for a bigger outing. But we also want you to get away from your desk. French researchers found that when you eat in stressful situations—and work qualifies as one of them—you subject yourself to a dangerous spike in cholesterol levels.

"Stress slows the rate at which fats are broken down, causing them to stay in the bloodstream longer," says Jean Dallongeville, M.D., the lead researcher of that study. Since these fluctuations can increase your risk of heart disease, having lunch with Mother Nature seems like a really good idea, don't you think?

Men and nature have a long, long history together, vestiges of which remain even in the urban world we live in today. Here's a case in point: In 1998, a woman wrote to Dear Abby complaining about the fact that her husband continually urinated in their backyard. He was over 50, college-educated, a successful businessman, and a resident of a nice neighborhood. Yet, like most men, he felt a primal urge to be near nature.

This one letter touched off a firestorm, with many women writing in to sympathize with the original complainant. Men wrote, too, defending their need to pee freely. One man even pointed out the environmental benefits—by avoiding one flush a day, a single man could conserve 1,000 gallons of water per year. According to this gentleman, if one-fourth of the men in the United States joined him, we'd save more than 4.5 billion cubic feet of water annually.

Whether it's territory marking or a simple need to cast off our societal constraints in some small way, outdoor whizzing proves that men and nature go together like urine and brown grass. We need to be free from concrete, shopping malls, and suits and ties on a regular basis.

How Nature Preserves

Natural environments have a remarkable way of firing up your zest for life and heightening your senses. This fact has even led to a branch of psychology called ecopsychology. "Being in nature—in a forest, at the beach, or just near the ocean—can have a pronounced effect," says Joel Robertson, Pharm.D., head of the Robertson Institute in Saginaw, Michigan, and author of *Natural Prozac*.

You know the feeling. It's when your worries and cares wash away with the outgoing tide, when your thoughts slow down but your sense of purpose seems clearer.

Your whole way of approaching the world changes. In one year-long study, researchers found that urban residents who lived near trees and grass found more productive ways to resolve family arguments and were less likely to be involved in violent disputes than were folks surrounded by concrete and asphalt. Unnatural environments contribute to mental fatigue, which understandably makes people irritable and more likely to fly off the handle.

There are other benefits to heading back to nature. Take sunlight. For those who are brought low by gloomy winter months and weeks of incessant rain, sunlight acts to lift the low-grade depression that can happen in those cases.

Going out of doors can also help you lose some extra flab. Studies show that exercising outside makes you subconsciously step up your tempo. You work harder without feeling it. "When you're inside, you tend to focus on your breathing and how miserable you may be feeling. But outside, you can ignore your body's reaction because you're distracted by your surroundings," explains John

Porcari, Ph.D., professor in the department of exercise and sports science at the University of Wisconsin in La Crosse. Whether you walk or jog, the end result will be a slimmer you.

Beyond the physical and emotional benefits, there's one other important reason for you to go someplace where the earth rises up to meet you: the spiritual benefit. Most Native American nations—and there are more than 550 tribal groups in North America—teach that everything on the planet has a spirit. According to this belief, you're not just part of everything that surrounds you, you're kin to it.

That's a feeling that you understand when you stand below the darkened sky, hearing nothing but the sounds of the forest and thinking that you're truly in a place that feels like home.

Acknowledge a Higher Force

Week 11 • Day 5

The Day's Task

Tonight is going to be a particularly special night. You're going to do something that you probably haven't done since you were a kid. Wait until the sun goes down and the stars come out in full force. Bundle yourself up if it's a chilly night, because you're going to be outside for a while. Find yourself a patch of good old solid ground. Lie on it.

With the earth at your back and the universe in your face, let yourself stare upward. Try to fathom the incredible distances you're looking at. Let the enormity of the universe settle in. Imagine the unimaginable. How did this happen? What kind of force brought this endless beauty into being?

Sit with these thoughts for a bit. Let them stretch your brain, trickle into your soul, and confound your sensibilities. You, friend, are looking at eternity.

Are we here to present what we think God is all about? Of course not. The purpose of today's experience is to get you thinking about the great mystery again, not to foist any kind of dogma on you.

We're here only to tell you how spirituality can help you, no matter what your concept of a higher force is. You say you want to live forever? Then get spiritual. Whether that means organized religion or not is up to you.

The world's major religions promise eternal life. They don't all agree, though, on exactly how we get from here to eternity. But in a nicely ironic twist, it turns out that spiritual beliefs may well delay our journeys into the unknown. Numerous studies have suggested that aspects of spirituality contribute to better health, better quality of life, and even longer life.

"There are at least 250 studies showing that people who follow some type of religious practice in their lives—and that almost always includes prayer—are healthier across the board compared to people who don't," says

WHAT IS SPIRITUALITY?

Spirituality deals with the big questions, that much is for sure. But what exactly *is* spirituality? That's one of the biggest questions of all.

A review of 250 articles and studies dealing with spirituality revealed that 75 percent of people defined spirituality as a personal philosophy of meaning. Spirituality is more than a passive belief system, though. It is also an inspiration that comes out as action. How do you know if you're acting spiritually? There are six traits that can tell you, says Krista Kurth, Ph.D., a specialist in spirituality in the workplace.

1. Your action is motivated by an internal attitude of love.
2. Your action involves giving or serving with no expectation of personal gain. We like to think of it this way: Would you still do it if nobody knew it was you?
3. The elements of compassion and humility are present.
4. The effort involves some degree of difficulty because it requires that you transcend your own narrow self-interest.
5. A conscious, ongoing process of growth and learning must take place in order for you to live more fully and express the spiritual aspects of life.
6. The action involves spiritual practices or other consciously performed rituals that require commitment, discipline, or effort.

If you were an old-time country farmer, you might sum it up like this: It all boils down to common decency. Use it, and you'll be a good man.

Larry Dossey, M.D., author of *Prayer Is Good Medicine*. "They go to the doctor less often. They consume fewer health dollars. They get sick less often."

Here are a few more items worth pondering.

- A large study of people in Maryland found that those who attended a place of worship once a week or more often had lower death rates from heart disease, emphysema, cirrhosis of the liver, and suicide than those who did not.
- A study of heart patients in San Francisco General Medical Center found that

those who were prayed for—without their knowledge—were less likely to suffer complications than those who were not.

- People with high blood pressures who meditated experienced significant drops in their blood pressures and needed fewer or no medications.
- Researchers found that patients with chronic pain who meditated experienced less severity of pain, less anxiety, less depression, and less anger. They were also more active.

Have we thrown enough facts your way? Have we convinced you yet that you need to cast your eyes upward a bit to keep your health from heading downward?

Making Prayer Work for You

It's hard to say how strongly a man has to believe in order for spirituality to make an improvement in his life. One of the major researchers in the field, Herbert Benson, M.D., of Harvard Medical School, asserts that you don't have to believe in God at all—or at least, not in the god defined by Western religions. That position may raise some eyebrows in religious circles, but it's safe to say that few religious leaders would question the proposition that any spiritual seeker can increase his connection with a higher force through prayer.

Prayer is perhaps most simply defined as having a conversation with a greater power. Call it God, call it Allah, call it universal karma, call it Moe—that's up to you. "It does not matter which God you worship nor which theology you adopt. Spiritual life, in general, is very healthy," says Dr. Benson.

Here are some basic strategies for putting the power of prayer to work for you, courtesy of Dale Matthews, M.D., associate professor of internal medicine at Georgetown University Medical Center in Washington, D.C., and one of the leading researchers in the health-religion connection.

Develop a relationship. The key to an effective prayer life, says Dr. Matthews, is developing a sense that you have an ongoing relationship with God (or whatever greater power you believe in). "If we conceive of God as a friend we can talk to anytime, about anything," he writes in his book *The Faith Factor: Proof of the Healing Power of Prayer*, "or if we meditate on the nature of God and his goodness, we are likely to find a deep sense of satisfaction and even joy in our prayer and in our lives."

Set aside some time. Prayer is like anything else that you do for yourself—it

GOD BY THE NUMBERS

Here are some facts that will show you how the people around you feel about spirituality.

- Twenty percent of all Americans say that they have had revelations from God in the past year; 13 percent say that they have seen an angel or sensed its presence.
- Eighty-eight percent of Americans say that religion is important to them; 82 percent of Americans believe that prayer can heal.
- Peale Center for Christian Living in Pawling, New York, gets more than 2,500 prayer requests by phone, fax, letter, and e-mail every week.
- Ninety-six percent of all Americans say that they believe in God or some form of universal consciousness; 72 percent believe in angels; 65 percent believe in the devil.

can get pushed aside by other commitments. Don't let it be. Many people like to start and end their day with prayers. That might be a good idea for you.

Pray on the run. The funny thing about God is that he's easier to take out than pizza. While specific prayer times may be the foundation of a healthy spiritual life, praying spontaneously—in line at the grocery store or while you're doing the dishes, for example—is a skill well worth cultivating, says Dr. Matthews.

Define prayer loosely. Many people get hung up the notion that praying means reciting passages out of a sanctioned religious text that's overflowing with words like *thee* and *thou*. Such prayer may be what you say in a house of worship, but it is rarely how you communicate or think in day-to-day life. When doing private prayer, set aside the script if it doesn't mean much to you, and speak in your own words. Say what you want to say. Ask what you want to ask. Imagine what you want to imagine. Prayer means having a private, intimate, honest, one-way conversation with a higher force that you can't see but that you believe exists. We can't say for sure, but we doubt there's anyone out there saying, "Hmmm, he missed a word in that line."

Find a mentor. If you're just getting into this, you may have a bunch of misconceptions about the whole God thing. You may find yourself disappointed if God doesn't speak to you from a burning bush or send an angel to help you find a parking spot. "Go under the wing of someone who is more experienced in the faith," suggests Dr. Matthews. You'll be able to bounce concerns off that person as well as seek advice.

Find a community. Want to know something really cool about becoming more spiritual? You'll find yourself part of a vibrant, diverse community. The health benefits of consistent participation in a supportive community, religious or otherwise, have been thoroughly documented. Not coincidentally, sharing the religious experience with others is a central element of most faith traditions. If you find traditional churchgoing too impersonal, you might find a more intimate sense of connection by joining a small scripture or prayer discussion group.

Meditating on Yourself

It's easy to see meditation as something that only mystics and mountaintop gurus do. But there really is no mystery here. Meditation is a great way to chill out and leave earthly worries behind for a while.

Meditation, or meditative prayer, is less about talking to God and more about listening. Prayer is sending the transmission out; meditating is tuning in the big cosmic station, or something like that.

Meditation is also a conscious attempt to still the ceaseless chatter that typically fills your head day in and day out. When you meditate, you shift to a less distracted, more peaceful, more spiritually connected state of being. Imagine, if you will, a person with a high-pitched voice sitting 2 feet away from you and talking nonstop all day. That's your normal brain. Meditation stuffs a sock in it.

Dr. Benson has observed a form of secular meditation that he calls the relaxation response. Learn to use this surprisingly simple technique, and you, believe it or not, will be meditating. Start with 5 minutes every day, then work your way up to whatever seems right to you.

Find a focus. The essence of meditation is training your mind to focus. Pick something to focus on—a word, your breathing, a piece of music, a formal prayer, or even a physical activity like jogging. The trick then is to keep your mind in watchful attention. Concentrate on your focus object. What is it like? Notice everything you possibly can about it.

Disregard interruptions. We said this was a simple technique, and it is. But that doesn't mean it's simple to *do*, and therein lies the challenge. Your mind is used to babbling away about whatever it wants. Everyday thoughts will intrude on your focus. Don't worry about it; simply guide your mind back to your focus every time you notice that it has strayed.

ACTS OF PURE KINDNESS

Reconnecting with a higher force is not some abstract notion that rattles around uselessly in your brain. It truly does inspire you to a greater sense of kindness toward those around you. If you want to act on that feeling, here are a few suggestions from *Random Acts of Kindness*, coedited by Dawna Markova, Ph.D.

Praise good work. When an employee at a business does something helpful, write to the person's boss to thank the boss for having such a wonderful employee.

Brighten a day. Randomly select someone's name from your address book and send that person a card.

Donate a dolly. Have your children sort through their toys and pick some that they'd like to donate to children in need.

Clean the street. Make a habit of picking up the first piece of trash that you see each day.

Feed the flock. Keep birdseed in your car on winter days and scatter it for the birds.

Thank a teacher. Writer a letter to a teacher you once had and tell him that he made a difference in your life.

Purchase a pick-me-up. Anonymously buy a mail-order gift for a friend or someone at work whose spirits need a lift. Be sure to include a note signed, "A Friend" so the recipient knows it's not a mistake.

Share the wealth. When going through a tollbooth, pay for the next car in line behind you.

God at the Laundromat

Spirituality is not something to be dragged out for church and then neatly tucked away on Sunday afternoon. Learn to make it part of your every waking moment. Take another look at the way you live your life and ask if it's in agreement with what you see spirituality to be.

There are a couple of traits that men are often trained to ignore but that might just be a big help along the path of spirituality. First, we are raised to discount our intuition, our inner voice. Second, we are taught to suppress our emotions.

If you want your spiritual development to have a chance of continuing unimpeded, you need to do some unlearning. Don't listen only to your rational mind, urges Krista Kurth, Ph.D., a specialist in spirituality in the workplace from Potomac, Maryland. Listen, too, to your inner urges, nudges, leanings, and whispers. Give yourself the chance to act on what you know in your gut is right.

Learn tolerance, patience, a sense of justice, a willingness to do what needs to be done. These are also gifts of your spiritual side. And remember the following words.

There are diversities of gifts, but the same Spirit.
There are differences of ministries, but the same Lord.
And there are diversities of activities, but it is the same God who works all in all.
(1 Corinthians 12:4–6)

Buy Into Manhood

The Day's Task

Here's a simple task: Pick the one adjective from the list below that you would most like people to use in describing you. Not too long ago, we at *Men's Health* Books put the same task before 1,000 middle-aged men from across America. We'll tell you the results in a little bit.

Athletic	**Reliable**	**Sexual**
Capable	**Resourceful**	**Spiritual**
Creative	**Respected**	**Strong**
Handsome	**Sensitive**	**Successful**
Intelligent		

Scientists have confirmed what we men have long suspected: We are cavemen living in a modern world. And Adrian Targett is the living proof.

DNA tests conducted by scientists at Oxford University in England in the spring of 1997 found that Targett, a history teacher, is a direct descendant of Cheddar Man, a 9,000-year-old skeleton found less than a mile from Targett's home in England.

"My wife says that's why I like my steak rare," quips Targett.

But Targett—and the rest of us red-blooded males, for that matter—has far more in common with his fossilized forefather than just a taste for red meat. "It's very difficult to find differences between someone who lived 10,000 years ago and someone at present," explains David Glenn Smith, Ph.D., professor of anthropology at the University of California, Davis. Dr. Smith is an expert in one of Cheddar Man's peers: Kennewick Man, a 9,300-year-old skeleton found in the state of Washington. "Emotionally and intellectually, we evolved to our present form a very long time ago," says Dr. Smith.

But make no mistake, we men proffer no apologies for our primitive wiring. We relish it. Manhood gives us ancient delights. We proudly bay at the moon. We drag our knuckles, grunt with glee, grab onto things that are conveniently at arm's length. We pursue the opposite sex. We compete. And, since time immemorial, we've more or less taught our sons to do the same.

We are imprinted with Pleistocene memories, says Dr. Smith, memories left over from the birth of mankind that make us act and respond much as our primitive ancestors did. But just as we hold the traits of a caveman, so did he have imbedded within him the genetic blueprint of a modern man. Ancient man had a noble, greater side, as do his sons of today.

"Men strive," says George H. Hartlaub, M.D., of the University of Colorado Health Sciences Center. "We always move, we always look for the better way. That is profound in us."

That drive has led men to scale Mount Everest simply because it's there and to descend to the ocean's floor to find the Titanic. It has inspired and informed Shakespeare's sonnets, Emerson's mystical meditations, and Chandler's hard-boiled prose. It has given us the Sistine Chapel, the Taj Mahal, and the Empire State Building. It has blessed us with lasting images of Babe Ruth at bat, Michael Jordan soaring to unimagined heights, and Muhammad Ali floating like a butterfly, stinging like a bee.

It is, in a very real sense, what makes us men.

Men in Modern Times

As much as we enjoy our male heritage, the simple fact remains that although we're virtually identical to our long-dead forefathers, the world around us bears little resemblance to theirs. We require an amazing number of skills to wend our way through modern life.

Famed science fiction writer Robert Heinlein put it this way:

A human being should be able to change a diaper, plan an invasion, butcher a hog, conn a ship, design a building, write a sonnet, balance accounts, build a wall, set a bone, comfort the dying, take orders, give orders, cooperate, act alone, solve equations, analyze a new problem, pitch manure, program a computer, cook a tasty meal, fight efficiently, die gallantly. Specialization is for insects.

While most of us aren't called upon these days to plan an invasion (except for the occasional midnight raid on the refrigerator) or pitch manure (though, sure, we

THIS WE KNOW

Some things are just hardwired into a man's makeup. We hold truths like these to be self-evident.

- Just because we're adults now doesn't mean we can't actively seek out the banana with the sticker on it.
- Our penises are *never* to be referred to as cute.
- The fashion czars be damned, paisley ties will never go out of fashion for the simple reason that nothing else hides food stains as well.
- A true barber never has the word *curls* in his shop's name.
- Just because we know how to replace a belt in a washing machine doesn't mean we know how to do the laundry.
- There are two kinds of women: the kind you suck your gut in for and the kind you don't.
- Iced coffee makes about as much sense to us as hot peanut butter.
- We're not being deliberately nasty when we leave the toilet seat up. If we were being deliberately nasty, we'd take it *off*.

pitch woo), you get the idea. No man is complete without a solid arsenal of guy skills to call his own. And no man should ever apologize for practicing these skills.

A Man's Man

"What we really want and need from our fathers, our teachers, our men friends is that they see us as manly—as a man's man, as a man among men," says Michael Kimmel, Ph.D., sociology professor at the State University of New York at Stony Brook. "That's very, very important to us. I think it's the crucial theme in masculinity."

We agree. But what exactly is that elusive quality known as masculinity? It may bring various hairy images to mind, but in reality it's a very fluid concept.

"Manhood means different things at different times to different people," Dr. Kimmel explains. "Manhood is neither static nor timeless." What *is* consistent, though, is that we men seem to continue to ask the hard questions and probe for what it means to truly be a man during moments of crisis and transition, whether personal or societal.

So where does that leave the state of manhood today? We're glad you asked. Ronald F. Levant, Ed.D., dean of the center for psychological studies at Nova Southeastern University in Ft. Lauderdale and author of *Masculinity Reconstructed*, asked that very same question in a study he conducted. Here is what he found out.

- Men have loosened up a lot on what behavior they consider appropriate for men only and women only. We guys now believe that males can enjoy needlecraft and wear bracelets without it threatening their masculinity. We will, however, tease the hell out of the guys who do that stuff.
- Men reject the old stereotype of the strong, silent type. Those in the study said that showing emotions such as fear, worry, and love for their fathers was perfectly acceptable. John Wayne, we love you, we miss you, but we don't want to be you.
- Men are no longer expected to always be studs, eager whenever an opportunity for sex comes up. We are more inclined to connect sex with intimacy.
- Men are beginning to realize that achievement isn't the only thing that matters, and we are more willing to share power and status with women. Plus, it's nice to have that extra paycheck.
- Men are still committed to the idea that masculinity and self-reliance are closely related, but now it's okay, for example, to ask for help with changing a tire. The guys in the survey disagreed with the statement "A man should never doubt his judgment."
- Men still value the traits of strength, courage, and aggression, but we discriminate between healthy and unhealthy forms of aggression.
- There are signs that men have "worked free enough of homophobia" to disagree fairly strongly with the statement that a man should end a friendship with another man if he finds out the other man is a homosexual.

This brings us to our daily task. Here, in order of the most- to least-selected adjectives, are the words the men we surveyed most wanted used to describe them: reliable, capable, respected, successful, creative, resourceful, intelligent, athletic, sensitive, spiritual, strong, handsome, and sexual.

We think that makes a pretty good statement about manhood today. We have nothing to be ashamed of, friend. That's the point of this chapter. This week has focused intensely on helping you define who you are in terms of family, work, even the cosmos. But when every layer of meaning and purpose is stripped away,

THE CRYING GAME

One of the reasons that women are more likely to shed tears than men has nothing to do with emotions. Biologically, women have higher levels of the hormone prolactin, which primarily helps in the production of milk. Crying is one way to release excess quantities of prolactin.

About 80 percent of men report that they never or hardly ever cry, while the same percentage of women say they cry on a regular basis. According to one study, men are eight times less likely than women to cry when they are yelled at and nine times less likely to cry at sentimental gatherings. We're also less inclined to use tears manipulatively.

When men do cry, it is more likely to be framed in terms of their roles of provider, protector, warrior, athlete, husband, father, and team player. Male tears are more inclined to express experiences of pride, bravery, loyalty, victory, and defeat. Tears are not just more probable in those circumstances, they're almost expected. "I don't think I would like a man who is incapable of enough emotion to get tears in his eyes," said General Norman Schwarzkopf, of Desert Storm fame.

ultimately, you are a man. And that alone is something that should make you proud.

In fact, now is a better time than ever to be a man. Ignore the whining and finger pointing that comes from various male-bashing corners. At no other time in history have we been as free to be exactly the kind of man we want to be. At no other time has the definition of manhood embraced so many meanings.

Enjoy it, revel in it, be proud of it, and go get 'em. We *Men's Health* guys would slap you on the backside if you were closer.

10 Ways to Prevent or Lower High Blood Pressure

1 **Shedding excess flab is an excellent starting point for preventing high blood pressure.** If you weigh too much, you have more of a risk of high blood pressure. Those extra fat cells make your heart strain harder to pump blood. Each day, the average healthy adult heart pumps the equivalent of 2,100 gallons of blood through a circulatory system some 60,000 miles in length. High blood pressure complicates the task and also makes it easier for plaque and other bits of blood debris to clog your arteries.

2 **Regular exercise is one of the best ways to help prevent high blood pressure.** Exercise relaxes your blood vessels, creating less resistance for your heart to push against. After exercise, your vessels are wide open and your blood pressure is down. One long-term study found that those involved in vigorous physical activity decrease their risks of high blood pressure by 20 to 30 percent. Aerobic exercise done for 40 minutes, three times a week or more is a big blood pressure reducer. That means activities like walking, bicycling, swimming, or running will likely work for you.

And, of course, exercise helps you get your weight down, so the benefits are doubled.

3 **De-stress.** High blood pressure is more formally known as hypertension. The "tension" refers to the vessel walls, but it could just as easily refer to an element of your life that increases your blood pressure: stress. When you're stressed, your body pumps out hormones that contract your blood vessels, elevating your blood pressure. If your life is stressful (whose isn't?) do something about it.

4 **Pay attention to certain vitamins and minerals.** The B vitamin folate is especially important for keeping blood pressure down. Potassium is a mineral that actually lowers blood pressure. You get it in your multivitamin and in bananas, dried apricots, prunes, spinach, potatoes, and cantaloupes. Also note that people with high blood pressure tend to have less calcium and magnesium. Don't be one of them.

Salt, on the other hand, is sodium chloride, a mineral sometimes associated with elevating blood pressure. Get out of the habit of pouring salt all over everything.

5 **Diet is key for healthy blood pressure.** No surprise there—diet is key for just about everything. In this case, though, researchers have done all the work for you, testing something called the Dietary Approaches to Stop Hypertension, or the DASH diet. The details are pretty much the same as every piece of diet advice you've been reading about: lots of fruits and vegetables, grains, low-fat dairy products, and less than 25 percent of total calories from fat.

6 **Garlic is great for just about anything related to your cardiovascular system, including blood pressure.** Garlic helps your body maintain adequate levels of an enzyme that prevents hypertension. So an easy way to lower your blood pressure is to eat a clove or two of garlic or take a garlic powder supplement every day. Do not use supplements if you're on anticoagulants or before undergoing surgery because garlic thins the blood and may increase bleeding. Do not use if you're taking hypoglycemic drugs.

7 **Eating fish lowers your blood pressure.** When overweight study subjects ate 4 ounces of fish every day, their blood pressures dropped by 6 points within 4 months. So replace some meat meals with fish meals.

8 **Healthier blood pressure is another reason to replace processed foods with natural, whole foods.** For example, the processed wheat in white bread causes a surge of insulin, which triggers a blood pressure rise for several hours. A study of 400 people at Tulane University in New Orleans found that those with the highest blood insulin levels were three times more likely to have high blood pressures.

9 **Hypertension is yet another reason to give up the smokes.** Smoking cigarettes boosts your blood pressure because the nicotine constricts blood vessels. Every time you light up, it raises your blood pressure by as much as 20 points for as long as 30 minutes. Light up 30 times a day, and your blood pressure is up a lot.

10 **Make sure you have your pressure checked.** One way to *not* lower your blood pressure is to ignore it. But it's easy not to think about it if you don't get yourself tested because high blood pressure is not something you feel. There are no symptoms. That's why a third of Americans with high blood pressure don't know it. Those do-it-yourself machines at drugstores can give you a ballpark figure, but the only way to get an accurate blood pressure reading is to see a health professional.

WEEK 12

PREPARE FOR A LONG FUTURE

Day 1

Get Those around You on Board

Day 2

Find a Good Challenge

Day 3

Assess Your Money Situation

Day 4

Fill Out Your Calendar

Day 5

Choose Your Vices

Day 6

Celebrate Your Long Life

Get Those around You on Board

The Day's Task

Gather your family and head outside for a 30-minute walk. Hoof it around your neighborhood at a pace that's brisk, but not so brisk that you can't talk easily. That's key because you're going to use this family activity to tell the gang about the ideas you've adopted from this book and the goals you've set to have a long and healthy life.

Tell them what you've learned about yourself, which changes you intend to make permanent, and why. Thank them for putting up with you for the past 11 weeks, and let them know that they are part of the reason why you are sticking to this program. Tell them how good you feel, both physically and mentally, after all this work. Next, make clear that you don't intend to make everyone miserable by preaching at them the gospel of health or forcing them to do what you do. But let them know that it would be great if they would join along as you turn these tasks into lifelong habits and that, at a minimum, you want their support.

If you have really been following this program for the past 11 weeks, it has undoubtedly been tough on your family. You've taken a lot of time for yourself, you've probably bored them all to tears by talking about health and your daily tasks, and your attention most likely has been more internally focused than it has been for years.

They deserve something in return. That something is a happier, healthier you. And that should be enough. But spoil them anyhow, with thanks, a good restaurant meal, some extra time together, even a vacation.

Just as important is to let them know what you plan to do as you move forward. Explain that you intend to keep eating differently or exercising regularly or spending a guys' night out every Thursday, or that you plan to run a 10-K race 3 months from now. They deserve to know your intentions and will probably be happy to give you encouragement.

Then comes the trickiest part: getting everyone to join you on your quest for longevity.

Bring In Family

Scenario: It's October and the health authorities predict that a raging flu season will strike soon. So Bob, always mindful of his good health, dutifully goes out and gets a flu shot to protect himself. Unfortunately, he can't persuade anyone else in his office to get a shot.

As the flu sweeps through town, more and more of Bob's coworkers succumb to it. The good news is that Bob still feels perfectly fine. The bad news is that with almost everyone else out sick, he has a harder time doing his job.

These past few months, like Bob, you've taken steps to make yourself stronger and healthier. You lift weights and jog. You eat right and take your vitamins. You keep your mind active with books and hobbies. But if you look around your house and see kids who fill their free time with television and a wife whose contribution to the dinner table consists of creamy casseroles or frozen pizza, you're pretty much up the same creek as Bob and his flu shot.

Going it alone, you have a harder time living a healthy life. You have not only less motivation to keep going but also a greater risk of being lured into slothful ways and poor eating habits. That's bad.

Here's what's worse: If you stay on your longevity track and are still going strong 30 years from now, it's going to break your heart to see your loved ones in decrepit shape or, even worse, in early graves.

That's why it's in your best interest and your family's to get them to join you in your longevity plan. The more health seekers you have surrounding you, the easier your quest for longevity will be.

Get Your Loved Ones Moving

Even if you're the only one in your household who will willingly break a sweat, or if you eat chicken breasts and broccoli while your family gorges on pizza and cake, it may still be possible for you to lead a healthy life. But it's not likely. "I think that would make it almost impossible to sustain the lifestyle, unless you absolutely have a will of iron—and even then it would be a struggle," says Patricia Esperon, a behavior therapist at the Duke University Diet and Fitness Center.

On the other hand, you can't foist your new way of life on your family and expect to get instant buy-in. Push them too hard, Esperon warns, and they'll likely resist your suggestions.

Instead, go gradually. As you talk with them, make it clear that you're not going to force them to change their ways but that you do expect them to encourage you and be open-minded in trying some of your health recommendations. That means that while they can still enjoy junk food, it's not going to be lying everywhere around the house, taunting you. While they can still watch TV, you're going to set limits on it and urge some outdoor activity each week.

Then, set an example of good exercise, nutrition, and time management, and your family will be likely to follow you, Esperon says. Remember, though, that you'll also have to contribute some effort—especially with your wife—unless you want to do all of your workouts in the doghouse.

For starters, make sure your exercise time doesn't cut into your other obligations around the house, like helping to take care of the chores or watching the kids. And since you have some loftier eating demands now, be sure to pull your weight in the kitchen. If your wife does most of the cooking, you can't very well expect her to suddenly start preparing unfamiliar foods or to fix one meal for the rest of the family and another for you. If you can't help her fix the meals because, say, you come home from work too late, at the very least help write out grocery lists and plan meals for the coming week, Esperon suggests. Or make meals on weekends that you can freeze and eat later in the week.

Make Your Workplace Fitter

Even if you have a family that's totally on board with your healthy lifestyle plans, you can still sabotage your longevity if you fall into coworkers' unhealthy habits. "If you're in a workplace where people are constantly bringing junk food in or they're providing pastries for you rather than healthier stuff, that's a big issue. If you can get your workplace to cooperate and make it a healthier environment, you're in a much better position," Esperon says.

Instead of suffering through business meetings where there are bowls of candy or boxes of doughnuts on hand, ask the person who brings in the refreshments to stock the room with some fresh fruit. If you're the boss man in your office, then demand it, Esperon suggests.

SWEAT WITH YOUR FAMILY

If you want to get your family to join you on your exercise kick, find creative ways to get them involved in a workout routine.

Your Kids

- If you ride a bike or run frequently and have a baby or toddler, take her along with you. You can buy all-terrain strollers with knobby tires that you can push as you jog. Or get a trailer that you can pull behind your bike. You'll not only increase your workout since you're pushing or pulling extra weight but also get your kid acclimated early to a lifelong habit of exercising.
- Once the kids get older, many aerobic activities can be turned into family time, from jogging to cycling to inline skating. Just be sure to set your pace according to the slowest family member. If that doesn't allow you a good enough sweat, use your kids as a warmup and speed up to get your own workout. This will work especially well at a circular route, like a track, where you can see each other periodically as you all go at your own speeds. As the little ones become stronger and faster, encourage them to keep up with you for longer periods.
- Get outdoors together every chance you get. Shoot hoops or play one-on-one soccer or pitch a few games of fantasy major-league baseball. Don't be one of those dads who just watch as their kids climb around the playground—join in. Take your children hiking or tree climbing. When it snows, go outside and stay there, throwing snowballs, building snowmen and igloos, sledding, or just walking and observing the snow-covered view.

What if you can't get the snacks changed to your liking? Take your own healthy fare, and sit more than an arm's length away from the junk. As your coworkers grow envious of the way you can walk up stairs without gasping, maybe they'll start eyeing healthier foods too. Okay, we don't really think they will either. But at least they won't drag you down.

Here are a few other ideas on getting your coworkers to join your longevity-promoting habits.

- Take a martial arts class together. You're never too old and kids are never too young to start.
- Use your kids as gym equipment. If they're big enough, let them hold your feet as you do situps. If they're small enough, let them sit on your back while you do pushups. Bench-press them and curl them if you can get a comfortable grip on them.
- Introduce your child to your gym. You don't want to have to keep an eye on your kid the whole time you're working out, nor do you want the little imp scampering around the equipment unattended. Just make extra trips to the gym from time to time to show him how the different weights work and what body parts they strengthen. If your kid is old enough to handle a light weight, supervise as he curls a dumbbell or bench-presses a barbell.

Your Spouse

If your family is just you and your wife, here are a few ideas to make exercise more fun for the two of you.

- If you're a faster bicyclist than she is, ride in a lower gear. This will slow you down to her speed and give you a great leg workout. If you're a faster runner, carry hand weights as you go. Or she can ride a bike alongside you as you run.
- Hit the gym together. Work out on equipment side by side, or take turns doing the same exercises and spotting each other, changing the weights as appropriate.
- Learn a new sport together. If you're both novices, you'll start out at the same skill level. Plus, you'll have a partner to practice with and motivate you.

- Start an impromptu sports team on your lunch hour. Find some like-minded individuals, lace up your sneakers, and hit the road for a few miles of jogging. Or take in your baseballs and gloves and play catch.
- If you have a company gym, find a workout partner for a lunch-hour or pre- or post-work exercise session. Develop some goals and help each other reach them.
- If your company cafeteria and vending machines don't offer enough low-fat foods and snacks, start a petition asking for them.

Find a Good Challenge

The Day's Task

It's time to bust out of a rut. Today, we're going to ask you to do something that is relatively easy but that has significant long-term ramifications. Get out a pad of paper, and make two lists. In the first list, itemize all the things you have always been curious about or interested in knowing more of but have never gotten around to studying. Perhaps you're fascinated with the history of dinosaurs or the Civil War or the writings of Ernest Hemingway or how to cook a good Chinese meal or how to play the saxophone.

In the second list, include all the physical feats you have always fantasized about but have never gotten around to doing. Maybe you dream about running a 10-K race or biking 100 miles or taking up skiing or bench-pressing your weight or climbing a 12,000-foot mountain.

Pick the one item from each list that appeals the most to you. Grab a calendar. Figure out what the date will be 6 months from today. Mark your calendar: that's the date by which you'll complete the easier of the two tasks. Go 3 months farther, and mark the date by which you will complete the second item.

Figure out exactly what it will take to fulfill these goals. Convince yourself that you are going to do it. You *will* do it. Tell your wife, your kids, whomever that you are going to do it. By telling someone, you make the goal even more real. Now, get started. And don't look back.

Riddle for the day: What do a herd of cows, a life without challenge, and poet Robert Frost have in common?

Answer: They choose a path each day.

Cattle follow the same route through the pasture, day in and day out, until they wear a groove in the grass. The familiar path is comforting, easy to follow, and not at all taxing on what little brains they have.

ROCK AROUND THE TIME CLOCK

As you seek new experiences from day to day, don't forget to challenge yourself in those 8-hour chunks of time that you call work. John Sena, Ph.D, coauthor of *Work Is Not a Four-Letter Word*, offers a few pointers on giving your job a jolt.

- Though it might sound like a bad idea to volunteer for more work, ask to cover some of a coworker's tasks when he's out of the office. It can shake up your normal routine—and it may make you glad that you have *your* job and not the other guy's.
- Watch for problems around the office that aren't being addressed and think of solutions. Ask to take on assignments that can teach you new skills.
- When you hit a lull during the day, read a professional magazine, journal, or other material relating to your work. You'll get a break from your normal tasks, and you may even learn the latest news before your boss does.

When our lives take predictable patterns—get up, work, exercise on the treadmill, eat supper, read the paper, sleep, get up, and so on—we can wear a groove right through the calendar. When we live that way, the rut we make in our lives isn't too different from that cow path.

As for Robert Frost, well, you knew this was coming: He wrote the poem "The Road Not Taken," in which the narrator looks at two roads leading into the woods and decides to head down the less-used route. "And that has made all the difference," he concludes.

Frost knew all about choosing a challenge. After dropping out of Dartmouth and Harvard, he wound up teaching and working on a poultry farm in New Hampshire. He tried to get publishers interested in his poetry, but found little success.

At the age of 38, he faced a momentous decision. He could head into middle age with his chickens. Or he could sell the farm, pack up his stack of unpublished poetry, and head to London with his wife and four kids to look for a more receptive audience. He followed the uncertain path, won four Pulitzer Prizes, became his country's unofficial poet laureate, and got to read his work at the inauguration of President John F. Kennedy.

We're certainly not telling you to chuck your job and write poetry (unless that's what you really want to do), but you should find a challenge each and every day that gives you a new reason to jump out of bed in the morning, whether you are starting a family and career or enjoying retirement. The daily gauntlets that you throw down for yourself will keep your mind and body honed to a razor's edge and can protect your health, happiness, and sanity.

Drive Your Train of Thought Off the Tracks

Imagine the blizzard of the century descending upon your town, covering the roads with 3 feet of snow and trapping you in your home. For days, you'd eat the same foods, breathe the same air, and stare lethargically at the same wallpaper. After enough time deprived of new stimulation, you'd likely fall prey to cabin fever.

That same process can happen to your life—no blizzard needed—when you slip into an easy yet mind-numbing routine. One year passes, then another. You get the hang of it; it feels good. No, not good, exactly. It feels *comfortable*. Decades pass. But your life remains at a sort of standstill. "The longer one is in a particular position or lifestyle, the more likely it is that the lifestyle or position will become habit," says David Abramis, Ph.D., psychologist at California State University, Long Beach. "And once something is habitual, it's harder to change."

But sometimes, a guy wakes up one morning and wonders what he's been doing all this time (it happens at a certain age). By golly, he'd better start living! But he ain't no Robert Frost. Instead of finding an outlet in poetry, he decides he needs a girlfriend, a red sports car, and an earring, in no particular order. When he gets it all out of his system, our guy can be left looking at a broken family, an empty savings account, and a sheepish face in the mirror.

Let's be clear: The idea is to shake up your routine before you hit the extremes of either falling into a slumber or feeling the need to turn your whole life on its ear. "You should be mixing time spent doing comforting, familiar things with time spent sprinkling in challenging new things," says Powell Lawton, Ph.D., senior research scientist at the Polisher Institute of the Philadelphia Geriatric Center. "It doesn't take a whole lot of zestful sprinklings to make life interesting."

Challenges do more than add a shot of jalapeño pepper to a bland burrito of a life. Research has shown that people who throw themselves into new activities often have better problem-solving skills.

Novel adventures can also keep your mind and body from deteriorating as you age. Challenges trigger the release of endorphins and other brain chemicals that lift your mood. And, as we explained in Week 7, mastering new skills—from learning a musical instrument to solving crossword puzzles—strengthens your brain by encouraging cells to make new connections.

The Way to Change

Think about what you did the past 5 Saturday nights. If you can't remember or did the same thing all 5 nights, you may be slipping into a rut, suggests Sidney B. Simon, Ed.D., author of *Getting Unstuck: Breaking Through the Barriers to Change*. You can attack your complacency with several different approaches: physical, over-the-top physical, and mental and creative.

Physical. A good place to start challenging your regular routine is at the gym. If you regularly do one exercise—running, for instance—a mix of sports can give you the cross-training you need to avoid injury and keep from burning out. Toss in activities that use different body parts, like using a rowing machine for your arms, bicycling for your legs, or swimming for everything. If you normally do just aerobic workouts, toss in some weight training. If you're a dedicated lifter, mix in some lung-busting aerobic exercise.

Of course, you don't have to make exercise a solitary pursuit. Join a martial arts class to build your coordination, focus, and ability to kick someone in the head. Hook up with a running club and make plans to run in a 10-K. Join a sporting league at your workplace, or ask about adult team sports at your local YMCA, chamber of commerce, or university.

Over-the-top physical. The next time you flip through the channels and secretly admire the young, facially pierced lunatics who put their butts on the line by rock climbing, skateboarding, and leaping from planes on snowboards, remember that you're never too grizzled to get up and join them. Here are some cases in point.

- "Banana" George Blair still water-skis in his mid-eighties—barefoot. Sometimes he does it with the tow rope clenched between his teeth. He learned to ski like this when he was 46. Oh, he skydives and snowboards too.
- Sam Gadless's 92-year-old legs hauled him across the finish line of the New York City Marathon in a little less than 8 ½ hours. He might have run it even faster if he hadn't lost several weeks of training time after he was hit by a car. He plans to be the oldest man ever to finish the race when runs he it again at the age of a ripe, old 94.

STARTING EASY

Sometimes, before you can face up to a big new challenge, you need to ramp up with some small ones. Here are simple, seemingly unimportant things you can do on any given day that can put you on the path to grander changes and goals.

- When you leave work, head in the opposite direction from your usual route. Find your way home while driving on as few of the roads that you normally use as possible.
- Go to the gym and do only unfamiliar exercises. Join a kickboxing or abdominal-workout class, or hop on that thigh-strengthening machine that you've never seen a guy use. Or ask a trainer for his favorite exercises and instructions on doing them right.
- Pick up an international magazine and read it from cover to cover, or find a foreign-language cable station and watch it for 15 minutes. Even if you have little idea what's going on, you can see what people in other cultures find interesting and entertaining. At worst, you might find a destination for your next big vacation.
- Go to an ethnic restaurant that you've never before tried. Ask the waiter to select an array of dishes that represents the best of the chef's work. If you want to keep it inexpensive, limit the choices to appetizers, soups, and salads.
- Go online to see if you can track down classmates from high school. When you succeed, send an e-mail telling them how great your life is.

- Earl V. Shaffer hoofed the whole Appalachian Trail, which runs more than 2,000 miles between Georgia and Maine, at the age of 29. But that wasn't the really impressive part. He did it again 50 years later, when he was 79.

If you don't know where to go to find high adventure, you may want to consider Outward Bound, a nonprofit educational adventure group. This program offers courses like backpacking, rock-climbing, sailing, and other outdoor activities. While they design the activities with an eye on safety, you're expected to join in the challenges. We know a veterinarian in his mid-fifties who ended his trip with a mile-long swim through the choppy Atlantic. At the beginning, it was everything he disliked. At the end, he knew he was ready for more challenges. For more information, write to Outward Bound, 945 Pennsylvania Street, Denver, CO 80203.

Mental and creative. When you think back on your education, which teachers captured your attention? The ones who shuffled you and your bored classmates through repetitive drills and fact-memorizing sessions? Or the ones who taught physics with wind-up toys and covered medieval literature by explaining the bawdier parts of *The Canterbury Tales*?

Now that you're an adult, you can choose to take only the classes that fire up your brain with cool and unusual challenges. Here are the kinds of evening courses that community colleges around the country are offering these days: "Acupressure Self-Care," "Secrets of the Wolf," "Basic Car Repair," "Starting an Investment Club," and "Be a Home Builder or Learn to Hire One." Pick up a course catalog from a university, community college, or extension campus in your area to see if they have anything that strikes your interest.

You could also spend your spare time learning a creative skill that you could use to impress your friends, like painting a life-size oil portrait of the Three Stooges, cooking a skillet of Thai chicken, or picking up a guitar at a party and wowing the crowd with a little Aerosmith.

Think these creative endeavors are beyond you? Maybe they are. But if you don't try, you'll never know. While we tend to think that only a gifted few have creative gifts like these, most of us have some degree of artistic abilities—we just need to develop them, says Dean Keith Simonton, Ph.D., professor of psychology at the University of California, Davis.

Check out the art, music, cooking, and drama opportunities that your local educational centers and art councils offer. And don't forget that your odds of meeting a nude model jump much higher when you're in an art class.

Assess Your Money Situation

The Day's Task

Contrary to rumors that it's the root of all evil, money is good. As much as we might have, there probably isn't one among us who wouldn't like to have more income so we could buy the bigger and better things we see all around us, and more important, so we could feel the sense of security that savings provides.

But let's say you do move up to a wealthier income bracket. Let's say you can afford that four-bedroom house with the posh furniture and the two-car garage filled with new sport-utility vehicles. Nice, except you're responsible for bigger bills, and your money issues become more complicated, requiring larger amounts of time and even more cash to resolve. Rich people worry about money as much if not more than their lesser-income brethren. They just lie awake in nicer beds. We don't want you lying awake at night; insomnia is unhealthy, and there are better things to do in bed. That's why tonight, you're going to set aside a good 3 hours to yourself. Tell your wife that this is the last time you will be asking for time to yourself, that this crazy program is just 3 days away from being done.

You might wish to brew up some coffee and pop up some microwave popcorn. Go sequester yourself in a place in which you have access to the family financial books. (If your wife is the family bookkeeper, you may wish to do this together.) We want you to do a handful of calculations in the next few hours. Don't get overly precise. They will all change in a week anyhow.

This is a health book, not a personal-finance book. But we are very serious about the need to discuss money here. See, there are two types of people in the world: those with peace of mind and those without peace of mind. You know who lives longer and more happily. And whether we like it or not, financial status plays heavily into this peace-of-mind equation, particularly in modern America, where materialism is a hobby, where work status is more important than community status, where we measure our successes more by what we own than by who we are.

You don't need money to be happy. You need to keep money in perspective to be happy—for your health, for your sanity, for your longevity.

We're not telling you that you shouldn't want nice cars, big houses, fine wines. If that's what you want, terrific. We just want you to be honest with yourself. In fact, if you meet with a financial planner, this is the point with which he will start as well. He'll ask about your personal values and priorities.

How important are vacations to you? How important is it for your kids to go to good colleges? Are you the type to live for today, or are you working toward a truly luxurious retirement? Honest answers to these questions are the foundations of a good financial plan. When making your financial goals, "you add in the numbers after the real groundwork has been done, and the real groundwork is figuring out who you are and what you want to be in life," observes Delia Fernandez, a fee-only personal financial planner in Los Alamitos, California. Trying to write a financial plan without first identifying her clients' values, she says, "is just running numbers for people who won't implement the plan."

Where Are You Now?

- Make a list of all the high-cost purchases and expenses that you will definitely be facing in the months and years ahead. This should cover new cars, college tuition for kids, major vacations, a new home, even care for your aging parents, if you feel that it is inevitable.
- Figure out how much money you owe in total on credit cards, car loans, and other short-term loans.
- Figure out roughly how much cash you spend per month on food, clothes, utilities, and entertainment.
- Determine how much money you have in nonretirement savings.
- It's no surprise what's next: Tally up your retirement savings.
- Finally, if you own a home, come up with a rough estimate of how much cash you would walk away with if you sold your home today. Remember that 10 percent of the sales price will go to real estate agents and expenses.

Next, take a good, hard, intuitive look at the big picture. What kind of shape are you in? Do you have investments or savings to cover your expected expenses?

Is anything out of whack? You don't need an expert to tell you this stuff. It should be pretty obvious.

The Simplicity of Money

People worry only about things they cannot control. But money is within your control, which is why worrying about money is unnecessary. We wish to make three simple but crucial points.

1. Managing money is far easier than you think.
2. Once you start doing it, you will probably enjoy it.
3. Once you start enjoying it, you are much more likely to achieve your goals.

To be smart about money, you don't have buy into any Wall Street hype, and you don't need a master's degree in business administration (nor need you hire someone who has one). All you need are simple resources: a middle-school-level knowledge of arithmetic, basic literacy skills, and a little bit of time. Most important is a money-friendly attitude, one that says, "I'm interested; I'm willing to put in an hour or two a week on this stuff; I'm willing to read a little to understand what my choices are."

We'll give you a road map to how to proceed, and you can take it from there. Once you feel that your accounts are in good shape, you only need to revisit these once a year for updates and restrategizing.

Step one: Self-assessment. You've already done a lot of this with today's task. But to take it to the next step, you need to come up with some more precise measures.

- Your net worth (basically, the value of all your property, savings, and investments, minus all the debts you owe)
- Your cash flow (how much money you have coming in per month and how much you spend in the same amount of time)
- Your asset allocation (what percentage of your financial investment is in stocks, what percentage is in bonds, and what percentage is in cash accounts)
- Your specific financial goals (where you wish to go and what is important to you, financially)

As mentioned, there are financial books galore that offer worksheets to calculate these. With these numbers, you can start working on the following.

Step two: A financial plan. This includes a budget for day-to-day spending and a savings-and-investment plan to make sure that all your long-term needs are covered.

Step three: A family business plan. Beyond the basic spending-and-saving issues are four key personal-finance categories that you need to manage.

1. Housing and transportation: They're what you spend the most money on.
2. Taxes: They are your duty, like 'em or not.
3. Insurance: Make sure that you are financially protected if something bad happens to your body or property. We're talking about coverage for health, home, car, and untimely death.
4. Retirement planning: You should already be saving for retirement; you should also be envisioning some of the specifics.

The net sum of all this work is peace of mind. You'll know where you want to go financially and materially, and that you are on the right path. You'll be surprised at how much stress will be alleviated once you get to this point. And that, friend, is even more important than money.

Fill Out Your Calendar

The Day's Task

If you don't have a calendar or day planner for this year and the next, go buy one. (Software versions are just fine.) Most guys use their calendars strictly for work. Beginning today, you will use yours for all aspects of your life. So if the daily logs stop at 6:00 P.M., it won't work.

Now, set aside about 30 minutes to mark down every meaningful event that you deem worthy of a time allotment. Include those dates that you selected 2 days ago as the deadlines for learning and doing something new. Budget an hour for home finances each week or month. If your wife wants the two of you to go vegetarian one week a month, note that as well.

Feel free to make plans for 5, 10, and 25 years down the line. Tape this separate piece of paper on the December page of your calendar. Figure out the first steps that you need to take, and enter those into the calendar. When December rolls around, remove your long-term goals and put them in next year's calendar.

What is time, really? One dictionary calls it "the measured or measurable period during which an action, process, or condition exists or continues."

In other words, time is a man-made thing. The six billion of us on this planet have agreed to use watches and clocks with hands that spin around at precisely the same pace (except when a battery wears out). The progression from seconds to decades is measured the same way by everyone, from a pig farmer in Missouri to a gondolier in Italy.

But some people get more done with their time than others do. Obviously, they don't squeeze more hours out of the clock. They just plan their activities well.

Today you become one of them. You do it by sitting down with a calendar and mapping out some of your future endeavors. You've now learned enough from the Longevity Program to add time to your life by increasing the number of years in your life. You've also learned ways to fill that time productively, especially this past week, as you've come up with family goals, personal challenges, and financial plans that you'd like to accomplish.

Commit to the Calendar

When we can think of nothing pressing to do on a tired evening or a lazy Saturday morning, that's usually what we do—nothing. We fall asleep, flip through the channels a few times, aimlessly surf the Web, or page through last week's magazine. Without noticing, we lose another chance to do something that's worthwhile or interesting enough to become a memory that will bring smiles to our weathered faces when we're old.

There are worse ways to lose track of time, though. You can forget that your anniversary at work is tomorrow, and therefore you lose a vacation day that you didn't use because it won't roll over into the next year. Or you could neglect to call grandma on her birthday or fail to set aside time for your kid's recital. Once these opportunities become missed chances, they slip into the past, and rewinding the hands on your clock won't bring them back.

So avoid these misadventures and missed adventures by heading them off with your calendar. Here's how, step-by-step.

1. Rustle up a little information to help you plan your calendar. Know how many vacation days and holidays you and your spouse have as well as kids' breaks from school. Rough out spaces on the calendar that would be good times to get out of town.
2. Mark down family stuff, and not just birthdays and anniversaries. Make note of your kids' activities that you need to attend. Put in ink all those family and individual goals you've set recently.
3. Schedule in blocks of free time for yourself. When you know that, say, you'll have the house to yourself next Tuesday evening, you can think about useful things that you can do with your time.
4. When you show up for a regular appointment, whether it's a haircut or a teeth cleaning, schedule the next visit before you leave. Promptly get this information on your calendar.
5. Think long-term. Mark important events on next year's calendar.

THE TIMES, THEY WERE A-CHANGIN'

If you have trouble keeping up with the events in your calendar, just be glad you didn't live a few millennia ago.

The ancient Romans followed a calendar that contained 355 days and was based on the cycle of the moon. Unfortunately, the calendar came up about 10 days short of a year in terms of the Earth's orbit around the sun, so in just a few years, what were supposed to be autumn months would actually fall during summer. To avoid this problem, the Romans were supposed to insert a special month into the calendar every 2 years, but sometimes they didn't get around to it.

By 46 B.C., Julius Caesar was fed up with not knowing what day it was, so he ordered an astronomer to come up with a new calendar. This new Julian calendar assumed that a real year lasted 365¼ days and made up for the fraction by throwing in an extra day every fourth February. To kick it off, the Romans started January 1, 45 B.C., in what would have been March on their old calendar.

However, the calendar was still a few minutes out of sync with the sun, and by the late 1500s, it was in error by 10 days. Pope Gregory XIII had another astronomer come up with a better plan. This star watcher tinkered with the length of the year, declared that everyone should skip 10 days in October 1582, and decided that a centennial year can only be a leap year when it is divisible by 400. Thus, 1900 wasn't a leap year, but 2000 was.

Most of the world now goes by this Gregorian calendar, though the Islamic and Jewish calendars are much different. But that's another story.

If you think that this is a lot to schedule, you're right. But as you've seen, planning is a must if you want to live an active life.

If you already use a computer at the office or at home, let it do the work. Certain software lets you input your plans and appointments for virtually the rest of your life, if you have the foresight and inclination to do so. And, minutes to months ahead of time, your computer can remind you of an upcoming event.

Best of all, if you still miss an appointment, you can just blame the computer.

Choose Your Vices

The Day's Task

Today's task sounds easy, but it takes brutal honesty. Isolate yourself for a half-hour this evening and list all of the habits you have that you suspect are not good for your mental or physical health. They can be small or large: a daily chocolate bar at work, a propensity for Internet pornography, an ESPN addiction, swearing too much, getting drunk every Friday, sneaking in a fast-food cheeseburger on your way home from work.

Ponder each thing on your list. Ask yourself, "Why do I do this? Do I need to do this? Does it really make me happy to do this?" Honestly weigh the pleasure that each habit provides against the risk it poses. Then make a decision, asking and answering the questions "Do I want to continue doing this? Am I willing to live with the consequences of it, short-term and long?" Don't be afraid to answer yes—this is an internal dialogue, and you can't lie to yourself. But don't be afraid to say no either, even if you realize that the habit will be hard to kick. (The truth is, making a firm conviction to change is half the battle.)

Crumble up your list and don't let anyone see it. But remember this dialogue. It may seem innocuous, but this very well could be the one task in this whole program that by itself can add many years to your life.

We can read all day long about how to avoid dangers to our health, but when we're faced with a tempting vice, we often have to think long and hard before saying no or, as the case may be, saying yes. After all, life *is* for living.

Let's face it, virtue can be boring. But what are the consequences of embracing an unhealthy vice? Truth is, it's hard to tell since many vices don't have immediate effects or clear links to specific health problems.

But we can make some general predictions of how likely a vice is to come back and bite you in the seat. We came up with a list of so-called vices that commonly tempt guys. With the help of Kenneth A. Goldberg, M.D., of the Male Health Center, we grouped them by how likely they are to cause you harm. Our classifications are "Go Ahead, If You Must" (these aren't too bad), "Yellow Light" (proceed with more caution), "Roulette" (it may or may not kill you), and "Write Your Will" (this one will end you).

Since everyone will weigh these vices according to his own moral code, we're only measuring them by their health effects. We're not necessarily condoning any of them; we're just acknowledging that sometimes temptation lures even the healthiest guy off his course.

One more thing: Pay attention to the frequency in which you engage in the vices listed here, since indulging them every day can have very different effects than giving in to temptation only occasionally.

Go Ahead, If You Must

Eating a blow-out meal. Say you get an unexpected 8 percent bonus at work this year. You and the lady hit the fancy Italian restaurant downtown, and you eat until it hurts. You make room for the breaded calamari, the chicken and shrimp in cream sauce over pasta, the freshly baked bread drenched in garlic and butter. You top off the whole thing with a dense slice of cheesecake.

This is a feast that would send Dom DeLuise staggering, yet we call this acceptable? Yes, but only because it's a special occasion. Keep your blowouts like this few and far between—less often than once a month. Afterward, repent like those sinners in Dante's *Inferno*. Immediately go back to your healthy eating style. You know the drill: low-fat meals with plenty of fruits, vegetables, fiber, and water.

Having a daily drink. Every night, you pour yourself a glass of red wine. As you eat dinner, you slowly sip it, savoring its rich aroma and the way it fills your head and belly with warmth.

In moderation, meaning no more than two glasses a day, red wine is good for you, hence its placement on this list. Though some of the benefits may come from the alcohol, it appears that wine in particular has extra-helpful substances, such as flavonoids, that hinder clotting in your blood and work as antioxidants, reducing your risk of heart disease and cancer. Cabernet sauvignon, a type of red wine, has high levels of the antioxidant resveratrol, which can further protect you against heart disease by raising your good cholesterol and lowering your bad cholesterol.

Just remember, *moderation* is the important word here. More is not better.

Smoking an occasional cigar. Once a month, after you drop your mortgage payment in the mail, you lean back in an easy chair on the back porch of your castle and puff on an extremely satisfying cigar.

Not smoking will always be a healthier choice than smoking. Even if you smoke cigars instead of cigarettes and you don't inhale the smoke and you do it only once a month, you'd be better off without it.

That said, if you must have some sort of smoking ritual in your life, cigars carry less risk for lung cancer than cigarettes, and the fewer cigars you smoke, the smaller the risk you face. If lighting one stogie a month is your only vice, you could pick far worse ones.

Yellow Light

Regularly bingeing on junk food. Every other Friday is your poker night. A royal flush is a long shot, but you know you can count on a few beers and a belly full of very tasty junk food.

You're starting to get into more serious abuses of your health. Let's assume your appetite for plastic-packaged food is similar to ours, and you eat the following over several hours as you play cards: seven breaded chicken nuggets, one-fourth of a large bag of tortilla chips and half of a jar of cheese dip, four fistfuls of M&M's and two handfuls of peanuts, all chased down by a couple of 12-ounce beers.

That equals roughly 2,970 calories. Keep in mind that a pound of fat equals 3,500 calories. So if you don't exercise off all that junk food, you can theoretically gain more than a pound a month just from your poker eating. If you do want to sweat it off, you'll have to jog for nearly 3 hours.

You've also blown the doors off the first two nutritional commandments of the American Heart Association, which are that you get no more than 30 percent of your calories from fat and no more than 10 percent from saturated fat. Worst of all, you've turned this kind of eating into a habit, a ritual. This will invite further abuses, bubba. Beware.

Being a sports fanatic. You follow your favorite sports team obsessively, crowing all day after a big win and becoming short-tempered and irritable after a heartbreaking loss.

Two studies on die-hard sports fans, one centered on college basketball and the other on a World Cup soccer game, found that when a team won, its fans' testosterone levels went up, and when a team lost, the fans' testosterone levels dropped. Elevated testosterone may make you depressed and aggressive. And you sure don't want your levels going down, either.

Wavering hormone levels aside, guys who aren't in control of situations tend to get stressed out. And no matter how hard you scream at your television, you're not in control of how your team plays. Besides, no one likes raving sports lunatics, other than other raving sports lunatics. Our final point is that sports nuts spend an awful lot of time watching television, during which time they're not only idle but they also pig out on food.

Our advice is to let your emotions fly over more important events, like finding a parking space. Keep sports in perspective. Set a goal that for every minute you spend watching sports, you'll spend a minute being physically active.

Getting drunk. Every couple of months, something like this happens: You see all these open bottles in front of you, one after another. You weren't raised to be wasteful, so you drink them. You become better-looking and funnier and your troubles melt away. The room starts to orbit rapidly around your head. You awaken sometime the next afternoon.

At this point, you're far exceeding that "moderate" glass of red wine at supper. When you suck down more than four alcoholic drinks in one sitting, cells in your liver start filling up with fat and turning yellow, according to Robert Swift, M.D., Ph.D., of Brown University's center for alcohol and addiction studies. Stop drinking, and your liver should return to normal in a few days.

But if you make this binge drinking a regular occurrence, your liver cells can die and turn to scar tissue. Your liver does many more important things than we have room to list here, so you don't want that to happen. Heavy drinking can also harm organs throughout your body, increase your risk of cancer in every body part from your mouth to your rectum, and contribute to a big red nose. Even just the occasional drunken night is rough on your body, sapping you of energy for the next day or two and throwing off your blood chemistry in a big way. It's just not worth it.

If you have to drink, don't have more than two a day. If you can't bring yourself to limit your drinking to that level, you need help from a doctor or qualified treatment program.

Roulette

Having casual sex. One night, you head to a singles' bar with the sole intent of meeting a nice young lady or, barring that, someone who will go home with you and help you warm your bed. You find the latter. During the course of events, no condom gives its life in your name.

So you got lucky with a one-night stand, huh? Maybe you got unlucky too. That's because you're now into the roulette category. At this point, we can't really tell you for sure what's going to happen.

Maybe that young lady is as pure as the driven snow and as free of infectious microbes as grandma's butterscotch cookies, and you'll walk away the next morning with nothing but pleasant memories. Or maybe she has just passed along one or more sexually transmitted diseases that will change your life as you know it.

In a time when our populace is awash in sexually transmitted diseases (STDs), from gonorrhea to AIDS, a single unprotected encounter is all it takes to set you up with a problem that could range from embarrassing, itchy, and curable to tragic, permanent, and possibly fatal. By one estimate from the early 1990s, you have about a 30 percent risk of catching an STD from one unprotected act with someone who's infected. Of course, some diseases are easier to catch than others.

The decision whether or not to engage in casual sex is within your control. But once you say yes, the health repercussions are most definitely not up to you. The bottom line is, carry condoms, and use them.

Driving fast. You live on a long, straight stretch of backcountry road where Sheriff Buford and his boys rarely come around. So you regularly relive your high school hot-rodding days as you blast your four-door family mobile down the road. Your seatbelt flaps freely in the breeze as the speedometer moves well past your father's age.

Maybe you'll fly home like a bat out of hell and emerge from your car cool and collected, feeling like Steve McQueen in *Bullitt*. Or maybe a deer will leap headlong into your windshield, causing you to flip your car a half-dozen times. Who knows what number will come up in roulette territory?

In 1998, nearly one out of three fatal crashes involved speeding, killing 12,477 Americans. To put this into perspective, during the previous year about 8,700 people between the ages of 15 and 44 died from homicide. Does your fear of dying in a speed-related car wreck come anywhere close to your fear of being murdered? Maybe it should.

As far as whether you should bother with your seatbelt, consider these numbers. Of the people involved in wrecks in 1998, the ones without seatbelts were far more likely to be ejected completely out of their vehicles. Seventy-five percent of those completely thrown from their vehicles died.

Those speed limit signs and seatbelts are there for a reason. Give them a try, lead foot. If you feel compelled to go fast, take up running.

Playing loud music. You regularly blast your stereo so loud that it startles birds 200 yards away.

Fortunately, this vice won't kill you, unless you're behind the wheel and it keeps you from hearing an oncoming train or is the trigger that sets off the maniac in the car behind you. Maybe one loud noise will be enough to make you lose your hearing. Or maybe it will take years of ignoring everyone's pleas to turn down the Van Halen. Maybe you'll get your full hearing back, and maybe you won't.

According to the Musicians Clinics of Canada, a stereo headset puts off about 95 decibels when its volume is halfway up. By comparison, a normal conversation is 60 decibels, and the sound of a chain saw is 100. Any prolonged racket above 85 can be damaging.

The hearing professionals at the clinic say you can safely listen to your headphones with the volume halfway up for about 5 hours a week. For every 3 decibels you turn it up, you can listen to it only half as often.

If you won't stop blasting your music, don't blame your friends if they don't want to repeat punch lines for you.

Write Your Will

Smoking cigarettes. You smoke half of a pack of cigarettes a day. We really don't have too much to say about this fatal vice that you don't see every day on a billboard.

You're not enjoying the occasional naughty vice. Since you're smoking every day, even a half-pack, you're a nicotine addict engaged in the number one preventable cause of death in America. With each puff you take, you suck in a fresh lungful of at least 43 cancer-causing chemicals. With each cigarette, you inch a bit closer to an unpleasant death, possibly after you enjoy smoking-induced impotence for a while. If a long, happy life is your aim, this vice isn't going to take you there.

Celebrate Your Long Life

The Day's Task

Welcome to the last day of the 12-week Longevity Program. We want you to celebrate. Surprise your wife with good champagne tonight, or enjoy whichever ritual you do when you feel like celebrating. You've done good. Relish this. Relish the fact that you're alive and able to sample the adventure and joys that this crazy world offers. Make a mental note of how many pleasures you will indeed sample in the years ahead. Then, go give a hug to those with whom you will be having many of these pleasures, and do whatever it takes to make them smile today as well.

We don't want to give you a big head, and we certainly don't want to sound sappy or like a kindergarten teacher. But consider this idea: Of all the billions of people who have ever lived or who will live someday, you represent the sole copy of *you* that the world will ever see. The combination of abilities, ideas, and knowledge that you're carrying around is the absolute only one of its kind.

You've been handed the gift of an entire life and the opportunity to use it as you see fit. You can spend your time chasing big goals: making a billion dollars, saving the environment, inventing a rounder wheel. Or you can exert your influence in a smaller sphere: running a charity fund-raiser, raising good kids, and being a solid husband and worker. Or you can sit on a sofa and do absolutely nothing of the slightest importance. That's what's great about life. It's a blank space that you get to fill however you choose.

Like all great deals, though, it's for a limited time only. You set out in life knowing you'll get to enjoy it but with the vague understanding that it will eventually come to a close after about 74 years, give or take.

The pessimist would ask why he should bother trying to stay healthy and live longer, since we're all facing the same end result, anyway. Why not just suck down that whole pizza and pitcher of beer, turn on the TV, and snicker at that jogger passing by outside?

Philosopher Thomas Hobbes, back in the 1600s, had some downbeat thoughts on mankind's place in the world, too, and he left behind at least one bummer of a quote about it. The life of man, at least as nature intended it, is "solitary, poor, nasty, brutish, and short," Hobbes believed. This guy, by the way, lived to the ripe old age of 91.

When he wrote those words, maybe life wasn't as much fun. People couldn't turn up the thermostat when they were cold, get a shot of antibiotics when they had a infection, or hop on a jet and fly to Brazil if they were in a Carnival mood.

But now we can do all those things and far more. And mankind has fought long and hard to win a longer life span in which to do them.

Keep Going to Keep Going

Look at a chart of our longevity, and you'll notice a very promising trend: The longer we live, the longer we can plan to live.

A newborn baby boy can look forward to 73.1 years of life. That's not shabby. A guy can fit plenty of living into that time, but he could use more.

On that boy's 25th birthday, he can expect to live to the age of 74.6.

When he turns 50 and his friends give him a bunch of black balloons, our friend can smile to himself and enjoy the thought that he now can plan to be finding fun when he's 77.2.

And when he turns 73, the original age at which he was statistically scheduled to expire, he can look forward to another 11 years of life.

You now know enough about longevity to keep you sailing through your birthdays, hungry for whatever the next year will bring you. Use all these extra days you're giving yourself for all they're worth. If you want to celebrate your life on every continent of the Earth, go for it. Hike on the trails. Surf on the waves. Look at the unfolding landscape from the highest skyscraper. Experience as much of it as you can.

But while you're enjoying your life, help others enjoy theirs too. Teach your kids, or someone else's, something that's worth passing along to their kids. When you find an error, correct it. When you find something that's broken, fix it. When you have a great idea, share it widely. The more you do, the more people you influence, the more of a legacy you leave behind, and the more you will become—in the truest possible way—immortal. That is the ultimate in longevity. Happy trails.

Index

<u>Underscored</u> page references indicate boxed text. **Boldface** references indicate photographs.

A

B

C

D

F

G

H

Q

R

S

T

U

V

W

X

Y

Z